Speech Science

An Integrated Approach to Theory and Clinical Practice

SECOND EDITION

Carole T. Ferrand
Hofstra University

PEARSON

Allyn and Bacon

Boston   New York   San Francisco
Mexico City   Montreal   Toronto   London   Madrid   Munich   Paris
Hong Kong   Singapore   Tokyo   Cape Town   Sydney

Executive Editor and Publisher: *Stephen D. Dragin*
Editorial Assistant: *Katie Heimsoth*
Marketing Manager: *Kris Ellis-Levy*
Managing Editor: *Joe Sweeney*
Editorial Production Service: *Walsh & Associates, Inc.*
Composition Buyer: *Linda Cox*
Manufacturing Buyer: *Linda Morris*
Electronic Composition: *Publishers' Design and Production Services, Inc.*

For related titles and support materials, visit our online catalog at www.ablongman.com.

Between the time website information is gathered and then published, it is not unusual for some sites to have closed. Also, the transcription of URLs can result in typographical errors. The publisher would appreciate notification where these errors occur so that they may be corrected in subsequent editions.

Library of Congress Cataloging-in-Publication Data
Ferrand, Carole T.
    Speech science : an integrated approach to theory and clinical practice / Carole T.
Ferrand. — 2nd ed.
        p. cm.
    Includes bibliographical references and index.
    ISBN 0-205-48025-X
    1. Speech therapy. 2. Speech disorders. 3. Speech. I. Title.
RC423.F474 2007
616.85'506—dc22   2006044541

Printed in the United States of America

10 9 8 7   11 10

*In loving memory of my mother, Anne Friedman
(1922–2000),
and my brother, Alan Friedman
(1948–2004)*

Contents

CHAPTER 11

Clinical Application

CHAPTER 12

The Nervous System   301

CHAPTER 13

Clinical Application

Brain Function Measures 367

Foreword

Together with the disciplines of language science and hearing science, speech science forms the theoretical framework for research and professional practice in the fields of speech–language pathology and audiology. Speech science has emerged into the forefront of the curriculum in speech–language pathology for several reasons.

First, over the past decades an explosion of new technology has expanded the scientific knowledge base in speech–language pathology and presently influences all aspects of teaching, research, and clinical practice. Second, the study of speech science provides the opportunity to introduce students to the objective measurement of many aspects of human communication behavior and to the translation of numerical information into meaningful interpretations of this behavior. This is a critical ability for students to develop. Increasingly, speech–language pathologists and audiologists in different settings (hospitals, rehabilitation centers, early intervention centers, nursing homes, schools, etc.) are required to use and interpret information from acoustic and physiological instrumentation in order to evaluate and treat individuals with various communicative disorders. A thorough understanding of the scientific basis of the instrumentation, as well as an appreciation of the clinical relevance of the information, is therefore essential.

Third, speech science is an excellent way of helping students to understand and appreciate the scientific method and the importance of hypothesis testing, data collection, and empirical observation. Too often, however, science and clinical practice have been considered disparate subjects. This division creates the erroneous impression that clinical decision making is divorced from a scientific knowledge base.

This text is unique in its attempt to unify concepts in speech science with the clinical application to communication disorders. Students are provided with an integrated approach to speech science that emphasizes scientific concepts in relation to clinical practice. The link between theory and application is supported by current research highlighting the different diagnostic and intervention applications of the scientific material. The integration of theoretical information with clinical application makes the information more easily accessible, less intimidating, and more relevant to students.

The book also clearly guides the student to understand the relationship between acoustics, speech production, and speech perception. Concepts are integrated and explained through a thorough discussion of the speech systems of respiration, phonation, articulation, and perception. Not only do students become well acquainted with the different speech systems and how they normally function, but they are also introduced to the way these systems have been studied and measured through various instrumental means. In line with the overall goal of this book, emphasis is placed on current acoustic and physiologic measurements that are typically employed for clinical purposes as well as for research, such as fundamental frequency and intensity measures, jitter, shimmer, spectrography, electroglottography, and so on.

Scientific concepts are presented within a narrative framework that facilitates understanding the material as an integrated and coherent body of knowledge. Students thus have a firm base from which to further expand their knowledge. Consequently, depth of content is provided without sacrificing readability, and the text remains student and instructor friendly. Dr. Carole Ferrand presents the information in an unusually readable, easy-to-follow manner. Students will appreciate her lucid and accessible writing style, as well as the clear illustrations of concepts. Professors will find the material in-depth and comprehensive and the review questions at the end of each chapter most helpful in stimulating classroom discussion.

Ronald L. Bloom, Ph.D.
Associate Professor and Chair
Speech–Language–Hearing Sciences
Hofstra University

Preface to the Second Edition

I have been gratified by the overwhelmingly positive response to the first edition of *Speech Science: An Integrated Approach to Theory and Clinical Practice.* Clearly, this explicit linking of theory and management has been appreciated by users of the text. I am grateful for the excellent feedback I have received from colleagues who teach Speech Science, as well as from students in bachelor's and master's programs in speech–language pathology and audiology.

This new edition complements and expands the material in the first edition in several important ways. First, two new chapters have been added: Chapter 12 presents a comprehensive yet targeted discussion of neuroanatomy and neurophysiology relevant to speech production. The chapter begins with descriptions of nerve cell structure and function and continues with examination of cortical and subcortical areas of the brain. The spinal and cranial nerves are described and related to speech production, and the chapter concludes with a discussion of principles of motor control. Throughout the chapter, a wealth of new illustrations help students to visualize important aspects of neurological structure and function in human communicative behavior. Following the format of the first edition, Chapter 13 then examines clinical applications of the material. Current brain imaging techniques are described, including computerized tomography, magnetic resonance imaging, functional magnetic resonance imaging, positron emission tomography, single photon emission computed tomography, and evoked potentials. Applications of these technologies to various communication disorders are discussed, including stuttering, Parkinson's disease, multiple sclerosis, and Alzheimer's disease.

Second, clinical case studies and associated questions have been added to each clinical application chapter to further reinforce students' appreciation of the connections between theory and clinical practice. Third, marginal notes have been added to focus students' attention on important points and to help them better retain the material. Finally, the compact disk that accompanies the text is designed to facilitate student understanding of the written and visual material. Interactive quizzes and labeling of illustrations help to highlight the important concepts, while crossword puzzles promote familiarity with terminology. Links to online resources are also included.

It is my sincere hope that instructors and students alike will continue to appreciate the book and will find the additional material to be valuable.

Carole Ferrand
Hofstra University

Acknowledgments

I am very grateful to my husband, Ted Ferrand, the most creative person I know, for his beautiful illustrations of neuroanatomy and neurophysiology in this second edition. The illustrations are designed to convey important details of brain structure and function without unnecessary visual details that could be overwhelming to students. I greatly appreciate the help of my colleagues in writing the clinical case studies and questions: Diane Slavin, Chair of the Department of Communication Sciences and Disorders at Long Island University, C.W. Post Campus; Wendy Silverman, Director of the Speech and Hearing Center at Hofstra University's Saltzman Community Center; and Rose Valvezan, Coordinator of Audiology at the Speech and Hearing Center.

My editor at Allyn and Bacon, Steve Dragin, has facilitated the revision process with a refreshing dose of good humor. I also appreciate the feedback from the users and reviewers of the first edition, as well as reviewers from the second edition—Richard D. Andreatta, The University of Georgia; Irene M. Barrow, Hampton University; Margie L. Gilbertson, Arkansas State University; Paul Milner, Bridgewater State College; and James R. Wicka, Worcester State College—whose helpful comments have been incorporated into the second edition.

chapter 1

Introduction

This book arose from my experiences in teaching speech science at both undergraduate and graduate levels over the past ten years. When I first started teaching the subject, I was surprised at how intimidated students were by the topic. It soon became clear that a key factor in alleviating their anxiety and promoting a positive learning experience was to demystify the subject by breaking the material into small, logically linked units and by making the organizational links between units of information explicit. Students are thus able to use the basic concepts as a scaffold upon which to extend their scientific knowledge. Careful structuring of the information helps students to grasp the material more easily, to retain the material beyond the next quiz or exam, and to integrate previously learned material with new concepts.

However, although this scaffolding approach facilitates student understanding of the material, it does not help students to appreciate the relevance of the subject. "After all" was the frequently heard comment, "I'm going to be a clinician, not a researcher. I don't need this stuff to do therapy." It became clear, over the years, that the way to help students to appreciate the relevance of the speech science material is to explicitly connect it to clinical practice. Once students understand the connection between "science" and "clinic," the false dichotomy disappears, and students begin to appreciate the necessity of using scientific means of establishing rationales for clinical procedures, evaluating the effectiveness of treatment strategies, increasing clinical accountability, and applying the products of science and technology to clinical practice. Indeed, a discipline can be evaluated on the scope and depth of its scientific basis.

The explosion of computer technology over the past few decades has had an unprecedented effect on all areas of speech science and speech–language pathology. Due to technological advances such as electron microscopy, magnetic resonance imaging, and ultrasonography, basic knowledge of the structures and functions of all systems involved in speech production and perception has expanded tremendously. The application of this scientific knowledge base to the diagnosis and treatment of communication disorders has resulted in dramatic changes and refinements. Acoustic, aerodynamic, and physiological instrumentations are rapidly becoming accepted tools in hospitals, rehabilitation centers, clinics, schools, and other settings in which human communicative behavior is of interest.

This book takes a systems approach to the scientific study of speech production and speech perception, focusing on the physiological and acoustic generation and measurement of verbal output. Rather than studying scientific concepts in isolation, concepts are explained in relation to the complex interactions of the physiological subsystems of respiration, phonation, articulation and resonance, and audition. This approach provides a framework for discussing the acoustic nature of speech in relation to the human capacity for producing and perceiving speech. In this way, the scientific concepts relate meaningfully to human communicative behavior.

Although a large part of the focus of this book is on information that can be obtained from instrumentation, there are four very important points that students should keep in mind. First, we cannot assume that there is a direct link between underlying anatomical and physiological factors and acoustic or other instrumental data. We make inferences from the data about the functioning of a system, but they are just that—inferences. Second, the information obtained from instrumentation may be objective, but a subjective component is always involved in the interpretation of the data. Different researchers, teachers, clinicians, and students may interpret data very differently, depending on prior experience, level of sophistication, and so on. Third is the need to be aware of the validity of the information obtained. A degraded or distorted signal can yield acoustic information that is not valid. Furthermore, some kinds of analyses may not be appropriate for particular disorders. For instance, the jitter measure has been found to have decreased reliability when used with people with severe voice problems. Fourth, acoustic and other instrumental data do not replace behavioral and perceptual information, but supplement it.

It is also important to keep in mind that speech production, although a complex process with many levels, is, in reality, one process. Respiration, phonation, and articulation are so closely interwoven that they really cannot be separated. The divisions and separate discussions of these systems are purely for convenience and ease of discussion. For example, subglottal pressure is discussed in the chapter on voice production, but, in fact, subglottal pressure is also influenced by actions of the supraglottal articulators.

As with any subject, not all topics can be included in the book. The domains included under the broad rubric of speech science are numerous, varied, and complex. An author must necessarily select the topics he or she feels are most important. I have selected those that, over my ten years of teaching speech science, have contributed most to students' understanding of speech science as a whole. The book focuses on acoustic and aerodynamic measurement, rather than on techniques such as videoendoscopy, stroboscopy, ultrasound, and magnetic resonance imaging. These are, of course, enormously important technologies that students need to be aware of, but they are beyond the scope of this book. Keeping this limitation in mind, the aim of the book is to provide comprehensive and in-depth coverage of speech science. The book also aims to tell a story, that is, to give context and shape to the narrative in a way that logically develops and furthers student understanding and retention of the material.

Overview of Chapters

The chapters are organized in accordance with the systems approach of this book and with the aim of the book, which is first to present more basic information and then to build on this information in a systematic manner. Chapter 2 presents a framework to help students to understand the basic information about the nature of sound. The first part of the chapter focuses on the physics of sound. The vibratory nature of sound is described and explained in detail, focusing on essential concepts of pressure, elasticity, and inertia. We then explore the properties of sounds that make them different from one another, such as frequency and intensity. An important section of Chapter 2 is the presentation of detailed information about waveforms and spectra and the different sorts of information that they provide. Following the presentation of basic acoustic material, a discussion of resonance is presented, with an emphasis on acoustic resonators. Characteristics of acoustic resonators are explored, such as bandwidth, cutoff frequencies, and resonance curves. These concepts are integral to the understanding of the vocal tract as an acoustic resonator, a topic that is covered in depth in Chapter 8.

Chapter 3 introduces students to clinical applications of the concepts presented in Chapter 2. Frequency and intensity variables that are typically used in clinical situations are discussed, with a clear explanation of their contribution in helping to assess and treat various breakdowns in speech production, as well as their importance in documenting clinical effectiveness. Variables such as speaking fundamental frequency, frequency variability, average vocal amplitude level, and dynamic range are highlighted, and the current use of voice range profiles is explained. The chapter concludes by examining some specific disorders in which the measurement of frequency and intensity variables has been helpful in clinical management of such problems as voice disorders and neurological disorders. Although following logically from the material presented in Chapter 2, some instructors may prefer to defer the information until the discussion of phonation in Chapter 8.

Chapter 4 presents a detailed discussion of the respiratory system. Relevant anatomy and physiology help students to understand how respiration generates the power supply for speech. An important part of the chapter is the detailed discussion of respiratory volumes and capacities, which students often have difficulty in visualizing, but which are crucial to an understanding of the ways in which we use the air supply for speech and other purposes. Another important section covers the differences between vegetative and speech breathing, an understanding of which is essential in clinical intervention of many speech-related disorders. Breathing patterns for speech are highlighted. The volumes, pressures, and flows that are the basis of speech production are delineated, and instrumental ways of measuring these aspects of respiration are presented, including plethysmographs and pneumotachographs for kinematic respiratory analysis.

Chapter 5 focuses on clinical application of the principles discussed in Chapter 4. Respiratory function is discussed in relation to several types of neurological disorders, such as Parkinson's disease, cerebellar disease, and cerebral palsy. Other problems are also mentioned in which respiratory function may be an issue, including cervical spinal cord injury, voice disorders, and hearing impairment. Following the organization of Chapter 4, important concepts dealing with volumes, pressures, airflows, and chest-wall shape are integrated into the discussion of the clinical management of respiratory problems.

Chapter 6 focuses on the phonatory system, beginning with anatomical and physiological information. Links with respiration are emphasized, including a discussion of phonation threshold pressure, the minimum amount of subglottal pressure needed to set the vocal folds into vibration. The human voice is described in terms of its nearly periodic nature, leading to a discussion of jitter and shimmer, commonly used instrumental measures of vocal function. A detailed exploration of vocal registers, focusing on the physiological and acoustic aspects of modal, falsetto, and pulse registers, is presented. Comparisons are made thereafter between normal and abnormal vocal qualities, such as breathiness and hoarseness. The acoustic and spectral features of these different qualities are described. Acoustic and other ways of measuring registers and quality are presented, such as harmonics-to-noise ratios and Lx waves obtained from electroglottography.

Chapter 7 applies the theoretical principles presented in Chapter 6 to clinical situations that have been described in the research literature. The many ways in which jitter measurement has been utilized with patients with different neurological disorders are described, including amyotrophic lateral sclerosis and Parkinson's disease. Other medical uses of jitter analysis include evaluating the effects of endotracheal intubation and patient response to chemotherapy for advanced laryngeal cancer and documenting the effectiveness of behavioral voice therapy for certain types of functional voice problems. Similarly, clinical situations in which electroglottography has been used are presented, for example, in documenting the effects of Botox injection on vocal production in spasmodic dysphonia and in comparing different types of treatment for increasing vocal intensity in patients with Parkinson's disease.

Chapter 8 concerns the articulatory system and resonance. The articulators of the vocal tract are described, and their contributions to the shaping of the sound wave are presented. To help students understand the way in which the articulators shape the sound wave and the connections between the respiratory, laryngeal, and articulatory systems, the articulators of the vocal tract, as well as the vocal folds of the larynx, are conceptualized as a series of valves that open and close to regulate the flow of air through the vocal tract. This leads logically to a discussion of the traditional classification system of consonants and vowels, based on the manner and location of valving of the pulmonary airflow through the glottis and/or vocal tract. Following the exploration of the structures and functions of the various vocal tract articulators, Chapter 8 integrates acoustic and structural information in a discussion of the application of resonance to the vocal tract. The characteristics of the vocal tract resonator are described, such as its being a quarter-wave resonator with multiple resonance frequencies, as well as its variable nature. An explanation follows of how the vocal tract filters the glottal sound wave, formalized in Fant's source-filter theory of vowel production. The commonly used measure of spectrographic analysis is presented, followed by a detailed explanation of the spectral characteristics of vowels and consonants. To put the sounds in the perspective of connected speech, the concepts of coarticulation and suprasegmental aspects of speech production are then discussed.

Chapter 9 focuses on the issue of speech intelligibility, emphasizing disorders that affect intelligibility. Problems in speech production are conceptualized in terms of the source-filter theory, with problems affecting the source function, the transfer function, or both. Acoustic measures of speech output, such as measures of vowel duration, vowel formant measurements, and spectral analysis of consonants, are shown to be important in determining the precise articulatory movements that contribute to reduced intelligibility in dysarthria, hearing impairment, phonological disorders, tracheotomy, and cleft palate. Physiological measurements of palatometry and glossometry are also discussed in relation to diagnosis and treatment of intelligibility problems.

The focus in Chapter 10 is on the auditory system. Similarly to the other chapters, information about the structure and function of the different parts of the ear is presented at the beginning of the chapter. Building on previously discussed concepts of sound transmission, the role of the middle ear in transducing air pressure vibrations into mechanical vibrations and transmitting these vibrations to the inner ear is described. The ability of the cochlea of the inner ear to perform a frequency analysis of incoming sounds is also presented. Following the description of hearing, the emphasis turns to the perception of speech, the process of recognizing speech sounds and assigning meaning to them. All the classes of sounds are described in terms of their acoustic patterns that form the basis for phoneme recognition. Concepts central to issues in speech perception, such as categorical perception, multiple cues in perception, and trading relations between acoustic cues, are integrated into the discussion of sound recognition. Research using synthetic speech is described in terms of its role in defining patterns of speech perception. A discussion of currently used instrumental techniques for the diagnosis and treatment of hearing problems focuses on immittance audiometry, otoacoustic emissions, and cochlear implants. The importance of immittance audiometry and otoacoustic emissions in the screening and evaluating of middle and inner ear function, particularly in infants, young children, and hard-to-test individuals, is emphasized. In particular, otoacoustic emissions are used in neonatal screening to increase the chances of early detection of hearing problems.

Chapter 11 turns to the issue of speech perception, which is discussed with reference to hard-of-hearing and deaf individuals, as well as children with recurrent middle ear infections, language and reading disabilities, and phonological deficits. The link between speech perception and higher level linguistic functioning is explored using the research literature.

Chapter 12 presents a discussion of neuroanatomy and neurophysiology relevant to speech production. The chapter begins with descriptions of nerve cell structure and function and continues with examination of cortical and subcortical areas of the brain. The spinal and cranial nerves are described and related to speech production, and the chapter concludes with a discussion of principles of motor control. Chapter 13 then examines clinical applications of the material. Current brain imaging techniques are described, including computerized tomography, magnetic resonance imaging, functional magnetic resonance imaging, positron emission tomography, single photon emission computed tomography, and evoked potentials. Applications of these technologies to various various communication disorders are discussed, including stuttering, Parkinson's disease, multiple sclerosis, and Alzheimer's disease.

Finally, Chapter 14 presents a discussion of the nature of models and theories to help students to understand the importance of conceptual and theoretical frameworks in testing ideas about systems and in predicting the behavior of systems under various conditions. A brief description of selected issues in speech production and the models and theories that have been proposed to explain these issues follows the general discussion. Similarly, selected issues in the area of speech perception are identified, followed by a brief description of some of the models and theories proposed to account for these findings.

chapter **2**

The Nature of Sound

chapter objectives | *After reading this chapter you will*

1. Understand how sound is generated by changes in air pressure.
2. Be able to describe dimensions of sound, such as frequency and period, pure tones and complex sounds, and intensity and amplitude.
3. Understand that the decibel (dB) scale is logarithmic and is based on a comparison of sounds to a standard reference sound.
4. Become familiar with the terms *reverberation, absorption, reflection,* and *interference.*
5. Understand the difference between waveforms and spectra.
6. Appreciate the concepts of resonance and acoustic filtering.

Sound occurs when a disturbance creates changes in pressure in a gas, such as air, or in a liquid or solid medium. The disturbance is caused by some kind of movement, such as a cup being placed on a table, a book falling on the floor, a tuning fork being struck, or the human vocal folds opening and closing. The pressure changes created by the disturbance are transmitted through the medium and may end up at a listener's ear, eventually to be perceived as sound. Because the human sound production and perception systems rely primarily on air, we will focus on sound in air, rather than in solids and liquids. Thus, to understand the nature of sound and the means whereby the human

7

sound producing and receiving systems work, it is essential to understand the behavior of air.

Air is a gas made up of countless numbers of molecules of various chemicals (oxygen, nitrogen, hydrogen, etc.). These molecules of air are not stationary, but constantly move around in random patterns, and at extremely high speeds. This random movement is called **Brownian motion**. As the molecules move around, these particles of air collide with each other and with whatever is in their path—walls, furniture, people, and so on. These collisions produce pressure.

Pressure (P) is a force (F) that acts perpendicularly on a surface area (A). The formula for pressure is P = F/A.

Air Pressure

Pressure is a force that acts perpendicularly on a surface. When you sit on a chair, for example, your body exerts a certain amount of downward force on the horizontal surface of the seat, generating a certain amount of pressure. If you were sitting on a sofa, the pressure you exert would be less, because the force would be spread out over a larger area. The force of any pressure, including air pressure, can move objects. For instance, air pressure acting on a tree moves the branches and leaves. Air pressure causes the hanging objects on wind chimes to collide with each other and create a pleasant sound. In the same way, air pressure acting on an eardrum can push it inward or pull it outward.

Measurement of Air Pressure

Pressure can be measured in various ways that incorporate the force exerted and the surface area on which the force is acting. When talking about the pressure needed to move the eardrum, for example, the unit of force is the **dyne** (d), and the unit of area is the square centimeter (cm^2). The dyne measures extremely small amounts of force, so it is suitable for measuring the tiny amounts of pressure acting on the eardrum to produce sound. Larger amounts of force over larger surfaces are measured with larger units, such as pounds per square inch (psi), which is a measure deriving from the traditional English system. The pressure of air in your car tires is probably around 30 psi, a much larger amount of pressure over a much larger surface area than the eardrum.

The MKS and cgs systems are metric systems. The MKS system uses larger units than the cgs system.

Dynes per square centimeter and pounds per square inch are commonly used measurements of pressure in the fields of speech pathology and audiology. However, more current measurement systems are based on the modernized metric system, the International System of Units (SI). In this system, pressure can be measured using either the **MKS system** or the **cgs system**. MKS and cgs are the abbreviations for three units of measurement: distance, mass, and time. M stands for meters, K for kilograms, and S for seconds. The letter c stands for centimeters, g for grams, and s for seconds. These two systems are related, but the cgs system uses smaller units for distance and mass than the MKS system. In the cgs system, the unit of measurement for pressure is dynes per square centimeter (dynes/cm^2), also called a **microbar**. One dyne/cm^2 equals 1 microbar. Force in the MKS system is measured in **newtons**, and pressure is measured in newtons per square meter (N/m^2), which is also known as a **pascal**. One N/m^2 is 1 pascal. This is a very large value, so for speech and hearing applications in which minute amounts of pressure are measured the micropascal (µPa) is used. One µPa is equal to one-millionth of 1 Pa. Most older texts use the dynes measure for pressure, although the current measure of choice among scientists is the pascal (or µPa). Both, however, are perfectly acceptable, and these measures are all equivalent. For example, the pressure of air in the atmosphere at sea level is 14.7 psi in the English system and around 1,000,000 dynes/cm^2 (1,000,000 microbars) in the cgs system.

Pressure can also be described by the amount of force it takes to move a column of liquid such as water or mercury in a tube. In this kind of situation, the unit of measurement is centimeters of water (cm H$_2$O). If you blow into a tube that is partially filled with water, the force of your breath exerts pressure on the surface of the water, which will therefore be displaced by a certain distance (see Figure 2.1). If you displace the water by 5 cm, you have exerted

> Some measures of pressure include pounds per square inch (psi), dynes/cm^2, microbar, micropascal, cm H$_2$O.

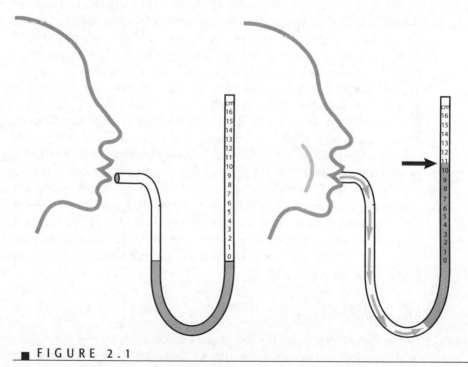

■ FIGURE 2.1
Measuring air pressure in centimeters of water.

■ TABLE 2.1

Units of Measurement of Air Pressure

Dynes per square centimeter	dyne/cm²
Pounds per square inch	psi
Microbar	µbar
Pascal	Pa
Micropascal	µPa
Centimeters of water	cm H₂O
Millimeters of mercury	mm Hg

enough pressure on the water to shift it by 5 cm, and the resulting pressure measurement is 5 cm H₂O.

Sometimes the liquid manipulated in this kind of measurement is mercury. In this case, the unit of measurement is millimeters of mercury (mm Hg). Barometers measuring pressure changes in the atmosphere use mercury. Hence the comment often used by weather forecasters that the barometer is rising (indicating that air pressure is increasing) or the barometer is falling (air pressure is decreasing). These different ways of measuring pressure are useful in describing different areas of the speech production process. Table 2.1 provides easy reference to the measurement terms and their units of measure.

Pressures can be generated in different locations and areas and can increase or decrease, depending on the specific circumstances. It is handy, therefore, to have a way of indicating the location or type of pressure. The scientific notation for pressure is P. When combined with a subscript, the type or location of pressure is indicated. For example, atmospheric pressure is written as P_{atmos}. At sea level, P_{atmos} is around 760 mm Hg, or 14.7 psi, or 1,000,000 dynes/cm². At higher altitudes, P_{atmos} decreases.

Pressure in different locations can be higher or lower than P_{atmos}. For instance, the pressure of the air inside a tire on your car is typically around 30 psi, considerably higher than P_{atmos}. Pressure that is higher than P_{atmos} is called **positive pressure** (P_{pos}). If you puncture your tire, the air leaks out, and pressure could decrease below P_{atmos}, say to 7 psi. Pressure below P_{atmos} is called **negative pressure** (P_{neg}). Note that P_{neg} is not the same as a vacuum. A vacuum refers to a total absence of air, and thus a total absence of pressure. The pressures within various locations within our body, such as our lungs ($P_{alveolar}$), tracheas (P_{trach}), and mouths (P_{oral}), play an important role in producing and perceiving speech.

Movement of Air

Because air is a gas, it moves in predictable ways. Molecules of air have a natural tendency to equalize, that is, to spread themselves around more or less equally. To achieve this equalization, air always moves from an area of high pressure to an area of lower pressure. The movement of air through a particular area in a certain interval of time is called **flow**. Flow is usually measured metrically in liters per second (l/s), liters per minute (l/min), milliliters per second (ml/s), or millimeters per minute (ml/min). The rate of flow, that is, how fast a gas is flowing, is known as **volume velocity**. Velocity refers to speed occurring in a particular direction. Thus volume velocity refers to the speed of a volume of air traveling in a certain direction.

The difference in pressure causes air to flow from higher to lower pressure. This difference is known as the **driving pressure**. Driving pressures in various areas of the human speech production system are crucial in generating speech. Another characteristic of air is that it can flow with various degrees of smoothness or turbulence. Air that flows smoothly, with molecules moving in a parallel manner and at the same speed, is called **laminar flow**. **Turbulent flow**, on the other hand, occurs when an obstacle in its way disturbs the flow. When this happens, the flow becomes less regular in its movement, resulting in little swirls, or eddies, of currents. These eddy currents result in random variations in the pressure of the air. Laminar and turbulent flow can be compared to water flowing in a river. When nothing disturbs the water, the flow is smooth, with the water molecules moving at the same speed. When rocks get in the way and the water flows around and over the rocks, the flow becomes turbulent, with little local water pressure changes. As with driving pressure, the smoothness or turbulence of airflow is an important aspect of speech production.

Driving pressure occurs when air flows from an area of higher pressure to an area of lower pressure.

Air Pressure, Volume, and Density

Another characteristic of air is that there is an inverse relationship between air volume and pressure and a proportional relationship between air pressure and density. **Volume** refers to the amount of space occupied in three dimensions; **density** refers to the amount of mass per unit of volume. As the volume of a particular enclosed space increases, the pressure of the air within that space decreases as long as the temperature remains constant. As the volume of the enclosed space decreases, the pressure of the air increases, given a constant air temperature. This relationship is known as **Boyle's law**, after the scientist who discovered it. Figure 2.2 shows this relationship, using the example of a container with a plunger in it. Each container has an equal amount of air, but the plungers are inserted to different depths, changing the volume. The farther a plunger is inserted, the smaller the volume of the container. However, because the amount of air within the container has not changed, the density of the air within the smaller space is increased. When density is increased, pressure is increased as

Boyle's law explains the inverse relationship between volume and pressure, given a constant temperature and density.

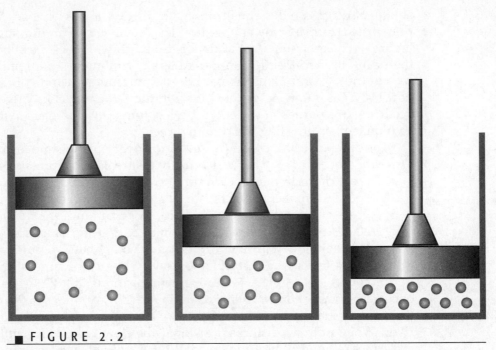

■ FIGURE 2.2

Air pressure and volume.

well, because the molecules collide with the surfaces and with each other more often and more forcefully.

Sound: Changes in Air Pressure

We have seen that air molecules move around, creating a relatively steady pressure. This relatively constant pressure that is around us at any particular place or time is called the ambient pressure (P_{am}). The P_{am} in the room where you are working could be the same as or different from the P_{am} in another room, or the P_{atmos}. For a sound to be generated, the constant P_{am} must be disturbed in some way so as to increase and decrease in a systematic manner. For changes to occur in the ambient air pressure, some force must disturb the air molecules from their usual random patterns of movement. A tuning fork provides an excellent example of the way in which P_{am} is changed by a disturbance and how this change results in sound (see Figure 2.3).

When you strike a tuning fork, its prongs, or tines, are set into vibration; they move back and forth (oscillate) very rapidly. As the tines vibrate, they set up a chain reaction in the air molecules in adjacent areas. As the tine moves

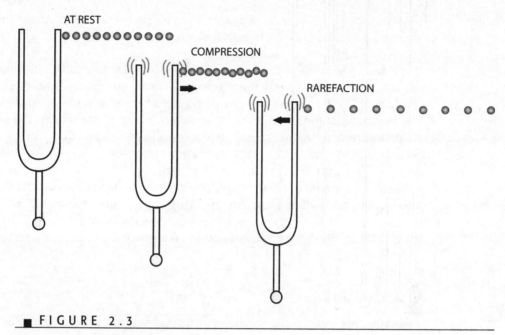

■ FIGURE 2.3

Compression and Rarefaction.

outward, it pushes against the air molecules closest to it. These molecules are displaced from their original positions and, in turn, push against their neighboring molecules, which push against their neighbors, and so on. When molecules have been displaced in this manner and are approaching and colliding with the next group of molecules, there is an increased density of air in that area. Increased density results in an increase of pressure. Thus, when molecules approach and collide, an area of positive pressure, known as **compression**, results.

However, the air molecules that have been displaced do not remain in their new positions, but swing back toward their original positions. As molecules down the line are displaced toward their neighbors, molecules that were earlier displaced are already returning to their original positions. However, the molecules returning toward their original positions overshoot their marks and swing farther away to the other side of their original positions. This results in increased distance between the two groups of molecules involved. There is now decreased density of air in the area between the two groups of molecules, resulting in a lower pressure, known as **rarefaction**.

Compression is an area of high pressure; rarefaction is an area of low pressure.

This process of increasing and decreasing distances between groups of molecules results in increasing and decreasing amounts of density and the corresponding increases and decreases in air pressure. The changes in pressure continue in a wavelike motion that travels, or propagates, through the air in an ever-widening sphere (see Figure 2.4).

If an ear is in the path of some of these shifting molecules, the compression of air moves the **tympanic membrane** (eardrum) inward slightly, whereas the rarefaction of air allows the tympanic membrane to move slightly outward. The tympanic membrane is therefore set into vibration through the changes in air pressure arriving at the ear. The vibration of the tympanic membrane sets bones within the middle ear into vibration. The vibration of these bones in turn sets the fluid in the inner ear into vibration, resulting in the stimulation of hair cells (nerve cells) in the inner ear. The triggering of the nerve cells generates a nerve impulse, which is conducted along the auditory pathway to the appropriate areas of the nervous system and is then interpreted by the brain as sound. Thus, the basic nature of sound consists of alternating increases and decreases in P_{am}.

Elasticity and Inertia

When air molecules are set into vibration by a disturbance such as a tuning fork being struck, they vibrate a tiny distance around their rest positions, eventually coming to a stop. Once the molecules have been disturbed, two forces in-

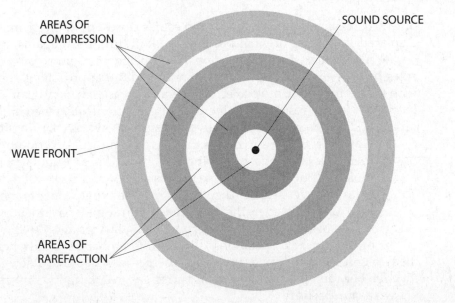

■ FIGURE 2.4

Compression and rarefaction radiating in all directions from a point source.

teract to keep them swinging back and forth for a while before they settle down again. These forces are **elasticity** and **inertia**. Elasticity is a restoring force; it refers to the property of an object to be able to spring back to its original size, form, location, and shape after being stretched, displaced, or deformed. The amount of restoring force depends on the extent to which the object is displaced. **Hooke's law**, which describes elasticity, states that the restoring force is proportional to the distance of displacement and acts in the opposite direction. Thus, the farther an object is displaced from its original location, the stronger the restoring force that pulls it back toward that position. All solid materials possess some degree of elasticity, and air and other gases behave as though they, too, possess elasticity.

Hooke's law states that the restoring force of elasticity is proportional to the amount of displacement undergone by the object.

After the fork is initially struck and the molecules have been displaced, they start moving back toward their rest positions due to elasticity. However, they do not immediately stop at their rest positions, but overshoot the mark, swinging out farther in the opposite direction. This overshooting is due to inertia. Inertia is a law of physics describing the tendency of matter to remain at rest or to continue in a fixed direction unless affected by some outside force. In the case of the air molecules, the outside force that overcomes the inertia is their inherent elasticity. In other words, due to inertia the molecules continue to overshoot their original positions until the restoring force of elasticity becomes stronger than the inertia and starts to pull the molecules back toward their resting positions again. Hence, the molecules swing back and forth through their original positions due to the interaction of elasticity and inertia (see Figure 2.5). This is handy, because it means that the original disturbance that is the source of the sound (in our example, the striking of the tuning fork) does not have to be reapplied in order for the sound to continue.

The vibration of the air molecules does not, however, last indefinitely. Because of the frictional resistance of the air, each time the molecules move back and forth around their rest positions, they do so with slightly less **amplitude**. Amplitude refers to the maximum distance away from rest position that the molecule is displaced, which is determined by the amount of energy involved in the movement. The decrease of amplitude, called **damping**, thus indicates a decrease in the energy of the sound. (We will discuss the concepts of amplitude and energy in more detail later in the chapter.) Damping finally causes the molecules to settle down once again at their original positions. At this point, no further changes in P_{am} occur, and, consequently, no further sound is generated.

Damping occurs due to friction and causes an object to vibrate with less amplitude.

It is important to realize that sources of sound cause changes in air pressure not just in one direction, but in all directions. Figure 2.4 shows how increases and decreases in air pressure radiate outward from the source in all directions. You can easily appreciate this fact by walking away from a person who is talking. Although the sound of his or her voice becomes softer as you

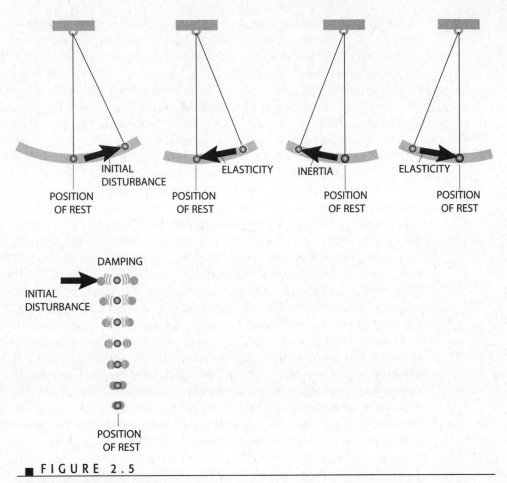

■ FIGURE 2.5

Elasticity, inertia, and damping.

move away, you are still able to hear it, at least for a while, no matter in what direction you move.

Wave Motion of Sound

A wave is a disturbance that moves through a medium. Once molecules have been set into vibration, each molecule (or group of molecules) does not, itself, travel long distances to get to a listener's ear. Rather, the molecules travel only a tiny distance around their rest positions before their motion dies away. What travels toward the listener's ear is the disturbance, that is, the changes in air pressure caused by molecular vibration. These compressions and rarefactions can propagate long distances, and these changes in air pressure affect the listener's ear. Waves, in general, are characterized by small motions of individual particles of the medium, resulting in changes of the medium being transmitted for long distances.

In the case of sound, the wave motion is longitudinal. The individual air molecules move parallel to the direction that the wave is traveling. Wave motion of water, on the other hand, is transverse; that is, the individual molecules of water move up and down at right angles to the direction that the wave is traveling. We are all familiar with the phenomenon of water rippling outward in widening circles when a stone is dropped into a pond. These ripples are the waves, consisting of water molecules moving up and down and transmitting the disturbance in all directions. In a very similar way, when a sound wave is generated by a tuning fork or other vibrating object, the air all around the fork is disturbed, so the changes in pressure radiate from the fork in all directions. The area of compression around the vibrating source is followed by an area of rarefaction, followed by another area of compression, another of rarefaction, and so on, spreading outward in a sphere. The outermost area of the sphere is called the **wave front**.

The wave front is the outermost area of the wave that is traveling spherically through the air.

The farther these changes in air pressure travel from the source, the more damped they become, because of the relationship of the wave front and distance. The area of the wave front is directly proportional to the square of its distance from the source. Because the total energy of a wave is constant, this means that the amplitude of the wave decreases as it gets farther from the source. In a large lecture hall, for example, the people closest to the speaker hear him or her most loudly, and the farther from the speaker an individual is sitting, the less loudly will the speaker be heard.

Characteristics of Sound Waves

Sound waves are characterized by many different aspects, such as their frequency and period, amplitude, velocity, and wavelength. Many characteristics of a sound wave can be shown on a **waveform**, which is a graph with time on the horizontal axis and amplitude on the vertical axis. This graph can be used to represent movement over time. For instance, the movement of the tines of the tuning fork can be shown, as can molecular movement generated by the tuning fork. A waveform also shows the corresponding increases and decreases in air pressure. See Figures 2.6 and 2.7.

A waveform is a graph with time along the horizontal axis and amplitude along the vertical axis that is used to represent pressure changes over time.

Frequency and Period   One back and forth movement of the molecule makes up one cycle of vibration. In other words, one cycle of vibration occurs when the molecule moves to a maximum distance away from its original spot, back toward rest position, moves to a maximal point in the opposite direction, and then back again to rest position. Cycles of

HIGHER

AMPLITUDE

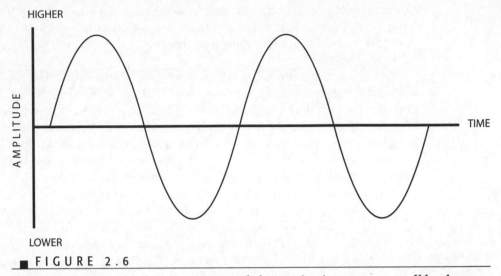

TIME

LOWER

■ FIGURE 2.6

Tine movement, molecular movement, and changes in air pressure can all be shown on a waveform.

Frequency refers to the number of cycles of vibration in one second, measured in hertz (Hz).

vibration, however, are typically thought of in terms of pressure changes, rather than in terms of individual movements of molecules. Acoustically, a cycle of vibration consists of an increase in pressure from P_{am} (compression), a decrease in pressure to P_{am}, a further decrease in pressure below P_{am} (rarefaction), and a return to baseline P_{am}. Cycles of vibration are measured in terms of time, typically in seconds. The tines of a tuning fork might vibrate at the rate of 100 **cycles per second (cps)**, causing the surrounding air molecules to vibrate at a rate of 100 cps as well. If this vibration eventually reaches a listener, that person's eardrum will vibrate at 100 cycles per second. The number of cycles per second at which objects (or air) vibrate is called **frequency**, and the unit of measurement of frequency is **hertz** (abbreviated **Hz**). Thus, a tuning fork vibrating at 100 cycles per second has a frequency of 100 Hz. The sound wave produced by the tuning fork, correspondingly, also has a frequency of 100 Hz, and the eardrum in the path of this 100 Hz sound wave would be set into vibration at 100 Hz. Frequency can also be expressed in terms of kilohertz (KHz); thus, 1000 Hz equals 1 kHz, and 2500 Hz equals 2.5 kHz.

The time that each cycle in a wave takes to occur is its period. Period and frequency are reciprocal, with the formula p = 1/F or F = 1/p.

We said that the frequency of a sound refers to the rate at which the source and the air molecules vibrate. We can turn this around and think of this rate of vibration in terms of the time it takes for one cycle of

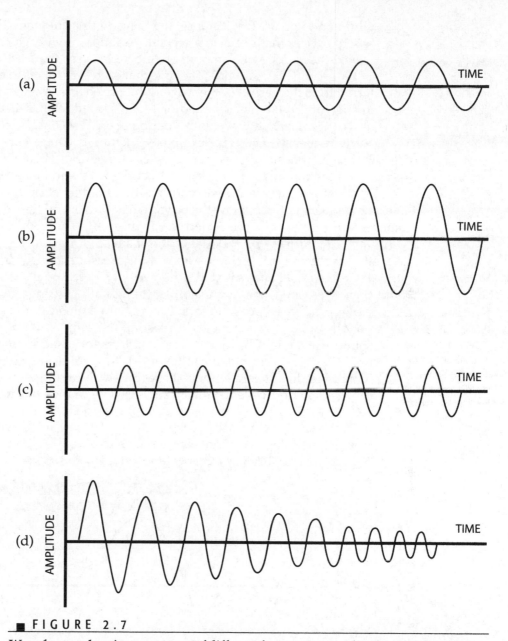

■ FIGURE 2.7

Waveforms whowing pure tones of different frequencies, amplitudes, and damping.

A periodic wave is one in which each cycle takes the same amount of time to occur. Such a wave can be assigned a pitch on a musical scale.

vibration to occur. For instance, the wave with a frequency of 100 Hz has 100 cycles that occur in a second. Assuming that each cycle in the wave lasts for the same amount of time, we can see that each must take 1/100 second (0.01 second). The time that each cycle takes to occur is referred to as the **period** of the wave, symbolized as t. A wave with a frequency of 250 Hz has a period of 1/250 second, or 0.004 second (t = 0.004 s). Similarly, a wave with a period of 0.002 second (1/500 second) has a frequency of 500 Hz. From these examples you can see that there is a reciprocal relationship between frequency and period. This relationship is expressed by the formula $F = 1/t$, where F is frequency and t equals period. If you know the frequency of a wave, you can figure out its period by putting a 1 over the frequency; if you know the period of the wave, you figure out its frequency by putting a 1 over the period (see Figure 2.8).

A wave in which every cycle takes the same amount of time to occur as every other cycle, and in which the extent of the pressure changes (i.e., the amplitude) is equal for all cycles is said to be **periodic**. Perceptually, such a wave would have a musical tone. For example, the vibrating string of a guitar or violin produces a periodic sound wave with a musical tone. However, not all sound waves have cycles lasting the same amount of time. A sound wave might have one cycle that lasts for 0.002 second, the next might take 0.003 second, the following 0.001 second, and so on. A wave in which individual cycles do not take the same amount of time to occur is called **aperiodic**. Perceptually, such a wave sounds like noise. If you

Cycles in an aperiodic wave take different amounts of time to occur. Such a wave sounds like noise.

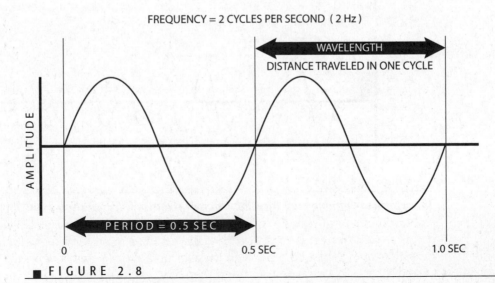

■ FIGURE 2.8

Frequency, period, and wavelength.

clap your hands or hiss through your teeth, you are producing an aperiodic sound wave, or noise.

Velocity and Wavelength   Sounds are physical phenomena, and they therefore obey physical laws, such as those governing motion and speed or the velocity of objects traveling through a medium. How fast the wave moves depends on the density and elastic properties of the medium through which it is moving. For instance, because water is more dense than air, sound travels about four times as quickly through water as it does through air and even faster than that in some solids such as steel. The speed of sound in air is around 331 m/s at 0°C (32°F), compared to 1461 m/s in water at 19°C. In a steel rod, sound may travel at a speed of 5000 m/s (Dull, Metcalfe, & Williams, 1960).

The speed of sound in liquids and solids is not affected much by temperature. In gases such as air, however, temperature plays an important part in how fast the sound travels. The warmer the air, the more quickly sound is transmitted. In fact, the speed of sound increases at the rate of about 0.6 m/s/°C (Dull et al., 1960). For example, the speed of sound in air at 0°C is 331 m/s, whereas at 20°C (68°F) it is 343 m/s (Durrant & Lovrinic, 1995).

Thus, two aspects of sound are related to time: period and speed. Period is related to the frequency of vibration, which in turn depends on the physical characteristics of the source. In general, the larger and more massive the source, the more slowly it will vibrate, and vice versa. Speed of sound, on the other hand, depends not on the frequency of the sound, but on the characteristics of the medium.

Sound waves not only occur at a certain frequency and are transmitted at a certain speed, but they also travel through space. The measurement of the travel of a sound wave is its **wavelength**. Wavelength refers to the distance in meters or centimeters covered by one complete cycle of pressure change. The wavelength of a sound is measured as the distance covered by the wave from any starting point to the same point on the next cycle. Frequency, period, and wavelength are closely related. The higher the frequency (the more cycles per second), the shorter in duration is the period and the shorter is the wavelength. The lower the frequency (the fewer cycles per second), the longer in duration is the period and the longer is the wavelength.

> Wavelength is defined as the distance covered by one complete cycle of pressure change.

Sound Absorption and Reflection   So far in our discussion we have talked about sound being transmitted through the air, without taking into account any objects or boundaries that sound waves might encounter in their travels. In fact, when sound waves come into contact with walls, ceilings, floors, and the like, they may or may not be transmitted through these boundaries. A sound wave that is generated, travels a certain distance, and then hits up against a boundary is called an **incident wave**. Incident waves may be transmitted, absorbed, or reflected.

In the case of a room with thick concrete walls, only a small amount of sound energy from the incident wave may be transmitted through the wall, whereas in a thin-walled room a lot of the incident wave's energy will probably be propagated through the wall. If all the energy in a sound wave is not transmitted, some portion of the sound not transmitted may be absorbed and some may be reflected.

Absorption is basically the damping of a wave, with diminishing changes in air pressure due to friction. Materials differ in the amount of sound energy they absorb. Typically, materials that are hard or dense and/or have smooth surfaces do not absorb much of the energy of the sound waves coming into contact with them. Materials that are soft and porous and/or have rough surfaces absorb a lot of the sound energy. Different materials, therefore, are used for different acoustic purposes. For instance, a special material, acoustic tile, is often put on ceilings specifically to absorb sound and prevent it from being transmitted. Often walls and ceilings in speech and hearing laboratories are acoustically treated in this way to absorb sound and reduce noise from the outside environment.

In **reflection**, some portion of the sound that is not transmitted or absorbed bounces back from the surface of the boundary and travels in the opposite direction of the incident wave. Similarly to absorption, the amount of reflection depends on the type of surface. A hard, smooth surface will reflect more sound than a soft or rough surface. This phenomenon is very similar to how a mirror works. A mirror is specially treated to have a hard, smooth surface. It therefore does not transmit or absorb light waves, but reflects them back into the environment, allowing the image to be seen.

Constructive and Destructive Interference   In general, physical objects cannot occupy the same space at the same time. Sound waves, however, can, because areas of high and low pressures can combine. Suppose that a tuning fork tuned to 100 Hz produces an incident sound wave that travels through the air, comes up against a wall, and is then reflected back toward the tuning fork. The tuning fork, in the meantime, continues to generate new incident waves 100 times per second. Thus, incident and reflected waves are combining with each other at any instant in time and space. This combining of waves is known as **interference**. The air pressure changes forming these two waves can interfere with each other in various ways. If the areas of compression and rarefaction of the two waves combine at exactly the same time and the same moment in space, the amplitude of the resulting wave will be doubled. This happens because when two areas of high pressure combine the resulting pressure is higher still. When two areas of low pressure combine, the pressure is further low-

All or part of a sound's energy may be absorbed (i.e., damped). Materials that are soft or rough and irregularly shaped absorb more of a sound's energy.

Reflection occurs when a wave collides with a boundary that is hard and smooth. All or a portion of a sound's energy may be reflected and travel back toward the source of the sound.

Interference occurs when two or more waves combine with each other. Constructive interference increases the amplitude of the resultant wave; destructive interference decreases the amplitude of the resultant wave.

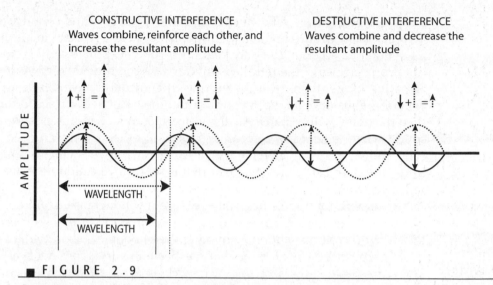

CONSTRUCTIVE INTERFERENCE
Waves combine, reinforce each other, and increase the resultant amplitude

DESTRUCTIVE INTERFERENCE
Waves combine and decrease the resultant amplitude

■ FIGURE 2.9

Constructive and destructive interference.

ered at that point. This produces greater deviations from normal P_{am} and therefore increased amplitude of the wave. Interference that results in increased amplitude is called **constructive interference** (see Figure 2.9).

If the areas of compression of one of the waves combine at exactly the same time with an area of rarefaction of the other wave, the amplitude of the resulting wave will be decreased, which is known as **destructive interference**.

Theoretically, it is possible for two sound waves with the same frequency to combine such that each compression of one wave is matched exactly with the corresponding rarefaction of the second wave; the resulting sound will be completely damped. This happens when an area of high pressure combines with an area of low pressure, causing the air molecules to equalize themselves in such a way that an area of normal pressure (P_{am}) results. Because sound consists of changes in air pressure, normal P_{am}, by definition, cannot be a sound.

Waves of different frequencies can also combine, and their areas of compression and rarefaction will not line up exactly. The amplitude of the resulting wave will therefore not be doubled, nor will the sound be completely eliminated. Rather, the amplitude of the sound will be changed in complex ways. This relative timing of areas of high and low pressure in waves is called **phase**.

Sound waves that combine and interfere with each other can affect the way that you perceive the sound. For instance, a sound can experience **reverberation**, meaning that it lasts slightly longer because of the interference. This happens when a reflected sound wave arrives at your ear slightly delayed in time compared with the arrival of the incident wave at the same point. The duration of the delay depends on the

Reverberation occurs when reflected sound waves extend the duration of an incident sound. Too much reverberation can interfere with communication by making phonemes overlap and blend together.

distance between the reflective surface and your ear. The sound wave must travel to the reflective boundary and return to your ear, delaying its arrival by a fraction of a second. You only hear one sound, but this sound is extended in duration because of the reflected wave arriving in time to keep your eardrum vibrating longer than it would with just the incident wave vibrating it. However, if the distance between your ear and the reflective surface is substantial, then the delay will be perceptually noticeable. In fact, in this case the reflected sound wave is heard as a separate sound, in other words, an echo. With an echo, the incident wave vibrates your eardrum, but your eardrum has time to settle down and stop vibrating before it is set into vibration once again by the reflected wave.

Reverberation can be desirable because it can increase the intensity of the incident sound reaching a listener. However, too much reverberation can interfere with communication by making the phonemes blend together and become garbled. This is an issue that has become very prominent over the last few years in educational settings. Many classrooms are overly reverberant because of the uncarpeted floor and bare walls that create multiple reflections of sounds. The more reflective the room, the longer the incident sound and reflections take to be absorbed and damp. This can hinder students in their understanding of the instructor's speech, which is particularly problematic for individuals with hearing disorders or other types of learning difficulties.

Pure Tones and Complex Waves   When molecules of air are set into vibration by an object such as a tuning fork, the way in which they vibrate has a certain regular, predictable pattern. Pendulums on grandfather clocks and playground swings move in the same way. We will use the example of a swing to illustrate this motion. When you push a swing, it moves away from you to some maximum distance. As it approaches this maximum point, it slows down and stops for an instant. It then reverses direction and starts moving back toward you. As

A pure tone is a sound with only one frequency, generated by a source vibrating in simple harmonic motion; complex sounds contain two or more frequencies and may be periodic or aperiodic.

it does so, its speed increases, and it reaches its maximum speed as it passes over its rest position. As it continues to move toward you, its speed decreases until the swing stops for an instant, and then, once again, it reverses direction. This regular, smooth, back and forth movement with its characteristic pattern of acceleration through the rest position and deceleration at the endpoints of the movement is called **simple harmonic motion** (SHM). Simple harmonic motion of an object such as a tuning fork generates the same smooth and even pattern of vibration of the air molecules around it, which in turn vibrate the tympanic membrane in simple harmonic motion. An object vibrating in SHM produces a sound wave that has only one frequency, called a **pure tone**. Perceptually, such a sound is heard as a rather thin, clear tone.

Other kinds of sounds, however, are characterized by waves that consist of more than one frequency, called complex waves (see Figure 2.10). Complex

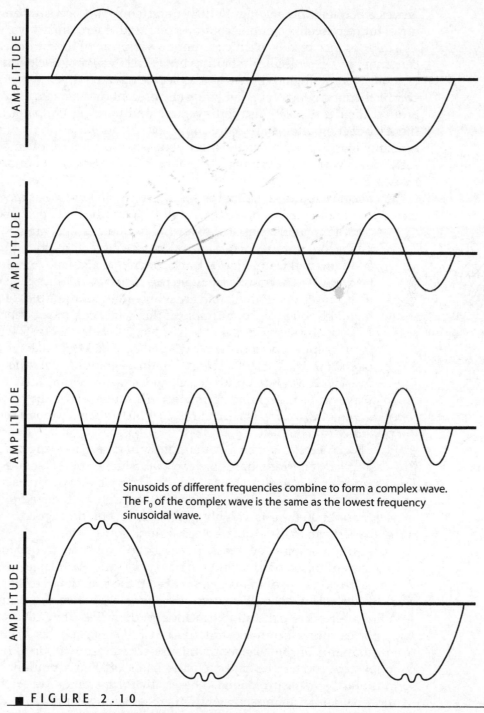

Sinusoids of different frequencies combine to form a complex wave. The F_0 of the complex wave is the same as the lowest frequency sinusoidal wave.

■ FIGURE 2.10

Pure tones combining to form a complex wave.

waves are much more common than pure tones and occur when sounds of different frequencies combine and interfere with each other in various ways. The interference results in a more complex vibration of the air molecules. One can imagine air molecules vibrating in SHM as walking back and forth in a regular even manner, whereas the molecules in a complex wave do a more complex "dance" involving all kinds of different movements as they vibrate around their rest positions. Both walking and dancing are patterned movements, but the patterns are more complicated and varied in dancing than in walking. Corresponding to the more complex molecular movement in complex sound waves, the tympanic membrane also vibrates in a more complex manner.

A **complex sound** is defined as a wave consisting of two or more frequencies. There are two types of complex sounds, periodic and aperiodic. Periodic complex sounds consist of a series of frequencies that are systematically related to each other. The lowest frequency of the sound is the **fundamental frequency** (F_0), and the frequencies above the fundamental are called **harmonic frequencies,** or just harmonics. The harmonics in a complex periodic sound are whole-number multiples of the fundamental frequency. For example, if the F_0 of a complex periodic wave is 100 Hz, the harmonics will be 200 Hz, 300 Hz, 400 Hz, 500 Hz, and so on. A complex periodic wave with an F_0 of 300 Hz will have harmonics of 600 Hz, 900 Hz, 1200 Hz, and so on. A complex periodic wave has a musical tone and sounds richer and more resonant than a pure tone wave. In fact, the more harmonics in a sound wave, the more resonant it will sound, and vice versa. Most musical instruments produce sounds that are periodic and complex.

> The fundamental frequency (F_0) is the lowest frequency in a complex periodic sound. Higher frequencies are called harmonics and are whole-number multiples of the F_0.

The harmonics in a complex periodic sound can be identified through a process called **Fourier analysis**. Jean-Baptiste Fourier (1768–1830) was a French mathematician who showed that any complex wave can be represented by the sum of its component frequencies as well as their amplitudes and phases. Fourier analysis is a highly complex mathematical procedure, which is typically performed these days by computer.

Aperiodic complex sounds also consist of two or more frequencies, but the frequencies in this kind of sound are not systematically related to each other. Rather, a broad range of frequencies make up the sound. For example, an aperiodic complex sound could contain all frequencies between 100 and 5000 Hz. Another aperiodic sound might include frequencies from 2000 to 4000 Hz. Such waves sound like noise, with no musical tone, such as steam escaping from a radiator or the sound of applause. There are two kinds of aperiodic complex sounds, differentiated on the basis of their duration. *Continuous* sounds are able to be prolonged, whereas *transient* sounds are extremely brief in duration. The steam hissing out from the radiator is continuous, whereas the sound made by a person hitting his or her hand on a desk is transient.

Speech as a Stream of Complex Periodic and Aperiodic Waves   We are now in a position to understand the basic acoustic nature of speech. When we produce speech sounds, we are actually producing different kinds of complex periodic and complex aperiodic sounds. All human sounds are complex, due to the nature of the source of the sounds. (This will be discussed in detail in later chapters.) Vowels are complex periodic sounds that have a musical tone; voiceless consonants are complex aperiodic sounds that are either transient (such as the stops /p/, /t/, and /k/) or continuous (such as the fricatives /f/, /s/, and /h/) and that sound like noise. Voiced stop and fricative consonants are a combination of periodic and aperiodic complex sound waves.

Visually Depicting Sound Waves: Waveforms and Spectra

Sound waves are invisible and intangible; the pressure changes are miniscule and cannot be seen. This could be a problem in understanding and working with sound, as sound is, by its nature, fleeting and insubstantial. Fortunately, there are graphic ways of representing sound waves that are extremely useful in helping to visualize the nature and characteristics of various sounds. One type of visual display is the waveform, and another is called a **spectrum**.

A spectrum is a graph with frequency along the horizontal axis and amplitude along the vertical axis. A line spectrum displays the frequency content of periodic sounds; a continuous spectrum displays the frequency content of aperiodic sounds.

Waveforms, as we have seen, are graphs that show time along the horizontal axis and amplitude along the vertical axis. The amplitude can represent the amount of whatever is being graphed. For instance, if a pen were attached to the tine of a tuning fork in such a way that as the tine moved the pen moved with it and traced a line on graph paper, the vertical axis of the resulting waveform would represent the distance that the tine vibrated around its rest position, and the horizontal axis would represent the time that the tine was moving. Now imagine that we attach a pen to an individual molecule so that when the molecule vibrated around its rest position a similar waveform would result. Now the waveform does not depict the motion of the tine of the tuning fork, but the amplitude of the motion of the molecule of air over time. When dealing with sound, typically what is represented on the waveform is not the tuning fork or individual molecule motion, but the changes in air pressure that result from molecular motion. So an acoustic waveform shows the amplitude of air pressure changes over time.

If we drew a line at around the midlevel of the graph, it would represent normal P_{am}, or baseline pressure. When the line goes above baseline, it represents an increase in pressure, that is, compression, and the height of the line at any point represents the amount, or magnitude, of increase. Similarly, when the line goes below baseline, it represents a decrease in pressure, or rarefaction, and again the depth of the line at any point represents the magnitude of decrease.

A waveform is useful in showing many different aspects of a sound. For instance, by counting the peaks in the waveform, we can calculate the frequency of the wave. Or, by measuring the time of each wave cycle, we can tell the period of the wave. Also, because the vertical axis measures the magnitude of pressure changes, it is easy to visualize the relative amplitude of the wave. Figure 2.7(d), for example, shows a wave that is damping.

Shape is another aspect of sound that is visible from a waveform (see Figure 2.11). A smoothly varying shape, a **sinusoid**, tells us that the wave is a pure tone, vibrating in SHM. If all the cycles in the wave repeat themselves in

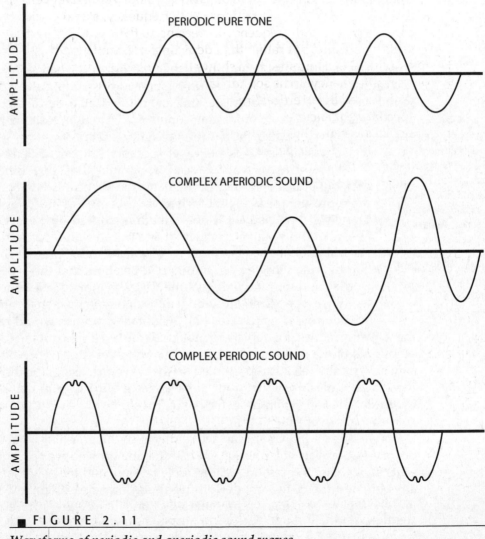

■ FIGURE 2.11

Waveforms of periodic and aperiodic sound waves.

a predictable fashion, the wave is periodic. If the cycles look different and take different amounts of time to occur, the wave is aperiodic. If the amplitude of the wave is decreasing over time, then the sound is damping. If the cycles in the wave repeat themselves in a regular way, but the shape of the wave is not sinusoidal (the cycles look more irregular in shape), then the wave is depicting a periodic complex sound. In this case, by counting the largest peaks we are able to determine the F_0 of the complex periodic sound. What cannot be seen from a waveform, however, are the harmonics of a complex sound.

To visualize harmonics, we need another kind of graph, a **line spectrum** (see Figure 2.12). A line spectrum also has a horizontal and vertical axis, but in this case the horizontal axis represents frequency, starting with low frequencies to the left, with frequency increasing to the right. The vertical axis represents amplitude, but rather than depicting amplitude of pressure changes, the amplitude in a line spectrum shows the amount of acoustic energy at each harmonic frequency of the sound. Each frequency in the wave, including the F_0, is represented by a vertical line, the height of which shows the amplitude of that specific frequency.

What is not evident in this kind of spectrum is time. The frequencies shown on a line spectrum are those that are present in a sound at one particular instant of time. Think of the difference between waveforms and spectra (singular: spectrum) in terms of a layer cake. A waveform would correspond to the entire uncut cake: You could determine the overall shape, the color of the frosting, the height of the cake, and the like, but you could not tell, without cutting the cake, what the inside was like. The line spectrum is analogous to one slice of cake. You can judge the internal section of the slice: its color, how many layers, whether there is jam or frosting between the layers, and so on, but from just the one slice, you could not tell about the overall shape of the cake.

You could also think of a spectrum as a snapshot of a person at one particular instant of time; a waveform corresponds more to a video, in which changes over time can be seen as the person walks around, performs different actions, and the like. A line spectrum can show equally well whether a sound is a pure tone (in which case it would have just one line) or a complex sound (more than one line). However, we would not be able to judge if the sound were damping or changing in other ways over time, because the overall amplitude of the sound over time is not shown.

A line spectrum is not used to represent complex aperiodic sounds, because these sounds are characterized by broad bands of frequencies. Rather than drawing individual vertical lines extremely close to each other, as would be appropriate for aperiodic complex sounds, we draw what is called the **envelope** of the wave as a horizontal line that is understood to connect all the component frequencies in the sound. This kind of spectrum is known as a *continuous* spectrum. As with periodic complex sounds on a line spectrum, the height of the

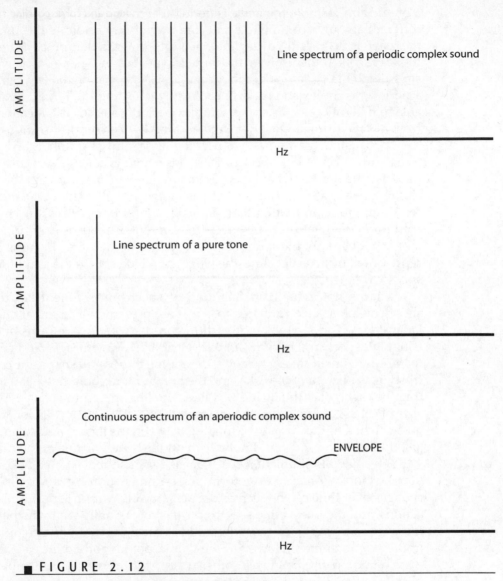

Spectra of periodic and aperiodic sounds.

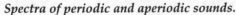

line at any frequency represents the amount of acoustic energy at that frequency. What cannot be seen from a continuous spectrum is the duration of the sound, so we cannot tell if the sound is continuous or transient. Figure 2.13 shows a waveform and the

Waveform of a transient aperiodic sound and corresponding spectrum

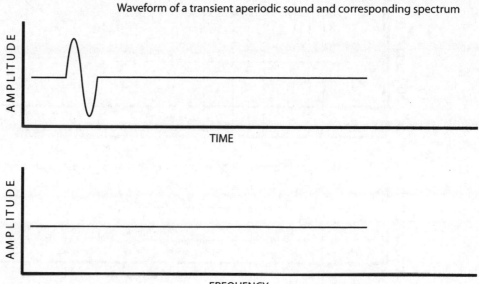

Waveform of a continuous aperiodic sound and corresponding spectrum

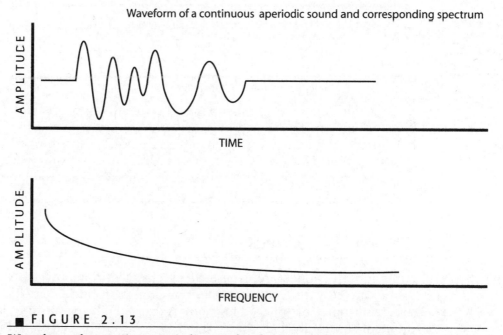

■ FIGURE 2.13

Waveform of a transient aperiodic sound and corresponding spectrum.

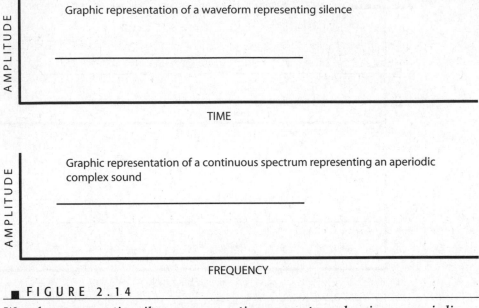

■ FIGURE 2.14

Waveform representing silence versus continuous spectrum showing an aperiodic complex sound wave.

corresponding spectrum of a transient and a continuous complex aperiodic sound wave.

It is very important to distinguish between waveforms and spectra, because the information they provide is very different. Figure 2.14 shows that a flat horizontal line on a waveform depicts silence, because the pressure is constant over time. However, a flat horizontal line on a spectrum would depict an aperiodic complex sound containing all frequencies in a certain range.

■ Attributes of Sounds

Although all sounds are generated by changes in air pressure, individual sounds are very different from one another. A high-pitched siren sounds very different from a low-pitched fog horn. A discreet whisper during class sounds different from a football cheer. The husky voice of a person with laryngitis sounds very different from that of a trained singer. We shall now explore the attributes of sounds that result in these kinds of differences, including frequency and pitch and amplitude, intensity, and loudness.

Frequency and Pitch

Frequency refers to the rate at which an object vibrates and is measured in hertz (Hz). Frequency is an objective measurement of a physical phenomenon. *Pitch,* on the other hand, is a psychological event. Pitch is how we perceive the sensation of sound as being high or low on a musical scale. You could say that pitch is the perceptual counterpart of frequency. Whereas frequency is measured in hertz, pitch is measured in **mels**. The mel scale is a perceptual, subjective scale that was constructed by having people subjectively decide whether tones of different pitches were higher or lower than others. A tone of 1000 Hz was selected as the standard tone and was called 1000 mels. A tone that was subjectively determined to be twice as high as this standard tone was called 2000 mels, one that was determined to be half as low was called 500 mels, and so on. Frequency and pitch are related. The rate at which an object vibrates determines how high or low the sound is perceived. In general, the faster the rate of vibration (the higher the frequency) is, the higher pitched the sound will be perceived. The slower the rate of vibration (the lower the frequency) is, the lower pitched the sound will be perceived. However, this relationship is not linear, as we will see later.

The frequency at which an object vibrates depends on its mass, length, and tension.

The frequency of a vibrating object depends on its physical characteristics, such as its overall size, length, thickness, and density; the material of which it is made and its stiffness; and so on. Typically, the larger the object or the more massive it is, the more slowly it will vibrate. A larger tuning fork with thicker tines will vibrate more slowly than a smaller fork with thinner tines. There are ways, however, of changing the rate at which an object vibrates. The three most important determinants of frequency are the length of the vibrating object, the mass of the object, and the tension of the object. If any one of these three characteristics is changed, the frequency will change in predictable ways. In terms of length, the longer the vibrating source, the more slowly it vibrates. Therefore, if we increase the length of whatever is vibrating, its frequency will decrease. For example, imagine that the chains of a swing hanging from a frame are a certain length so that, when the swing is pushed, it will swing back and forth (i.e., one cycle of vibration) exactly twice per second, resulting in a frequency of 2 Hz. By inserting more links in the chains, the length is increased, and the swing will move back and forth more slowly, perhaps at 1.5 Hz. Conversely, by removing links from the chain, the length is decreased and the swing now speeds up to, say, 2.5 Hz.

Mass is also important in determining the frequency at which an object will vibrate. The more massive an object, the more slowly it vibrates, and vice versa. For instance, the swing in our example vibrates at 2 Hz when no one is sitting on it. When a child sits on the swing, this adds mass, and the swing now moves back and forth more slowly, perhaps only once per second (1 Hz). The greater the mass is of the person sitting on the swing, the more the decrease in the rate of vibration. In the same way, decreasing the mass of a vibrating object will increase its rate of vibration.

Finally, the tension, or stiffness, of a body plays an important part in determining its frequency of vibration. The more tense or stiff, the quicker is the rate of vibration. The looser, or more relaxed the object, the slower is the rate of vibration. This principle can be easily seen with a rubber band. If a rubber band is held loosely at either end and plucked, it will vibrate at a certain rate. If the band is stretched more tightly, it becomes stiffer and more tense, and its frequency increases when it is plucked. Note, however, that when the elastic band was stretched it became longer, and, as we have just seen, objects that are longer generally vibrate more slowly than shorter ones. But, although the elastic band is longer when it is stretched, its mass per unit of area has been decreased, so although it is longer, it is now skinnier as well. In other words, there is the same amount of material in the elastic band, but it has been stretched out over a greater distance, and its cross-sectional area is less. The increased tension on the band and its decreased mass per unit of area cause it to vibrate more quickly. This interaction between length, mass, and tension to determine frequency is extremely important in the production of voice, as we will see in later chapters.

Human Range of Hearing   The range of frequencies that humans are capable of perceiving is around 20 to 20,000 Hz. Frequencies below this range are called **subsonic**, and frequencies above this range are **supersonic**. This range is really very limited. Some animals can perceive sounds well below 20 Hz, such as elephants, who make use of these subsonic sounds in their communication. Some birds, such as pigeons and chickens, can also perceive exceedingly low-pitched sounds that would be inaudible to humans (Gill, 1995). On the other hand, dogs can hear sounds well above 20,000 Hz, which is why dog whistles actually work: The whistle emits an extremely high-frequency sound that is inaudible to humans, but audible to dogs. Bats, too, are well known for their use of very high-frequency sounds to locate objects in space. Humans tend to hear best those frequencies that are in the middle of their range, around 1000 Hz (1 kHz) to 4000 Hz (4 kHz). Sounds that are above or below this midrange are not as easily perceived by the human auditory system. Conveniently, most speech sounds fall within this range.

Amplitude and Intensity

Amplitude   The term *amplitude* refers to either the amount of motion of a vibrating object or the amount of pressure change generated by the motion of the object. With reference to molecular movement, amplitude refers to the dis-

Amplitude refers to the magnitude of pressure changes in a sound and is measured in microbar or micropascals.

tance that the molecules are displaced from their rest positions during vibration. When talking about sound, it is more common for amplitude to refer to the measurement of the pressure changes that constitute sound. Like frequency, amplitude is a measurement of a physical phenomenon—the pressure changes that occur in the air as sound is propagated through it. Because amplitude is related to pressure, it is typically measured in dynes per square centimeter (dyne/cm^2) in the cgs system or micropascals (µPa) in the MKS system.

Intensity   To understand intensity, we first need to appreciate the concepts of energy, work, and power. Scientifically speaking, energy is the capacity of an individual or an object to perform work. Work is defined as a push or a pull that moves an object a certain distance. Energy and work, although related, are not identical. If you push as hard as you can against a building, you have probably expended energy, but no work has been done (unless, of course, you have actually managed to move the building). Energy is measured in **ergs** in the cgs system or **joules** (J) in the MKS system. One erg is the amount of work done when a force of 1 dyne displaces an object by 1 centimeter (Denes & Pinson, 1993). One joule is a force of 1 newton acting through a distance of 1 meter.

Intensity refers to the power of a sound and is measured in W/cm^2 or W/m^2. Intensity is the square of amplitude.

Power refers to the amount of energy expended in a given time and is measured in **watts** (W). One watt equals 1 joule per second or 10 million ergs per second. Power is easy to understand in terms of your own level of energy and how quickly you expend it. If you take a leisurely bike ride, you expend energy at a certain rate. Perhaps you can go on for several hours before fatiguing. If you are practicing for a race and you ride as fast and hard as you can, you may expend the same amount of energy in a much shorter amount of time. Even though you used up the same amount of energy for each ride, the powers would be different because of the different rates at which you expended the energy.

Intensity refers to power (i.e., the amount of energy expended in a second) measured over a particular area, usually square meters or square centimeters. Thus, the unit of measurement of intensity is watts per square centimeter (W/cm^2). You can think of intensity as the amount of energy or power required to generate a certain output, whether the output is sound or some other form of energy, such as light. For instance, light bulbs are available that produce different intensities of output (with light, the output is measured in units called lumens). A light bulb that uses less energy produces a less intense light than one that uses more energy. A 40 W light bulb uses 40 W to generate a certain light output. Such a light bulb gives off a less bright light than a 75 W light bulb. The same is true of sound intensity. If your stereo speakers use 10 W of power, you will hear a certain loudness of sound. If you have really large speakers designed to produce 30 W, the sound output will be much greater.

It is clear that there must be some kind of relationship between amplitude and intensity, which are physical measurements, and loudness, which is how your ears perceive the intensity generated by the degree of pressure change. The greater the amplitude and intensity, the louder the sound that is heard, and vice versa. Similar to frequency, this relationship is not linear. A sound must be 10 times more intense before it becomes twice as loud, but it must be 100 times as intense before it becomes three times as loud (Dull et al., 1960). A perceptual scale for loudness was developed in a similar way to the mel scale for pitch. A 1000 Hz tone of a particular intensity served as the reference for loudness. The scale that resulted from matching sounds of varying frequencies and intensities to the 1000 Hz tone is called the **phon** scale.

Amplitude and intensity (sound power) are related to each other. The greater the amplitude, the greater the intensity that is generated in the sound wave. However, intensity increases much more rapidly than does amplitude. Mathematically, intensity is the square of amplitude. In other words, if a sound wave has a certain amplitude with a corresponding intensity level and the amplitude of that sound wave is doubled, the intensity of the wave will not be doubled; it will be increased by the square of the increase in amplitude, so the intensity will be quadrupled (increase of 2^2). If the amplitude is increased by a factor of 5, the intensity will be increased by a factor of 5^2 (i.e., 25). Thus, it takes only small increases in air pressure changes to generate much larger increases in sound intensity.

Decibel Scale   The **decibel (dB) scale** is designed to measure sounds in a way that takes into account the amplitudes and intensities of sounds in relation to how we perceive sounds. The decibel scale is named after Alexander Graham Bell. It is abbreviated with a lowercase d, which stands for deci, or one-tenth, and an uppercase B, for Bell. A decibel is thus one-tenth of a bel, which is a large unit of measurement of sound intensity based on the logarithm of a ratio.

The human auditory system is sensitive to an enormous range of intensity levels. From the softest sound that a person can hear to the loudest sound, which produces a feeling of pain in the ears, is a range of around 1 trillion intensities. Trying to deal with huge numbers like this on a *linear* scale would be unwieldy and confusing. The decibel scale is *logarithmic*, which has the effect of compressing the trillion intensities into a scale with far fewer levels. This compression occurs because of the essential difference between linear and logarithmic scales. A **linear scale** is one in which units are the same distance from each other, and units can be added or subtracted (see Figure 2.15). For example, a ruler is a linear measure. A ruler has distances marked off on it, typically in inches (in.), centimeters (cm), and millimeters (mm). A distance of, say, 10 mm between

The decibel (dB) scale is a logarithmic ratio scale that compares the amplitude and/or intensity of any sound to a standard reference sound.

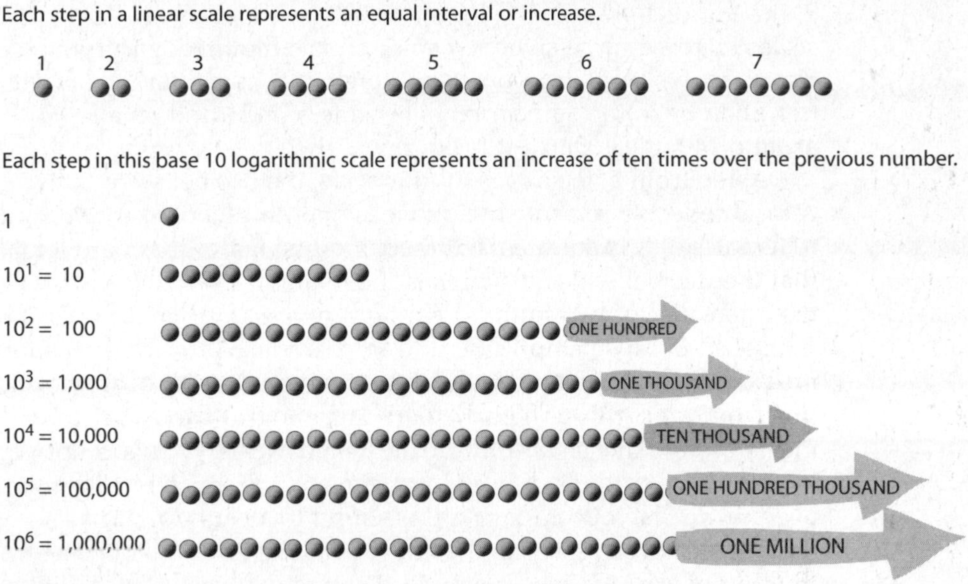

Each step in a linear scale represents an equal interval or increase.

Each step in this base 10 logarithmic scale represents an increase of ten times over the previous number.

■ FIGURE 2.15

Linear versus logarithmic scale.

two points on the ruler is ten times greater than a distance of 1 mm. Put another way, the distance between 2 and 3 in. is exactly the same as the distance between 8 and 9 in., which is exactly the same as the distance between 4 and 5 in. Thus, successive units are always the same distance from each other. Temperature scales are also examples of linear scales, with the distance between units indicating equal increments of temperature increase or decrease.

Logarithmic scales, on the other hand, contain units that increase by greater and greater amounts as we go up the scale. These units cannot be added or subtracted because they are not equal. A logarithmic scale has several components. The first is a base, such as 2 or 10. A logarithmic scale with a base of 2 indicates that each successive unit increases by a factor of 2. With a base of 10, each unit increases by a factor of 10. The number of increases on a logarithmic scale is indicated by the exponent, or power (not to be confused with power as it relates to energy). A base is raised to some power. A base of 10 raised to the first power, or with an exponent of 1, is 10^1. 10 multiplied by 1 is 10. A base of 10 raised to the second power equals 10^2. In this case you multiply the base by itself 2 times. 10 times 10 is 100. Similarly, 10 raised to the third power is 10^3. Multiply base 10 by itself 3 times, and you get 10 times 10 times 10, equaling 1000. Particularly with base 10, the exponents are often used by themselves with the understanding that this is the power to which 10 must be raised in order to equal the original number. This exponent is then called the log. For example, the log of 100 is

2, the log of 1000 is 3, the log of 10,000 is 4, and so on. Thus, whereas linear scales increase successively by some equal amount, logarithmic scales increase by successively greater amounts. Therefore, a huge number of units of intensity (a trillion or so) on a linear scale becomes condensed on a logarithmic scale to around 140 units (Durrant & Lovrinic, 1995).

Aside from being a logarithmic scale, the decibel scale is also a **ratio scale**. A ratio reflects a relationship between quantities. For example, a ratio of males to females of 2:1 indicates that there are two males for every female. The ratio that the decibel scale measures is the relationship between the amplitudes or the intensities of two sounds. Why is it necessary to make these kinds of comparisons? Because amplitude and intensity are physical measures, we could measure the precise amplitude or the precise intensity of any sound. However, this would not give us a particularly meaningful value. Say that a sound were measured to have an amplitude of 0.045 dyne/cm^2. This is not very revealing information, in terms of how loud you actually perceive the sound to be. We need some way of comparing this sound to a sound that has a known amplitude and intensity level so that we can tell if it is higher or lower in intensity. In other words, we need a standard sound that can serve as the basis of comparison for all other sounds. This is the basis for the decibel scale.

The decibel scale is a ratio scale; it compares any target sound with a **standard reference sound**. This standard reference sound has a specific amplitude of 20 μ Pa (0.0002 dyne/cm^2, or 0.0002 microbar, μbar) and a specific intensity of 10^{-12} W/m^2 (10^{-16} W/cm^2). In the perceptual domain, a sound with this amplitude and intensity indicates the softest sound of a particular frequency that a pair of normal human ears can hear 50 percent of the time under ideal listening conditions. Perceptually, this is known as the **threshold of hearing**. (Baken [1996] pointed out that the human threshold of hearing at 0.0002 μbar is equivalent to 0.000000204 cm H$_2$O, demonstrating the extraordinary sensitivity of the human auditory system.) On the decibel scale, a sound of this level is indicated by 0. Keeping in mind that the decibel scale is a ratio scale, 0 dB does not mean that there is silence, but that the sound in question has the same intensity and amplitude as the standard reference sound. It is also possible to have a negative number on the decibel scale; this just means that the sound in question has an amplitude and intensity less than that of the standard reference sound.

The formula to derive the intensity or amplitude of a target sound (I_1 or P_1) in relation to a standard reference intensity or amplitude (I_0 or P_0) is based on the logarithm of a ratio, or the bel. The formula for intensity is $N(bels)=\log_{10} I_1/I_0$. This means that the number of bels is equal to a logarithmic scale of base 10 on which the target intensity level (I_1) is divided by the reference intensity level (I_0). However, because the bel is a large unit, most applications in acoustics use the deci-

The standard reference sound has an amplitude of 20 micropascals and an intensity of 10^{-12} W/m^2. It corresponds to 0 dB.

The threshold of hearing indicates the softest sound of a particular frequency that a pair of normal human ears can hear 50 percent of the time under ideal listening conditions. This corresponds to the standard reference sound on the dB scale.

bel, which, as noted previously, is one-tenth of a bel. Thus, the formula for intensity in decibels (dB) is $N(dB)=10 \log_{10} I_1/I_0$. Say, for example, the target intensity I_1 is 100 times the reference intensity I_0. We know that the log of 100 is 2. Multiplying 2 by 10 gives 20, so a sound that is 100 times as intense as the reference sound has a value of 20 dB. In the same way, a sound that is 1000 times as intense as the reference sound will have a dB value of 30 (the log of 1000 is 3; multiply 3 by 10), a sound that is 10,000 times as intense as the reference will be equal to 40 dB, and so on. The standard reference for intensity is 10^{-12} W/m². Substituting this value for I_0, intensity level is expressed as the formula: $IL(dB)=10 \log_{10} I_1/10^{-12}$ W/m².

> The formula for intensity is $IL(dB) = 10 \log_{10} I_1/10^{-12}$ W/m².

A similar formula is used for amplitude, or sound pressure level (SPL). The only difference is that instead of multiplying the log by 10, it is multiplied by 20, because of the relationship between intensity and amplitude (recall that intensity is the square of pressure). The formula for SPL is $SPL(dB) = 20 \log_{10} P_1/P_0$. We know that the reference for amplitude is 20 micropascals, so $SPL(dB) = 20 \log_{10} P_1/20 \, \mu Pa$. It is very important to keep in mind, however, that the difference in the equations for intensity and pressure does not mean that a sound with an IL of 30 dB has an SPL of 60 dB.

> The formula for amplitude is $SPL(dB) = 20 \log_{10} P_1/20 \, \mu Pa$.

The decibel unit is dimensionless unless it is anchored to a referent. In other words, if you say that a sound has a decibel level of 32, even though we know this number is in comparison to 0 dB the information is meaningless, because the number lacks a referent. By analogy, if someone told you that Sue is twice as tall as Mary, you still would not know how tall either of them was, despite the comparison between them. Therefore, it is important when using the decibel scale to specify whether amplitude or intensity is being measured. When amplitude is measured, the units on the decibel scale are referenced to sound pressure level (SPL). For intensity, the units are referenced to intensity level (IL). Thus, it is clear that a sound of 32 dB SPL has a certain amplitude in relation to the standard amplitude reference of 20 μPa; a sound of 32 dB IL has a certain intensity in relation to the standard intensity referent of 10^{-12} W/m².

Zero on the decibel scale means that there is a one-to-one ratio of the two sound intensities or amplitudes of the sounds being compared. A unit of 1 dB corresponds to an intensity ratio of about 1.26:1. That is, the higher intensity is 26 percent greater than the lower one (Denes & Pinson, 1993). Thus, a 1 dB step in intensity corresponds to about a 26 percent change. Perceptually, the decibel is the smallest change in sound intensity that an individual with normal hearing can perceive (Durrant & Lovrinic, 1995). Each step in the decibel scale corresponds to a more or less equal increase in a person's perception of loudness, even though the actual pressure and power differences increase dramatically (Borden, Harris, & Raphael, 1994). Since the decibel scale is logarithmic, a 1 dB step at the threshold of hearing will be a very tiny change. At the intensity level for normal conversational speech, however, which is around 60 dB

IL, this 26 percent intensity change for 1 dB is 1 million times greater than the 1 dB change at the threshold of hearing.

Since intensity is the square of amplitude, a 100-fold increase in intensity corresponds to a 10-fold increase in amplitude. A 10,000-fold increase in intensity corresponds to a 100-fold increase in amplitude (Denes & Pinson, 1993). Because of this correspondence between intensity and amplitude, the same decibel level can refer to values of both intensity and amplitude. Decibel IL always equals decibel SPL as long as equivalent reference pressures and intensities are used (Speaks, 1992). For example, 60 dB IL equals 60 dB SPL, 78.5 dB IL equals 78.5 dB SPL, and so on. By analogy, a pound of feathers equals a pound of lead, despite the different materials of which they are composed.

Very specific mathematical relationships have been worked out between intensity, amplitude, and the decibel scale. In terms of intensity, any doubling (or halving) of sound power results in an increase (or decrease) of 3 dB. Increasing (or decreasing) intensity by a factor of 10 corresponds to an increase (or decrease) of 10 dB. In terms of amplitude, a doubling (or halving) of sound pressure corresponds to an increase (or decrease) of 6 dB. A ten-fold change in sound pressure corresponds to a change of 20 dB. Also note that doubling (or halving) sound power increases (or decreases) both IL and SPL by 3 dB, whereas doubling (or halving) sound pressure increases (or decreases) both IL and SPL by 6 dB.

■ TABLE 2.2

Familiar Sounds and Sound Levels

SOUND	SOUND LEVEL (dB SPL OR IL)
Threshold of hearing	0
Normal breathing	10
Rustle of leaves	20
Very soft whisper	30
Quiet residential community	40
Department store	50
Normal conversation	60
Inside moving car	70
Loud music from radio	80
City traffic	90
Subway train	100
Loud thunder	110
Amplified rock and roll band	120
Machine gun fire at close range	130
Jet engine at takeoff	140
Space rocket at blast-off	180

Source: Durrant & Lovrinic (1995).

Advantages of the Decibel Scale   One important advantage of using the decibel scale is that huge ranges of intensities are condensed, because of the logarithmic nature of the scale, into around 140 units on the decibel scale. Another advantage is that the relationship between the decibel scale and absolute values of pressure and intensity is very similar to the physiological function of the human auditory system. A change in intensity that is just barely able to be perceived near our hearing threshold is produced by a 1 dB change in the stimulus. As the sound intensity level increases, the intensity change that produces a just perceivable change in loudness continues to be about 1 dB, although the absolute intensity change increases. Table 2.2 provides examples of decibel levels that correspond to the perception of some familiar sounds.

Auditory Area   With a knowledge of frequency, amplitude, and intensity, we are now in a position to examine the human range of hearing in terms of both frequency and intensity. We noted that humans can perceive frequencies from around 20 to 20,000 Hz. The human auditory system is also equipped to perceive an enormously wide range of intensities. However, the intensities that humans are sensitive to depend on the frequency of the sound. The human auditory system is more sensitive to sounds in the midrange of frequencies than to those that are very low or very high. Frequencies in the midrange can be perceived when they are less intense, whereas a very low or very high frequency sound needs to have much more intensity in order to be perceptible to humans. A sound in the middle of the range, say 2000 Hz, requires an intensity of around 11 dB to be just audible (threshold of hearing), whereas a sound with a frequency of 125 Hz requires an intensity of 47.5 dB. According to the ANSI Standard (1969) for audiometers, Table 2.3 shows frequencies and intensities at the threshold of hearing for normal ears.

Although the threshold of hearing changes depending on the frequency of the sound, any frequency with an intensity of 130 dB will cause a sensation of

■ TABLE 2.3

Frequencies and Intensities at the Threshold of Hearing (Normal Ears)

FREQUENCY (Hz)	INTENSITY (dB)
125	47.5
250	26.5
500	13.5
1000	7.5
2000	11.0
4000	10.5
8000	13.0

The auditory area is the complete range of human hearing in terms of frequency and intensity bounded by the threshold of hearing and the threshold of pain.

pain in the ear. This level is known as the **threshold of pain**. Thus, some frequencies have a wider range of intensities at which they can be perceived, whereas others have a more limited range between the threshold of hearing and the threshold of pain. For example, a person with normal hearing would be able to just barely perceive a 1000 Hz tone with an intensity of 7.5 dB and would feel pain in the ear when that tone had an intensity of 130 dB. However, a tone with a frequency of 125 Hz would be just barely audible at an intensity of 47.5 dB, but would still cause pain at an intensity of 130 dB. People with hearing impairment are sensitive to smaller ranges of intensities. For example, a hearing-impaired individual may be only able to detect a 1000 Hz tone when it has an intensity of 60 dB and may find the sound painfully loud at an intensity of 90 dB.

■ *Resonance*

Free and Forced Vibration

Vibration of an object can occur freely or by force. An object that is vibrating freely does so without interference at a rate determined by its physical characteristics, including its mass, tension, and stiffness. Whenever this particular object is set into vibration, it will always vibrate at its own specific frequency.

Natural or resonant frequency refers to the rate at which an object vibrates freely and depends on its physical characteristics.

This is free vibration, and the frequency at which the object vibrates is called its natural or **resonant frequency** (RF). Free vibration demonstrates the natural response of a vibratory system (Durrant & Lovrinic, 1995). For example, a swing, when pushed, will move back and forth at a certain rate, say twice per second. Its RF is thus 2 Hz, and this is the rate at which the swing will always move as long as its physical characteristics remain constant.

Forced vibration refers to the fact that the vibrations from one object can set another object into vibration if the RFs of both objects are reasonably close to each other. You have probably had the experience of hearing or seeing the pictures hanging on your walls rattle when a car with a particularly loud stereo goes by. If the vibrations generated by the stereo are close to the RF of the wall, the wall will be set into vibration, causing the rattling of the pictures. Or maybe some part in your car starts to rattle in sympathy with the engine noise as you turn the key in the ignition. Here, too, the vibration of the engine may be close in frequency to some other part of your car, which is then forced to vibrate in sympathy with the engine noise. Another example of resonance is portrayed in cartoons in which a singer hits a particularly high note and suddenly a wine glass shatters. This, too, is an example of forced vibration. The glass has its own specific RF. When the singer hits a note that is close to the glass's RF, the glass is set into vibration. If the amplitude of vibration is great enough, the glass shatters as it vibrates.

The phenomenon of how the vibration generated by one object forces another object into vibration can be explained using the example of two tuning forks with identical frequencies. When one fork is struck and vibrates and is then brought close to the other fork, the vibrations from fork 1 push against fork 2, and eventually set it into vibration. When tuning fork 2 begins to vibrate, the resulting sound from both tuning forks is louder than the sound generated by tuning fork 1 alone. Using a swing as an analogy, if you push a swing very gently, the first push will hardly move the swing from its rest position. If you keep giving gentle pushes, after a time the swing will start to move, and the more pushes you give it, the greater distance back and forth the swing will move. The timing of the pushes is very important, however. To get the swing to move, the push has to be timed with the movement of the swing toward you, when it has reached its maximum amplitude, and just before it starts swinging back to its rest position. Timed like this, the swing's amplitude will increase. If you push the swing as it is still moving toward you, its amplitude will be decreased rather than increased. If you push the swing just as it is passing over its rest position on its way toward you, it will stop. In this analogy you are acting as tuning fork number 1, and the swing corresponds to tuning fork number 2.

Essentially, what happens with the tuning forks is constructive interference. Because the two tuning forks have the same frequency, each small vibration arrives at exactly the right moment so that areas of compression and rarefaction combine constructively and the amplitude of the resulting wave increases. Tuning fork 2 has not created the original sound, just as in the swing analogy the swing has not created the original movement. Instead, tuning fork 2 is vibrating in response to the vibrations of tuning fork 1. In the analogy, the swing is set into vibration in response to your pushing.

Another example of forced vibration is the situation in which we set the tuning fork into vibration and then press its stem against a table top. In this case, the fork forces the table top to vibrate at the fork's RF, even though the RF of the table top is different from that of the fork. Since the table has a much larger vibrating area than the tuning fork, forcing the table top to vibrate in sympathy increases the amplitude of the resulting sound wave.

The wave that forces a resonator into vibration is called the applied frequency or driving frequency.

In resonance, an object is forced to vibrate in response to the vibrations of another object. In the example, tuning fork 1 creates the original sound, and tuning fork 2 resonates the sound, making it louder. Tuning fork 1 supplies the driving or **applied frequency**, and tuning fork 2 is the **resonator**. The closer the RF of the driving force is to the RF of the resonator, the greater will be the amplitude of the response of the resonator.

Types of Resonators

There are two types of resonators, mechanical and acoustic. For a **mechanical resonator**, the actual object itself is set into vibration, for instance, tuning fork number 2 or the table in our examples above. Another type of resonator is a container filled with air. Such a container is an **acoustic resonator** and is enormously important in the production of speech.

Acoustic Resonators   A volume of air enclosed in a container can resonate. When a sound wave is applied to the air in the container, the air is compressed and rarefied. Because air has elasticity, the air inside the container pushes the compressed air out again. If another sound wave reaches the container at the same time that the compressed air is being pushed out, constructive interference causes an increased amplitude of the sound wave, as long as the applied frequency is close to the RF of the enclosed air. The RF of the air-filled container depends to a great extent on its volume. A smaller volume of air resonates at higher frequencies, whereas a larger volume of air resonates at lower frequencies.

A container filled with air acts as an acoustic resonator that selectively filters applied frequencies.

Many musical instruments are acoustic resonators in which the air is set into vibration through the action of some other vibration. A good example is a guitar. The body of the guitar is a container with a round hole in the middle, filled with air. The strings are stretched across the body of the guitar. When you pluck the string, you create a sound by setting the string into vibration. This sets air particles in the vicinity of the string into vibration, causing pressure changes to spread in all directions. Some of the pressure changes go into the body of the guitar through the hole and force the air within the body, as well as the body itself, to vibrate. The air vibrates with the greatest amplitude at frequencies close to the frequency at which the string is vibrating. The string creates the driving frequency, and the air in the body resonates at this frequency. Due to constructive interference, a much louder sound is created. If the string were not stretched across the guitar, but you just held it and plucked it, a very soft sound would result. Forcing the air in the guitar to vibrate with greatest amplitude at the frequency of the string results in a much greater loudness.

Acoustic Resonators as Filters

One reason that acoustic resonators are so important for speech is that they act as filters by filtering some frequencies out of a sound, while allowing others to remain. Let us use as an illustration of acoustic filtering a tube that is perfectly cylindrical along its length. This tube is an acoustic resonator because it is filled with air, and it has a RF of, say, 500 Hz. If you were at one end of this tube and another person were at the other end, and you whistled at different pitches, with each pitch having the same intensity, the other person would hear some pitches more loudly and some less loudly. The frequencies closest to the tube's RF of 500 Hz would be heard the loudest. The farther from 500 Hz the frequency of your whistle is, the more softly the other person would hear the sound. There might even be some pitches that the person would not hear at all.

In this example the effect of resonance is to amplify those frequencies that are closest to the tube's RF and damp or attenuate those frequencies that are farther away from its RF. The whistle close to 500 Hz is similar to the RF of the tube, and so the sound is amplified. The farther away the frequencies of the whistle to the RF of the tube, the more the sound is attenuated or damped. Thus, the resonator acts as a filter by amplifying and transmitting those frequencies close to its own RF and attenuating or preventing frequencies farther away from its own RF from being transmitted. This filtering property of acoustic resonators is one of the fundamental ways in which we produce different sounds.

Bandwidth   Not all acoustic resonators are perfectly symmetrical, like the tube in our example. Some containers are irregularly shaped or even change their shape. The shape and other physical characteristics of the container, such as whether it is closed at both of its ends, open at both ends, closed at one end and open at the other, and so on, determine the **bandwidth** of the resonator (see Figure 2.16). Bandwidth refers to the range of frequencies that a resonator will transmit. A symmetrical tube like the one in our example will only transmit a narrow range of frequencies. Our tube could have a bandwidth of 100 Hz. This means that it would transmit those frequencies within 50 Hz of its RF on either side. Frequencies between 450 and 550 Hz would be transmitted and amplified, whereas those frequencies below 450 Hz and above 550 Hz would be damped. This kind of resonator is said to be **sharply** or **narrowly tuned**.

> The bandwidth of a resonator is the range of frequencies that it will transmit.

> A sharply tuned resonator has a narrow bandwidth; a broadly tuned resonator has a greater bandwidth.

A narrowly tuned system responds slowly to the driving frequencies. In other words, the amplitude of an applied vibration grows slowly until it reaches its greatest level. A narrowly tuned resonator is also lightly damped. In other words, once it has been forced into vibration, the vibrations take a relatively long time to fade away.

Resonators that are more complex and irregular in shape tend to have wider bandwidths. An irregularly shaped container with an RF of 500 Hz might have a bandwidth of 400 Hz. Thus, frequencies between 300 and 700 Hz would be transmitted, whereas those below 300 Hz and above 700 Hz would be attenuated. Such a resonator is more **broadly tuned**. A broadly tuned system will respond very quickly to the applied frequencies, but the vibrations will also fade more quickly. A broadly tuned resonator is heavily damped. Broadly tuned systems are common in speech and hearing applications and

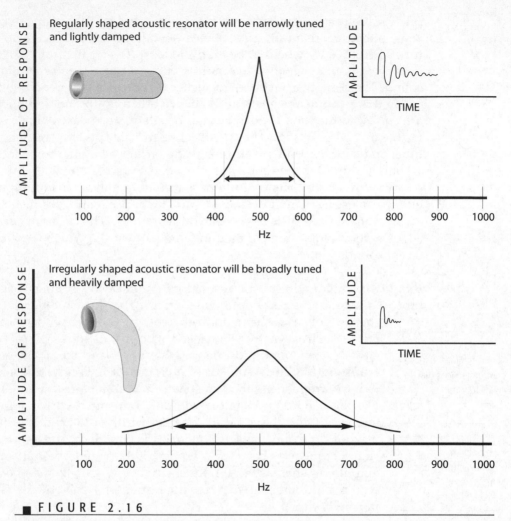

■ FIGURE 2.16

Bandwidth.

include the diaphragms of microphones, earphones, and loudspeakers, as well as our eardrums and vocal tracts.

Cutoff Frequencies   Resonant systems seldom have a clearcut point above which frequencies are amplified and below which they are attenuated. Instead, frequencies are transmitted with increasingly less efficiency as the driving frequency becomes farther removed from the RF of the system, until the amount of acoustic energy that is transmitted is so small as to be basically nonexistent.

A numerical value has been developed to describe the point at which the resonant system is considered to be unresponsive. This is the point where the intensity transmission is reduced by one-half and is known as the **cutoff**

The point at which a resonator becomes unresponsive to an applied frequency is called the cutoff frequency.

frequency. Remember that a reduction in intensity of one-half is equivalent to a decrease of 3 dB. Therefore, the frequency at which the intensity is 3 dB less than the peak intensity of the RF is the cutoff frequency and is also, therefore, called the 3 dB *down point*. Another way the cutoff frequency can be stated is in percentage form. The 3 dB cutoff corresponds to a percentage of 70.7. In other words, any frequency within the resonator's bandwidth will generate an output whose amplitude will be at least 70.7 percent of the amplitude of the vibrations caused by the frequency closest to the RF of the resonator.

Resonance Curves   The way in which a resonator vibrates in response to any applied frequency can be described by a graph known as a **resonance** (or filter) **curve**. This curve is also called the **transfer function** of a resonant system. If we apply different frequencies to a resonator and each frequency has the same amplitude, the resonator will be forced into vibration by each of these applied frequencies. However, the applied frequencies closest to the RF of the resonator will cause the largest vibrations. The sounds that are used to set a resonator in motion are known as the input to the resonator. The way in which the resonator vibrates in response to these sounds is known as its output for a given input, and it is this input–output relationship that is shown on a resonance curve. Another way of stating this relationship is that a resonance or filter curve shows the frequency response of a resonant system.

A resonance curve, also called a transfer function, is a graph with frequency on the horizontal axis and relative amplitude on the vertical axis. It depicts the response of a resonator to any applied frequency.

As Figure 2.17 shows, the greatest amplitude of response occurs at the RF of the system. Frequencies far from the RF have been filtered, so their

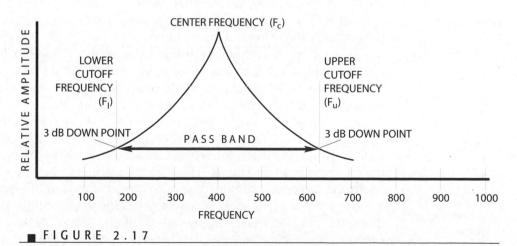

■ FIGURE 2.17

Cutoff frequency response and passband of resonator.

amplitudes are less than the amplitude at the RF. Thus, this resonance curve describes how the amplitudes of the various component frequencies of the sound wave are affected by the resonator or, to put it slightly differently, how the spectrum of a sound is changed when the sound is resonated with this particular system. It is important to keep in mind that this curve is not a sound wave, but describes the frequency response, or transfer function, of the resonator.

Parameters of a Filter   All resonators, or filter systems, have certain characteristics. These include the natural or resonant frequency, the upper cutoff frequency, the lower cutoff frequency, the bandwidth, and the attenuation or rejection rate.

The natural frequency is also called the **center frequency** (F_c). This is the resonant frequency of the system that results in the greatest amplitude of vibration of the resonator. The center frequency depends on the physical characteristics of the resonator, such as its length and shape. In the example earlier, the center frequency of the tube was 500 Hz.

> The natural or center frequency is the resonant frequency of a system that results in the greatest amplitude of vibration.

The **upper cutoff frequency** (F_u) is the frequency above F_c at which there is a 3 dB less amplitude of response of the resonator than that at F_c. The **lower cutoff frequency** (F_l) corresponds to the frequency below F_c where the amplitude is decreased by 3 dB. Because a 3 dB decrease in amplitude corresponds to a halving of amplitude, both F_u and F_l are also called the 3 dB down points, or the **half-power points**.

The bandwidth, or **passband**, refers to the frequencies between F_u and F_l, that is, the range of frequencies that the resonator will transmit. The bandwidth can be broad or narrow, depending on the physical characteristics of the resonator. The rate at which the resonator's amplitude of response is attenuated is known as the **attenuation rate**. (It is also referred to as the **roll-off rate**, the **rejection rate**, or the **slope**.) This parameter describes how rapidly the resonator decreases in its amplitude of response to different frequencies and is measured in decibels per octave. Slopes can range from shallow to steep. A slope of less than 18 dB/octave would be considered fairly shallow. A filter with an attenuation rate between 18 and 48 dB/octave is moderately steep, while filters with cutoffs greater than 90 dB/octave are extremely steep (Rosen & Howell, 1991).

> Attenuation rate refers to the rate at which the resonator's amplitude of response is attenuated. It is also called the roll-off rate, rejection rate, or slope.

Types of Filters   Different types of filters are suitable for performing different types of functions. Three kinds of filters are commonly encountered in speech pathology and audiology. First is a **low-pass filter**, which passes acoustic energy below a specific upper cutoff frequency. Acoustic energy above the F_u is attenuated at a particular rejection rate. Frequencies below the cutoff frequency are passed through the system well, while those above the cutoff frequency are attenuated. Second is a

> A low-pass filter passes acoustic energy below a specific upper cutoff frequency; a high-pass filter transmits energy above a specific lower cutoff frequency.

high-pass filter, which passes energy above a designated lower cutoff frequency. Energy below F_l is rejected at a particular attenuation rate, while acoustic energy above F_l is transmitted through the system. Third, a **band-pass filter** passes energy in a particular range of frequencies between an F_l and an F_u. Energy outside this range is rejected at a specific attenuation rate. A band-pass filter is a combination of low-pass and high-pass filtering. The low-pass filter transmits energy below the F_u, while the high-pass filter transmits energy above the F_l. The vocal tract is an example of a band-pass filter.

s u m m a r y

- Sound consists of increases and decreases in air pressure caused by the movement of a source, such as a tuning fork.
- Sound waves are characterized by different dimensions of frequency, period, wavelength, amplitude, and intensity.
- Sound waves can consist of one frequency (pure tone) or many frequencies (complex waves).
- Sound waves can be visually depicted on waveforms and spectra.

- Amplitude and intensity of sounds can be measured conveniently on the decibel scale.
- Resonance involves forced vibration in which an object or container of air is set into vibration by the action of another vibration.
- Acoustic resonators may be sharply or broadly tuned, with different center frequencies and upper and lower cutoff frequencies.

r e v i e w   e x e r c i s e s

1. Use an example other than a tuning fork to explain how sound is generated. Describe the forces involved in generating, maintaining, and damping vibration.
2. Define and explain the terms *reverberation*, *absorption*, *reflection*, and *interference*.
3. Discuss the following statement: "Speech is a stream of periodic and aperiodic complex sounds."

4. Describe the decibel scale and explain its major advantage in measuring sound intensity.
5. Discuss the concept of resonance and explain how an acoustic resonator acts as a filter.

chapter 3

Clinical Application
Frequency and Intensity Variables

After reading this chapter, you will

1. Be familiar with frequency variables often used in clinical situations, such as average F_0, speaking F_0, F_0 variability, and maximum phonation frequency range.

2. Be familiar with amplitude variables often used in clinical situations, such as average amplitude, amplitude variability, and dynamic range.

3. Understand the relationship between the measurements of frequency, intensity, and the voice range profile.

4. Appreciate the importance of F_0 and amplitude measurement in the diagnosis and treatment of voice disorders.

5. Understand the application of frequency and amplitude measurement in communication disorders.

An understanding of the basic nature of sound and of the important dimensions of sound, including frequency and intensity, allows speech–language pathologists and audiologists to apply this knowledge in the diagnosis and treatment of many different communication problems. Norms have been developed for many acoustic variables related to human voice and speech production, including various aspects of frequency and intensity. Norms are available for different age groups, including infants and toddlers, school-age children, and adults at different stages of life. These objective normal values form a scientifically based body of knowledge against which the voice and speech characteristics of individuals with various communication disorders can be compared, such as functional and organic voice disorders, neurological problems, and speech problems related to hearing impairment.

These kinds of comparisons are invaluable in clinical situations. They help to refine the process of differential diagnosis by providing information about aspects of speech production that may not be detected or processed by human ears, but that offer important clues about a patient's condition. Objective measures are vital also to validate a clinician's perceptual judgments of disordered voice and speech. In addition, they offer a starting point for rehabilitation and provide an objective means of assessing the patient's progress. Objective acoustic measures not only supplement the clinician's therapeutic skills, but also strengthen clinician accountability, which is a crucial issue in health care management. More and more, third-party payers such as insurance companies and HMOs will only pay for benefits if it can be shown that the treatment is effective. Objective measures are invaluable in providing this kind of supporting information about the patient's progress.

However, a word of caution is in order. Although norms, in general, provide a valuable basis of comparison, abnormal data do not always indicate a pathology, even when they exceed typical values. It is important, therefore, for clinicians and researchers to critically evaluate the information obtained and to supplement it with information from other sources.

Vocal Frequency and Amplitude

When people talk, their vocal folds open and close to produce vibration, resulting in a complex periodic sound with a certain fundamental frequency (F_0) and amplitude. As with any complex periodic sound, the F_0 is perceived as the pitch of the sound, and the amplitude is perceived as its loudness.

Vocal fold vibration gives rise to numerous aspects of vocal F_0 and amplitude that can be measured by way of acoustic instrumentation. A commonly used instrument in university speech and hearing clinics, rehabilitation centers, schools, and hospitals is the Visi-Pitch, made and distributed by Kay Elemetrics. This is a computer-based **transducer** fitted with acoustic hardware and software. A person speaks into an attached microphone, which changes, or *transduces*, the acoustic signal into corresponding electrical signals. The hardware and software digitize the signal, converting it into a format that the computer can process. The Visi-Pitch calculates F_0 and relative amplitude over time, and displays these on a monitor. Variables related to F_0 and amplitude can then be determined, such as the average and range. Other instruments are also commercially available for acoustic measurement of voice F_0 and amplitude.

Frequency Variables

F_0 variables that are very commonly used in the clinical situation include average F_0, F_0 variability and range, and maximum phonational frequency range.

Average Fundamental Frequency   The F_0 measured in a particular task, such as sustaining a vowel, reading aloud, or conversational speech, is averaged over the speaking time of that task. When average F_0 is measured in an oral reading or conversational speech task, it is often referred to as the person's speaking fundamental frequency (SFF). Many speech scientists have examined the average F_0 in different age groups and across both sexes. Table 3.1 shows some of the values for average F_0 that have been derived using various types of acoustic instrumentation.

Looking at the table, you can see a systematic pattern of F_0 values that vary according to age level and sex. Infants in the first several years of life have a very high F_0, from around 350 to almost 500 Hz. In musical terms, this is from around the F an octave above middle C to the B almost two octaves above middle C. This high F_0 is the result of the infant's very short and thin vocal folds, which have a very rapid rate of vibration. As the baby

> Average fundamental frequency (F_0) refers to the F_0 measured in a particular speaking task, averaged over the speaking time of that task.

■ **TABLE 3.1**

Average F_0 for Different Age Groups Reported in the Literature

AUTHOR(S)	AGE GROUP	MALES	FEMALES	RACE
		(HERTZ)		
Robb & Saxman (1985)	11–25 (mos)	357	357	
McGlone & Shipp (1971)	13–23 (mos)	443	443	
Eguchi & Hirsh (1969)	3	298	298	
	4	286	286	
	5	289	289	
Awan & Mueller (1996)	5–6	240	243	W
	5–6	241	231	AA
	5–6	249	248	H
Weinberg & Bennett (1971)	5	252	248	
	6	247	247	
Wheat & Hudson (1988)	6	219	211	AA
Ferrand & Bloom (1996)	3–6	256	246	
	7–10	237	253	

■ TABLE 3.1 *continued*

AUTHOR(S)	AGE GROUP	MALES (HERTZ)	FEMALES	RACE
Sorenson (1989)	6	251	296	
	7	288	258	
	8	229	251	
	9	221	266	
	10	220	229	
Pederson et al. (1990)	8.6–12.9		256	
	13–15.9		248	
	16–19.8		241	
Bennett (1983)	8.2	234	235	
	9.2	226	222	
	10.2	224	228	
	11.2	216	221	
Fitch (1990)	21–26	109	210	
Kent (1994)	20.3	120		
	47.9	123		
	73.3	119		
	85	136		
Hollien & Shipp (1972)	20–29	120		
	30–39	112		
	40–49	107		
	50–59	118		
	60–69	112		
	70–79	132		
	80–89	146		
de Pinto & Hollien (1982)	18–25	229		
Morgan & Rastatter (1986)	20–24		228	
Pegoraro Krook (1988)	20–29		195	
	30–39		195	
	40–49		191	
	50–59		182	
	60–69		181	
	70–79		188	
	80–89		188	
Russell et al. (1995)	65–68		181	
Brown et al. (1996)	21–33	136		
	20–22		189	
	40–54	128		
	42–50		186	
	69–87	134		
	65–89		175	
Honjo & Isshiki (1980)	69–85	162	177	

Values for postlingual children and adults are for conversational speech or oral reading. Some studies included race as a factor: white (W), African American (AA), Hispanic (H). Unless otherwise stated, ages are in years.

Note: Some values have been rounded to the nearest whole number.

grows, his or her vocal folds lengthen and thicken, with a corresponding decrease in F_0. From around age 3 to 10 years, both males and females have an average F_0 of approximately 270 to 300 Hz. After puberty, the average F_0 for males drops markedly, while that for females remains essentially the same or may decrease slightly. Again, these F_0 patterns are related to growth factors. At puberty, the male larynx enlarges considerably, and the vocal folds become longer, thicker, and more massive, with a corresponding dramatic drop in F_0. A girl's larynx and vocal folds also enlarge somewhat during puberty, but not to the same extent as a boy's. By age 20, the average F_0 for males is around 120 Hz, while for females the average F_0 is approximately 100 Hz higher than males, at 220 Hz.

Average F_0 remains fairly stable for adult males and females until the sixth and seventh decades, when males' average F_0 typically increase due to age-related degenerative changes that occur within the larynx, including a thinning of the vocal folds. Because objects that are thinner and less massive vibrate more quickly than those that are more massive, the thinning of the male's vocal folds produces an increase in vocal F_0. Older women, on the other hand, tend to develop more massive vocal folds due to hormonal changes. Thus, the F_0 of older women tends to decrease with age.

These age- and gender-related values for average F_0 are vitally important in clinical situations. First, they tell us that we cannot judge F_0 the same way for young children and adults, or for younger adults and older adults, or for adult males and females. Second, they provide an objective basis for evaluating the appropriateness of an individual's pitch level. That is, is it normal or too high for their age and gender or too low for their age and gender? So, if we are interested in judging if a person's pitch level is adequate, why not just listen to her or him and rate the pitch according to what we hear? The answer is that subjective, perceptual methods of assessing pitch are unreliable. Although F_0 and pitch are related, how we perceive pitch also depends on the interaction of frequency, intensity, and other properties of the sound. In addition, the human auditory system responds more easily to some frequencies than others. For example, pitch changes at lower frequencies are usually perceived much more easily than changes at higher frequencies. Raising F_0 from 100 to 200 Hz results in a much greater change in perceived pitch than going from 3000 to 3100 Hz (Baken, 1996). Thus, a pitch level that is heard as abnormal may be due to the speaker's actual F_0, vocal intensity, or other factors. Therefore, to make a clinical decision about whether or how to treat an individual with a pitch disorder, objective acoustic measurement of the person's F_0 is critical. Quantifying a speaker's F_0 levels and comparing his or her SFF to established norms for speakers of similar age and sex will help the clinician decide whether the perceived abnormality really does result from an F_0 problem, or whether (and what) other vocal factors are involved.

Frequency variability is the range of F_0s used in conversational speech measured either in terms of standard deviation of F_0 or pitch sigma.

Frequency Variability   People constantly change their F_0 levels as they speak to reflect different emotions, different types of accenting and stress of syllables, and different grammatical constructions. These F_0 changes contribute to the overall melody, or prosody, of speech. For instance, the sentence "Peter's going home" can be said either as a declarative statement or as a question. As a declarative, the F_0 level drops at the end of the utterance, whereas for a question the F_0 level rises at the end of the utterance. The prosody of a sentence also is influenced by the mood of the speaker. There are likely to be many more F_0 changes, and more extensive changes, when the individual is wildly excited that Peter's going home than when the speaker is depressed by Peter's plans. Acoustically, these F_0 changes correspond to frequency variability. A certain amount of frequency variability is desirable in a speaker's voice, depending on the individual's age, sex, social situation, mood, and so on. This variability is something that speakers of a particular language in a particular culture intuitively recognize. Too much or too little frequency variability sounds wrong and can indicate a functional, organic, or neurogenic voice problem.

F_0 variability is measured in terms of standard deviation (SD) from the average F_0. Standard deviation is a statistical measure that reflects the spread of scores around the average score, so standard deviation of F_0 reflects the spread of F_0 around the average F_0. When this variability is measured in hertz, it is called F_0SD. F_0SD in normal conversational speech is around 20 to 35 Hz. F_0SD is likely to increase when the speaker is excited or agitated. Sometimes F_0SD is converted to semitones. When the frequency variability is discussed in semitones rather than hertz, it is called **pitch sigma**. Pitch sigma for normal speakers during conversation should be around 2 to 4 semitones for both males and females (Colton & Casper, 1996).

Another measure of F_0 variability is the range, which is the difference between the highest and lowest F_0 in a particular sample of speech. The range can be expressed in hertz, or it can be converted to semitones and octaves. Table 3.2 displays F_0 range information for different age groups.

An interesting trend emerges from the numbers in Table 3.2. The infants (11 to 25 months) have by far the greatest range of frequencies. This is not surprising, because their vocalizations include a wide variety of nonwords, such as squeaks and squeals and cries. From around age 3 years, when children have mastered speech, to just before puberty, the range of F_0 used in normal conversational speech is around 150 to 200 Hz. The range decreases further in the adult years. From approximately age 7 years on, females tend to use a wider range of F_0 than males. This may be a sociocultural rather than a physical phenomenon. Ferrand and Bloom (1996) compared F_0 ranges in various age groups of boys and girls. The 7- to 10-year-old boys in their study had a narrower range than the 3- to 6-year-old boys. The range of the 7- to 10-year-old girls, however, was as wide

■ **TABLE 3.2**

F_0 Ranges for Spontaneous Speech for Males and Females in Selected Age Groups Reported in the Literature

AUTHORS	AGE GROUP	MALES (HERTZ)	FEMALES	RACE
Robb & Saxman (1985)	11–25 (mos)	1202	1202	
Ferrand & Bloom (1996)	3–4	202	190	
	5–6	214	199	
	7–8	158	203	
	9–10	151	180	
Awan & Mueller (1996)	5–6	186	214	W
	5–6	204	190	AA
	5–6	185	164	H
Benjamin (1981)	Younger adults	64	95	
	Older adults	78	101	
Fitch (1990)	21–26	46	77	

Some authors provide race information for white (W), African American (AA), and Hispanic (H) groups. Age is in years unless otherwise stated.

Notes: (a) Some values were derived by subtracting minimum from maximum frequencies. (b) Some values have been rounded to the nearest whole number.

as for younger girls. The authors suggested that boys, a few years before puberty, start to imitate the prosodic patterns of adult males, who tend to use fewer pitch levels than females and who also, in general, avoid dramatic pitch shifts.

F_0 variability, whether expressed in semitones, F_0SD, or F_0 range, is an important indicator of normal or disordered speech. In the clinic situation, it is very common for a person with a voice or speech disorder to demonstrate a reduced F_0 range. This is particularly true in many neurological problems, such as vocal fold paralysis or Parkinson's disease. F_0SD is also often used diagnostically to determine how well a person is able to control her vocal fold vibration. When a speaker prolongs a vowel, there should be very little F_0 variability in her production, because the goal is to produce the vowel with as steady an F_0 as possible. In this type of task, F_0SD should be low, around 3 to 6 Hz. A figure higher than this may indicate that the speaker has difficulty in controlling the frequency aspects of vocal fold vibration.

Maximum Phonational Frequency Range   **Maximum phonational frequency range** (MPFR) refers to the complete range of frequencies that an individual can generate, as opposed to the F_0 variability measure, which refers to the range of F_0 a person generally uses in connected speech. MPFR has been defined as the range of frequencies from the lowest tone that the person can sustain to the highest, including **falsetto**, which refers to a very high range of

The complete range of F_0s that an individual can generate from lowest to highest is called the maximum phonational frequency range.

frequencies (Baken, 1996). MPFR is often measured in semitones or octaves. A range of around 3 octaves is normal for young adults, while older adults may show a decrease in range. In terms of hertz, the lowest frequency that adult males are able to produce is around 80 Hz, and the highest is in the 700 Hz range (Colton & Casper, 1996). Adult females produce, on the whole, a low F_0 of approximately 135 Hz, with a high level that can reach over 1000 Hz. Trained singers, of course, are able to produce an even higher F_0 than this. Kent (1994) provided normative MPFRs in semitones for individuals from age 8 years to late adulthood. The lowest value of 24.3 semitones was demonstrated by older men in poor health; the greatest range of 41.4 semitones was shown by teenaged boys. Most values fell between these extremes, in the range of 30 semitones, or 2.5 octaves.

The MPFR is a useful measure because it reflects both the physiological limits of a speaker's voice (Colton & Casper, 1996) and the physical condition of the person's vocal mechanism and basic vocal ability (Baken, 1996). In fact, it has been shown that, for normally speaking adults, neither age nor sex greatly affects MPFR. What does affect this value is physical condition. Older subjects in good health tend to have larger MPFRs than younger subjects in poor physical condition. Thus, a clinician may suspect that a voice problem exists in a speaker who has a reduced MPFR.

Amplitude and Intensity Variables

Similarly to frequency variables, the voice amplitude that a person can generate is often an important indication of the normalcy or pathology of the vocal apparatus. Several common measurements of amplitude include the average amplitude level, amplitude variability, and dynamic range. Amplitude variables are typically measured in dB SPL (0.0002 dyne/cm^2). It is important to keep in mind that the voice amplitude that a person can generate depends strongly on the vocal F_0. We will talk more about this relationship between frequency and amplitude when we discuss the voice range profile.

Average amplitude level refers to the overall level of amplitude during a speech task.

Average Amplitude Level   Like average F_0, average amplitude refers to the overall level of amplitude during a speech task such as oral reading, conversation, or sustaining a vowel. Perceptually, this corresponds to the loudness that the individual generates during the speech activity. Amplitude level varies depending on the speaker's situation. A person's average amplitude level will be much lower during a soft conversation in a classroom and much higher when cheering at a football game. Normal conversational speech usually ranges between 65 and 80 dB SPL, with an average SPL in the general range of 70 dB for adult males and females (Baken, 1996). Children seem to use similar amplitude levels as adults. Amplitude levels do not depend on age as much as do frequency levels, although there is some evidence that amplitude may be decreased slightly in older individuals.

Clinically, a reduced amplitude level is strongly indicative of speech disorder, particularly those resulting from neurologic disease. Parkinson's disease, for example, is typically characterized by very low vocal amplitude, because the afflicted person has great difficulty in opening his or her vocal folds widely enough and closing them. Also, weak vocal amplitude is a large part of the problem in *alaryngeal speech,* that is, speech produced without a larynx after an individual has the larynx removed due to cancer. Obtaining acoustic information in these kinds of cases is vital for diagnosis and intervention purposes. Similar to the measurement of average frequency, measurement of average amplitude provides a basis of comparison for the patient's voice before, during, and after therapy. Identifying the specific amplitude levels that a patient is able to generate for various speech tasks can help the clinician determine whether a particular treatment strategy is producing the desired effect or whether a different strategy should be tried.

Amplitude Variability   During any conversation, amplitude varies depending on the speaker's mood, feelings, the message he or she is conveying, the stress and accenting of syllables and words, and so on. Titze (1994) remarked:

> Loudness variation is an important part of phrasing in speech. It serves as a punctuation, the setting apart of words, phrases, sentences, and paragraphs. In addition, loudness variation is used to emphasize . . . or to get attention. In poetry, rhetoric, and song, large variations in intensity are used to dramatize emotions, to convince someone of a point of view, or simply to entertain. (p. 246)

Changes in amplitude related to the speaker's mood, situation, feelings, and so on contribute to amplitude variability.

As with F_0, amplitude variability is expressed as a standard deviation, measured in dB SPL. Standard deviation of amplitude for a neutral, unemotional sentence is around 10 dB SPL. The greater the speaker's level of excitement or enthusiasm, the greater the variability is likely to be. Because amplitude variability is such an important marker of emphasis, emotion, and the like, a reduced ability to vary loudness can be highly upsetting. Not much research exists regarding amplitude variability in different age groups. However, many different communication disorders are characterized by such reduction in amplitude variability, including those resulting from organic and neurologic causes. In general, people who have reduced average amplitude levels also have problems with amplitude variability. As with frequency, the ability to vary amplitude is what imparts dynamism and interest to a speaker's voice. Individuals who lack this ability, for whatever reason, tend to sound flat and monotonous.

Dynamic range refers to the range of vocal amplitudes a speaker can generate from the softest phonation that is not a whisper to the loudest shout, measured in dB.

Dynamic Range   Dynamic range is similar to phonational range. It relates to the physiological range of the vocal amplitudes that a speaker can generate, from the softest phonation that is not a whisper to the loudest shout. A normal adult female should be able to produce a minimum level of around 50 dB and a maximum of approximately 115 dB SPL; the figures for normal adult males should be slightly higher (Coleman, Mabis, & Hinson, 1977). Depending on frequency, the minimum dynamic range should be around 30 dB SPL. A restricted dynamic range may prevent a person from using stress and emphasis patterns appropriately, reducing the flexibility of spoken language. Although amplitudes above and below the 60 to 80 dB range are not normally used for conversational speech, the ability to raise one's voice is important for special occasions that demand higher levels of loudness (Sulter, Schutte, & Miller, 1995). The dynamic range depends on the F_0 produced and tends to be greatest for F_0 in the midrange and less for F_0 that is much lower or much higher.

Voice Range Profile   The voice range profile (VRP, also called a *phonetogram* or F_0 **SPL profile)** is a graph that plots a person's phonational range against his or her dynamic range. Dynamic range is plotted on the vertical axis in dB SPL, and F_0 is plotted on the horizontal axis in hertz. See Figure 3.1.

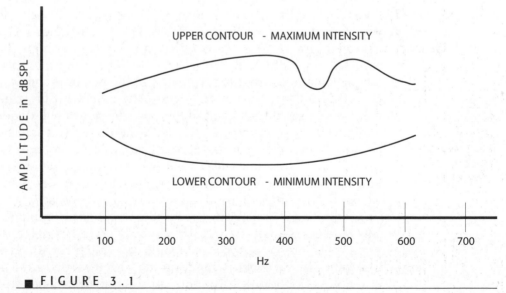

■ FIGURE 3.1

Voice range profile.

To generate the profile, the speaker phonates a vowel at various F_0 levels. At each F_0 level, the individual produces the softest and loudest sounds that she can. This results in two contours. The upper contour shows maximum intensity at each selected frequency, and the lower contour shows minimum intensity at each frequency, giving a good indication of normal frequency and amplitude relationships in the human voice.

VRPs have a characteristic shape, reflecting some physiological quirks of the human voice production system. The shape is roughly similar to an oval, with narrower endpoints and a more expanded midportion. This shape results from the typical relationship between the range of frequencies and amplitudes that we can generate. Humans have a far greater dynamic range in the middle of the frequency range, whereas the dynamic range shrinks considerably at very high or very low frequencies. In the middle of the frequency range, an individual can generally vary the intensity by 20 to 30 dB, whereas at the ends of the frequency range the person might only be able to vary intensity by a few decibels (Titze, 1994).

> The voice range profile is a graph that plots a person's maximum phonational frequency range against the dynamic range with F_0 on the horizontal axis in Hz and dynamic range on the vertical axis in dB SPL.

Another feature of the shape is the dip that is usually seen in the maximum intensity upper contour at around 390 Hz for men and 440 Hz for women (Sulter et al., 1995). This dip reflects a drop in maximum intensity that occurs when speakers without any voice training go from their usual conversational speech frequency range to the much higher falsetto range. Trained singers show a considerably reduced dip, indicating a smoother transition between these ranges.

The VRP can be thought of as a snapshot of vocal fold behavior at one moment in time (Aerainer & Klingholz, 1993). This picture gives very useful information for several reasons. First, a VRP can help to determine the physiological limits of any individual's voice, because the dynamic and phonational frequency ranges are directly related to the person's ability to control the vocal folds (Sulter et al., 1995). A person who has difficulty in achieving normal frequency and amplitude ranges will demonstrate a constricted or compressed VRP, with the upper and lower contours closer together than normal. Second, this kind of graph can show the impact of treatment or surgical intervention on an individual's voice. An expanded VRT after treatment would show graphically that the patient's phonational and/or dynamic range has increased.

> The voice range profile can be used to compare an individual's vocal characteristics before and after treatment.

Useful clinical information can also be obtained by determining where the graph falls in terms of frequency. For example, Behrman, Agresti, Blumstein, and Sharma (1996) presented the case of an 11-year-old girl with a voice problem whose presurgery frequency range on the VRP extended from 440 to 987 Hz. Pictorially, her VRP was shifted to the right, to the higher frequencies. Table 3.1 shows that average F_0 for an 11-year-old girl should be somewhere between 220 and 250 Hz. Presurgery, this child was unable physiologically to achieve the normal frequency levels for her age and sex, and her pitch was correspondingly abnormally high. Postsurgery, her frequency range on the VRP shifted to the more normal values of 196 to 494 Hz, shown as a shift to the left on the VRP. Perceptually, too, her pitch level sounded much more appropriate for an 11-year-old girl. In this case, the VRP provided compelling objective evidence that the surgery had been successful.

Another use of VRPs is to compare the vocal characteristics of different groups of speakers. In comparison to adults, for instance, children demonstrate a somewhat compressed VRP. Children's upper contours are lower and their lower contours are higher than those of adults. This is a graphical and objective demonstration that children are not able to generate as high or as low amplitudes as adults, most likely due to the different structural and physiological characteristics of the vocal folds in children and adults (McAllister, Sederholm, Sundberg, & Gramming, 1994). VRPs also show differences between trained and untrained voices. Sulter and colleagues (1995) looked at differences in VRP features in males and females with and without vocal training. Untrained women obtained an average F_0 range of around 157 to 1223 Hz. Vocally trained women obtained a range from around 128 to 1320 Hz, showing a wider range at both the lower and higher ends of the frequency range. Vocally trained men obtained an average range from around 74 to 785 Hz, whereas their untrained counterparts had a range from 86 to about 688 Hz. Plotting this information on a VRP showed that not only do trained singers have wider phonational ranges than nonsingers, but they are also able to phonate at lower intensities over almost the entire frequency range.

Breakdowns in Control of Vocal Frequency and Amplitude

So far we have been discussing in a theoretical way the various dimensions of sounds, including those of F_0 and amplitude. These measurements are extremely valuable when dealing with breakdowns in the control of frequency and amplitude, as often occurs in voice and neurological disorders.

Voice Disorders

Patients with voice disorders are very commonly seen in hospitals, clinics, private practice, nursing homes, preschools, and elementary and secondary schools. Individuals of any age, including infants, can exhibit voice disorders.

Voice disorders can result from numerous and varied causes, including vocal abuse, organic problems such as benign tumors or cysts on the vocal folds, neurological problems such as stroke or progressive degenerative diseases (e.g., Parkinson's disease), trauma such as car accidents and gunshot wounds that affect the larynx, and numerous others. Voice disorders result in problems related to frequency and amplitude. In terms of frequency, speakers may use a range of F_0 that is too low or too high for their age, sex, and build; may produce a restricted range of F_0 (i.e., speak in a monotone); may demonstrate frequency breaks, in which the voice shifts F_0 involuntarily and abruptly; or may demonstrate **diplophonia**, which occurs when each vocal fold vibrates at a slightly different rate, resulting in the perception of two pitches simultaneously. Often a combination of these frequency control problems exists. Amplitude problems include using a habitual amplitude level that is too high or too low, producing a restricted range of amplitudes (i.e., monoloudness), or having sudden involuntary and inappropriate amplitude changes. Often, frequency and amplitude problems occur simultaneously in various combinations.

Before sophisticated computerized equipment was widely available, clinicians used to rely solely on their subjective, perceptual impressions of the person's voice in making a diagnosis of the voice problem. However, with current instrumentation it is not only important but easy to supplement this perceptual information with more objective and quantifiable information about the acoustic characteristics of the speaker's voice. This kind of information is invaluable for making finely tuned diagnoses about the problem, detecting early changes in speech and voice that are not apparent perceptually, making intelligent decisions about treatment options, and assessing the outcomes of treatment. Treatment options and results can be compared and validated. For instance, some kinds of voice problems related to emotional stress are often treated by teaching the individual to reduce tension in the larynx. However, until recently, there was little evidence that this kind of treatment actually works. To determine the effectiveness of tension reduction treatment techniques, Roy, Bless, Heisey, and Ford (1997) audiorecorded 25 patients pre- and posttreatment and analyzed these voice samples both perceptually and acoustically in terms of F_0. The patients' F_0 values in connected speech changed from the pretreatment session to the posttreatment sessions, reflecting a decrease in laryngeal tension. These acoustic data provide objective support for the effectiveness of this particular kind of voice therapy.

In addition, the precise measurement of F_0 can help the clinician to make decisions about voice parameters that are difficult to verify perceptually. For example, a person with vocal nodules typically demonstrates a voice that sounds low-pitched, hoarse, and breathy. Before acoustic instrumentation was commonly used, many clinicians treated this problem by having the patient use a higher pitch level. Often, however, the low pitch that is heard does not

> Voice disorders can result from numerous causes such as vocal abuse, neurological disorders, infections, trauma, etc.

correspond to a lower than normal F_0. In other words, the patient's F_0, when objectively measured, is actually within normal limits, but is perceived as lower due to the influence of other factors, such as rate of speech and the hoarseness itself. Because the speaker's F_0 is within normal limits, treatment focusing on changing the F_0 is not indicated. Thus, this acoustic information signals the clinician to choose a more appropriate treatment strategy based on the physiological functioning of the vocal folds. This kind of precise measurement, then, can help the clinician to avoid implementing ineffective treatment plans.

Other uses of F_0 measurement help in making medically related decisions. For instance, Orlikoff, Kraus, Harrison, Ho, and Gartner (1997) used F_0 as an indication of how a cancerous tumor on the vocal folds responded to chemotherapy. They measured "comfortable" F_0 plus variability in F_0 during speaking situations in patients with advanced laryngeal cancer before each of three cycles of chemotherapy. They found a link between the reduction or elimination of the cancerous growth and the F_0 measures. F_0 variability increased when the growth was reduced, indicating that the patients had increased their vocal flexibility. These frequency measures were helpful in documenting both the extent of the laryngeal impairment resulting from the cancer and the effectiveness of the chemotherapy.

> Measurement of vocal frequency and intensity variables can help to make medically related decisions.

Frequency and intensity characteristics have been used as a yardstick for successful voice restoration in people who have had their larynx removed due to cancer and who use different methods of alaryngeal speech (speech produced without a larynx). One such type of voice production is called **esophageal speech**. This is voice produced by vibrating a certain part of the esophagus, rather than the vocal folds in the larynx. Speech produced in this way typically is much lower in F_0 and amplitude than normally produced speech.

Clinicians have traditionally judged the effectiveness of esophageal speech partially in terms of its frequency and amplitude. Historically, speech pathologists have characterized proficient esophageal speech as having a higher F_0 and higher amplitude level than poor esophageal speech. Slavin and Ferrand (1995) tested this assumption by acoustically analyzing the speech of esophageal speakers who were all judged perceptually as being highly proficient speakers. The average frequency for the entire group of speakers was 69 Hz, considerably lower than the normal values for adult speakers presented in Table 3.1. However, Slavin and Ferrand (1995) found that these individuals clustered into four groups, with each group characterized by a different frequency and amplitude profile. For instance, individuals in one group had higher than average mean F_0 and greater frequency variability than the group mean. Speakers in a different group had lower mean F_0 and less frequency variability. A third group of speakers obtained an F_0 around 69 Hz, but these individuals had relatively high amplitude levels (around a 70 dB SPL). Understanding that different patterns of frequency and amplitude characterize individual esophageal speakers can allow clinicians to be more flexible in choosing rehabilitation strategies geared to the individual's specific anatomical characteristics and communication needs.

Neurological Disorders

A voice or speech problem can often be the first sign of a more generalized neurological disorder. This was shown in a classic study on voice and speech symptoms in patients with Parkinson's disease (PD) by Logemann, Fisher, Boshes, and Blonsky in 1978. They found that 89 percent of these individuals showed a voice problem. Indeed, almost half of this number had shown a voice problem as the first sign of the neurological disease. Other neurological disorders that tend to affect speech and voice production include amyotrophic lateral sclerosis (ALS), multiple sclerosis (MS), Huntington's chorea, and many others. Strokes, brain tumors, and traumatic brain injury also contribute to voice and speech problems. Over the past ten to fifteen years, much information has been collected regarding the acoustic characteristics of voice that often result from these disorders. This information is used to plan, carry out, and evaluate different types of therapy regimes.

Acoustic measures can provide objective validation of perceptual judgments of voice pitch and loudness characteristics.

In 1975, Darley, Aronson, and Brown made voice history by conducting a large-scale study to investigate the voice and speech characteristics of patients with various kinds of neurological problems. They characterized these problems in terms of perceptual parameters of voice and speech, such as problems with pitch (too high, too low, monotone) and loudness (too loud, too soft, monoloud), and derived different profiles of vocal characteristics for different disorders. See Table 3.3.

Recently, researchers have begun to supplement these perceptual dimensions of vocal function with more objective information. For example, acoustic

■ **TABLE 3.3**

Perceptual Characteristics Related to Pitch and Loudness in Some Types of Dysarthria

TYPE OF DYSARTHRIA	PERCEPTUAL CHARACTERISTICS OF VOICE
Ataxic	Monopitch, monoloudness, inappropriate bursts of pitch and loudness, equal and excess stress
Flaccid	Low pitch, monopitch, monoloudness
Hyperkinetic	Involuntary variations in pitch and loudness
Hypokinetic	Monopitch, monoloudness, reduced loudness
Spastic	Low pitch, monopitch, reduced stress

Source: Based on Darley, Aronson, and Brown's (1975) classification.

analysis of F_0 and amplitude has revealed that patients with PD tend to show higher than normal F_0 lower standard deviations of frequency and amplitude, and decreased phonational and dynamic ranges (Gamboa et al., 1997). In addition, speakers with neurological problems are less able to use F_0 effectively to distinguish between declarative and interrogative sentences. Normal speakers in a study by LeDorze, Ouellet, and Ryalls (1994) showed an average difference of 83 Hz between the final syllables in the same utterance produced as a declarative and as an interrogative sentence. Subjects with neurological problems produced an average final syllable difference of only 25 Hz.

Acoustic analysis of fundamental frequency and amplitude may detect early changes in voice production due to neurological disease even before such changes can be heard perceptually.

These kinds of acoustic data support the perceptual impressions of restricted pitch and loudness ranges, which are the common complaint of patients with PD and other neurological disorders. Furthermore, these measures have the added advantage of quantifying the precise degree of loss of frequency and intensity range compared to normal.

Acoustic analysis of F_0 and amplitude can also serve to detect early changes in voice production due to neurologic disease, even before such changes can be heard perceptually. This has been shown in patients suffering from amyotrophic lateral sclerosis (ALS). In this disease, the patient's voice becomes progressively weaker. F_0 and amplitude levels decrease over time, and eventually the person becomes completely unable to produce voice and speech. Research has demonstrated that patients with ALS who sound perceptually normal have a much smaller frequency range than normal, 16.4 semitones compared to 22.7 semitones (Silbergleit, Johnson, & Jacobson, 1997). This smaller frequency range may be an indication of early signs of laryngeal weakness affecting the laryngeal muscles. Knowing that weakness is present despite the normal-sounding voice, clinicians can offer intervention at early stages of the disease in order to maintain the patient's vocal function for as long as possible.

Another important factor in ALS that has been revealed by acoustic analysis is that the vocal characteristics of patients are not uniform, but vary greatly from patient to patient. Measurement of mean F_0, standard deviation of F_0, plus F_0 and amplitude contours during sustained phonation and production of phrases show that, although changes in F_0 seem to be present consistently in patients with ALS, some speakers have lower than normal F_0 levels while others are higher than normal. In addition, some but not all individuals with ALS exhibit a reduced range of F_0 during connected speech (Strand, Buder, Yorkston, & Olson Ramig, 1994). This information is critical in planning effective therapy tailored to each individual's particular voice and speech defects. With this knowledge, therapy procedures can be planned that focus on normalizing or maintaining vocal function as much as possible for the individual. Another benefit is that the same instrumentation used to obtain diagnostic data can then be used for visual feedback and motivation during therapy.

Clinical Study

Background

Jaime is a speech–language pathologist in an elementary school, which is part of a large school district. An important part of her job is to screen all entering kindergartners in the school district for any speech or language problems. She recently acquired a Visi-Pitch (Kay) and is eager to implement a new screening protocol that she developed for identifying possible voice disorders in the children.

Acoustic Measures

Jaime's protocol includes several F_0 and intensity variables, including average F_0, SFF, and average intensity. For average F_0, the child is asked to hold the vowel /a/ for 5 seconds; SFF is taken from a picture description task. Average intensity is also taken from these activities. During these activities, Jaime also listens carefully to the children's voices and rates them perceptually.

After screening 150 children (87 girls and 63 boys), she is able to obtain means for these different acoustic measures. Jaime did not think it was necessary to separate the data for the girls and boys and obtained all her information from the averages for all the children. The average F_0 for /a/ for all the children was approximately 248 Hz; SFF yielded an average of 242 Hz. Average intensity was 59 dB. Based on these normative values that she derived, Jaime was able to identify several children whose means fell outside of these ranges. For example, Peter obtained an F_0 of 224 Hz for /a/, 215 Hz for his SFF, and an average intensity of 77 dB. This was consistent perceptually with his low-pitched and somewhat loud voice. Emma's values were 258 Hz for /a/, 254 Hz for SFF, and 56 dB for average intensity. Jaime was surprised about the F_0 measures, because perceptually, Emma's voice sounded extremely low-pitched for her age. Emma was also hoarse and complained that her throat was sore. Both of these children were referred to an ENT for a laryngeal exam.

Clinical Questions

1. What are the possible advantages and disadvantages of using this kind of instrumentation in conjunction with traditional perceptual methods of screening?
2. What may be the advantages and/or disadvantages of Jaime's using her own normative data to make comparisons, rather than using values from reported literature?
3. Should the values of these two children have been compared to the single group averages that Jaime derived from the screenings? Why or why not?

4. What could account for the lack of consistency between the perceptual and acoustic results in Emma's case?

summary

- Frequency measures typically used in clinical settings include average F_0, speaking F_0, F_0 range, and maximum phonational frequency range.
- Typically used amplitude measures include average amplitude, amplitude variability, and dynamic range.
- The voice range profile plots a person's maximum phonational frequency range against his or her dynamic range at dif-ferent frequencies and acts as a snapshot of phonatory behavior.
- Frequency and amplitude variables related to voice use are used in clinical situations to make diagnostic decisions, supplement perceptual judgments of voice, and assess outcomes of treatment.
- Neurologic diseases are often characterized by problems in the control of vocal frequency and amplitude.

review exercises

1. Identify three clinical situations in which the measurement of frequency and amplitude variables might be useful, and explain why.
2. Discuss the rationale for the development of separate average F_0 and F_0 variability norms for men, women, and children.
3. Explain why the voice range profile can be considered as a snapshot of phonatory behavior.
4. What are two major advantages in measuring frequency and/or amplitude variables in individuals with voice problems?
5. Explain how frequency and amplitude measures can serve to detect early laryngeal changes in neurological diseases.

chapter 4

The Respiratory System

chapter objectives

After reading this chapter, you will

1. Be familiar with the anatomy and physiology of the respiratory system.

2. Understand how the lungs move due to pleural linkage.

3. Appreciate the different lung volumes and capacities and their relationship to speech breathing.

4. Be able to describe the four differences between life breathing and speech breathing.

5. Understand the air pressure and flows involved in respiration.

6. Know how speech breathing patterns develop over the lifespan.

With an understanding of basic acoustics and a good idea of the clinical relevance of these acoustic concepts, we turn now to a discussion of how the human speech production system is finely suited to generating acoustic outputs, that is, speech. To appreciate the acoustic capacities of the system, we need to understand the structure of the components of the system, how they work, and how they fit together and interact in complex ways to generate the end product of speech. The subsystems that are involved in speech production and perception include the respiratory system, the phonatory system, the articulatory system, the auditory system, and the nervous system.

The ability to speak depends on a steady outflow of air that is vibrated by the vocal folds to produce a basic sound, which is then further modified by the articulators to generate the specific speech sounds of whatever language is being spoken. Without this outflow of air, there would be no speech. The subject of air—how we get it into and out of our lungs; how we change our breathing patterns when we breathe for speech, rather than for purely vegetative, life-sustaining purposes; the pressures and flows of air in different locations of our bodies as we breathe and speak—will be our concern in this chapter. First, however, we need to discuss how we are able to breathe at all. That is, we will describe the structures of the respiratory system that enable us to perform this most necessary function of life. This will provide a framework for further exploration of the mechanics of respiration in relation to normal and disordered speech production.

The Structure and Mechanics of the Respiratory System

The respiratory system can be divided into the **pulmonary system** and the **chest-wall system** (Hoit, 1995). The pulmonary system includes the lungs and airways, and the chest wall system is made up of the rib cage, abdomen, and diaphragm. The pulmonary system can be further subdivided into two parts, the **upper** and the **lower respiratory systems**. The upper respiratory system (URS) includes the oral and nasal cavities and the pharynx. The lower respiratory system (LRS) includes the larynx, the bronchial system, and the lungs. We will focus only on the LRS below the larynx in this chapter (the larynx will be discussed in Chapter 6 and the URS in Chapter 8). Keep in mind that many structures of the respiratory system, including the larynx, oral cavity, and nasal cavities, are involved not only in breathing, but in phonation and articulation, as well as in swallowing. This multipurpose organization of structures and systems is wonderfully efficient and is made possible by an extraordinary degree of control and coordination by the nervous system.

> The pulmonary system consists of the lungs and airways; the chest-wall system is made up of the rib cage, abdomen, and diaphragm.

Structures of the Lower Respiratory System

The lower respiratory system (LRS) is made up of the **trachea**, **bronchi**, **bronchioles**, **alveoli**, and lungs. The trachea, bronchi, and bronchioles are often referred to as the **bronchial tree**.

> The upper respiratory system includes the oral and nasal cavities and the pharynx. The lower respiratory system includes the larynx, bronchial tree, and lungs.

Bronchial Tree   The bronchial tree consists of a branching system of hollow tubes that conduct air to and from the lungs. Similar to a tree, the bronchial system begins with a larger tube (the trunk of the tree, in the analogy), which then divides into smaller and smaller tubes (the branches and twigs). Directly beneath the larynx lies the trachea (Figure 4.1), corresponding to the trunk of the tree in the analogy. This is a hollow tube, about 11 cm long in adults and approximately 2.5 cm in diameter. The trachea is made

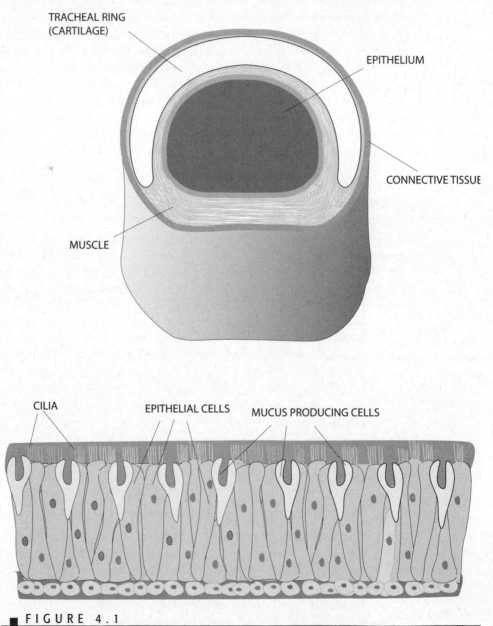

■ F I G U R E 4 . 1

Cross section of the trachea and enlargement of the epithelial layer.

up of sixteen to twenty rings of cartilage, which are closed in the front but open in the back. Between the cartilages and forming the back wall of the trachea is smooth muscle, and overlying the cartilages and muscle is a mucous membrane. This combination of cartilage and smooth muscle allows both great flexibility and support for the trachea. The support prevents the trachea from collapsing when negative or positive pressures operate inside it.

On the inside surface the trachea is lined with a layer of **epithelium**, from which protrude millions of tiny hairlike projections called **cilia**. The cilia continuously move in a wavelike motion. As they slowly move downward, they pick up particles of dust, pollution, bacteria, and viruses. As they quickly move upward, this material, held together in a sticky blanket of mucus, is forcefully expelled into the throat and swallowed or coughed out. Thus, the cilia act as a filtering system to clean the air going into the lungs.

The trachea splits into two branches called **mainstem bronchi** (singular: bronchus). Each mainstem bronchus is slightly less than half the diameter of the trachea. The right bronchus enters the right lung, and the left bronchus enters the left lung. Each mainstem bronchus gives off **secondary**, or lobar, **bronchi**, which supply the lobes of the lung. Each secondary bronchus, in turn, gives off **tertiary**, or segmental, **bronchi**, which go into various segments of the lungs. The structure of the bronchi is very similar to that of the trachea, being composed of rings of cartilage, as well as membrane and smooth muscle. The tertiary bronchi keep on branching into smaller and smaller tubes.

Eventually, the bronchi branch into tiny terminal bronchioles, which at this point lose their cartilage and are composed of only smooth muscle and membrane. The terminal bronchioles branch into **respiratory bronchioles**. As we see in Figure 4.2, there are numerous subdivisions of the bronchial tree, beginning with the trachea down to the final, tiny respiratory bronchioles (24 subdivisions according to Zemlin, 1998; 28 subdivisions according to Seikel, King, & Drumright, 1997).

With each successive subdivision into smaller branches, the total surface area of the smaller branch is larger than that of the next larger branch (Seikel et al., 1997). This provides an enormous amount of surface area for respiration. At the end of the line, the respiratory bronchioles open into **alveolar ducts** (see Figure 4.3). Each alveolar duct leads to an alveolus, which is a microscopic, thin-walled, air-filled structure. There are millions of alveoli in the lungs, with estimates ranging from around 300 million to 750 million in the adult lung (Sebel et al., 1987; Seikel et al., 1997). The alveoli participate in the exchange of oxygen and carbon dioxide that is the basis of respiration. Each alveolus is surrounded by a dense network of tiny blood capillaries. Within each alveolus is a substance called **surfactant**, which keeps the alveoli inflated by lowering the surface tension of the walls of the

The trachea divides into mainstem bronchi, which in turn branch into secondary bronchi, tertiary bronchi, and bronchioles.

Respiratory bronchioles open into alveolar ducts, leading into alveolar sacs. Alveoli are involved in the exchange of oxygen and carbon dioxide.

Alveoli are kept in an inflated state by a substance called surfactant.

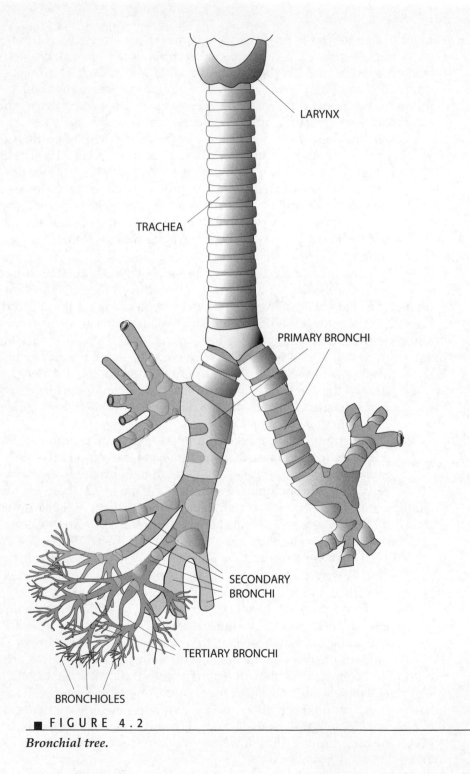

LARYNX

TRACHEA

PRIMARY BRONCHI

SECONDARY
BRONCHI

TERTIARY BRONCHI

BRONCHIOLES

■ F I G U R E   4 . 2

Bronchial tree.

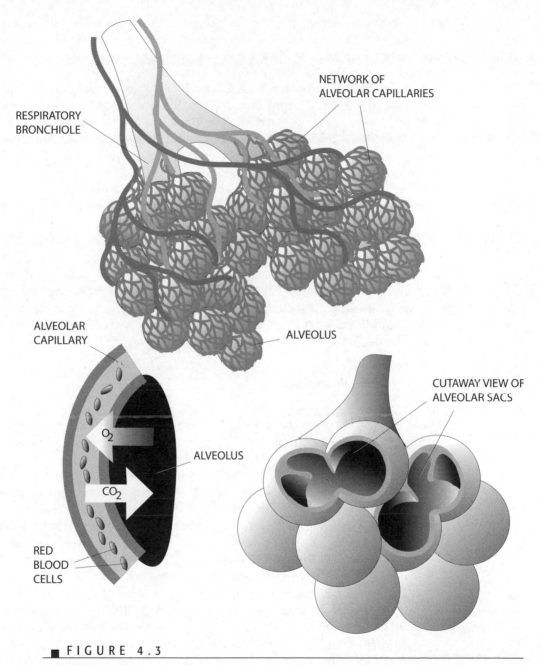

RESPIRATORY
BRONCHIOLE

NETWORK OF
ALVEOLAR CAPILLARIES

ALVEOLAR
CAPILLARY

ALVEOLUS

CUTAWAY VIEW OF
ALVEOLAR SACS

O_2

CO_2

ALVEOLUS

RED
BLOOD
CELLS

■ FIGURE 4.3

Alveolar sacs.

alveoli, thus preventing them from being pulled inward during inspiration. This substance is often lacking in premature infants, contributing to serious respiratory problems. The alveoli and the capillaries are extremely thin-walled, allowing for the easy exchange of gases between them.

The bronchi, bronchioles, alveoli, and blood vessels make up the interior structure of the lungs. The millions of alveoli in the lungs contain air, making the lungs very porous and elastic. The lungs are not symmetrical. The right lung is larger than the left and is composed of three lobes, which are separated by grooves. The left lung is smaller than the right, to make space for the heart on the left side. The left lung is therefore composed of only two lobes. The lungs in the newborn infant are a pinkish color, while the effects of environmental pollution and other toxins such as cigarette smoke contribute to a grayish or blackish color in adults.

The lungs are housed in the **thoracic cavity** (thorax) (Figure 4.4). This cavity is bounded by the sternum and rib cage on the front and sides, the spinal column and vertebrae at the back, and the diaphragm muscle at the bottom. Many muscles attach to the rib cage and to the pectoral and pelvic girdles. The lungs are thus well protected and are maintained in an airtight fashion. In a healthy, uninjured individual, the only way that air can get into and out of the lungs is through the bronchial tree.

Muscles of Respiration

The muscles of respiration (Figure 4.4) can be thought of as either participating fully in the respiratory process or as helping in the process as the need arises. Our respiratory needs differ, depending on the kind and level of our activity. For instance, just breathing quietly as you read a book requires less oxygen than running a mile. You would need to use fewer muscles for quiet breathing than for running. Many muscles can potentially be involved in respiration, and the more active you are, the more of these muscles you will use. We will also see that vegetative (life-sustaining) breathing involves coordinating different muscles and patterns of muscle activity than breathing for speech.

Probably the most important respiratory muscle is the **diaphragm**. This is a large, dome-shaped muscle that stretches from one side of the rib cage to the other. It attaches along the lower margins of the rib cage, the sternum, and the vertebral column (Seikel et al., 1997). This muscle makes up the floor of the thoracic cavity, as well the roof of the abdominal cavity. This position makes it extremely sensitive to the shifting around of the abdominal contents, which plays an important role in breathing, particularly for speech. In its relaxed state, the diaphragm is shaped like an inverted bowl, in which position the middle portion extends somewhat upward. When it contracts, the diaphragm flattens out, with the

The diaphragm is a large dome-shaped muscle stretching from one side of the rib cage to the other and helps to regulate the volume of the thoracic cavity.

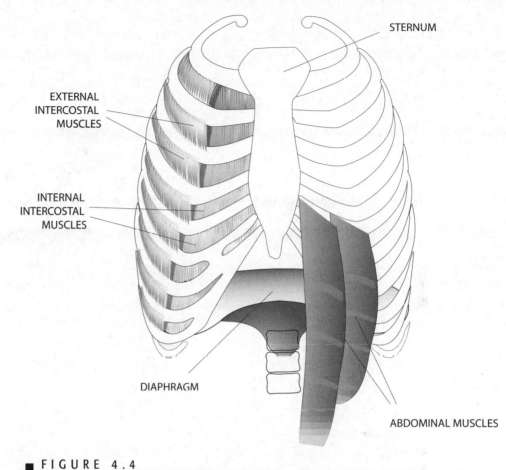

STERNUM

EXTERNAL
INTERCOSTAL
MUSCLES

INTERNAL
INTERCOSTAL
MUSCLES

DIAPHRAGM

ABDOMINAL MUSCLES

■ FIGURE 4.4

Thoracic cavity and major muscles of respiration.

middle portion lowering. Thus, when the diaphragm contracts, the volume of the thoracic cavity is increased in a vertical direction. See Figure 4.5.

Another very important set of muscles for respiration is the external **intercostals**. There are eleven pairs of external intercostals, and, as the name implies, these muscles run between the ribs. They originate on the lower surface of each rib, and the fibers course downward at an oblique angle to insert into the upper border of the rib below. When these muscles contract, they elevate the entire rib cage and increase the volume of the thoracic cavity in the front-to-back and lateral directions.

The internal intercostals are similar to the external intercostals. Like the external intercostals, there are eleven pairs, running from the lower

The eleven pairs of external intercostal muscles run between the ribs and pull the rib cage upward and outward during inspiration.

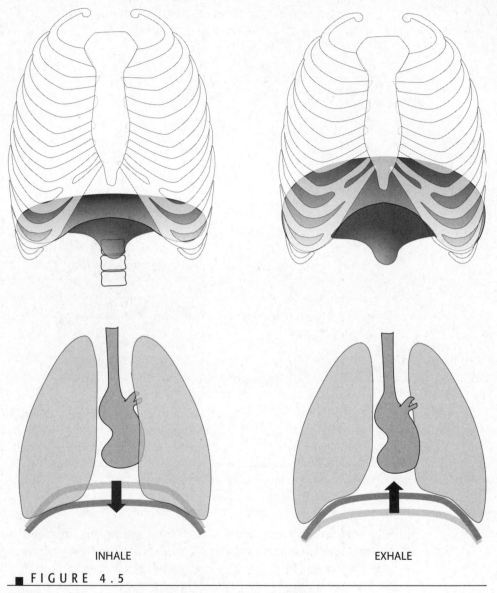

INHALE   EXHALE

■ FIGURE 4.5

Position of diaphragm for inhalation and exhalation.

margin of the rib above to the upper margin of the rib below. However, the internal intercostals are deep to the external intercostals and, while they run at an angle, the angle is opposite in direction to that of the external intercostals. This cross-laced effect (Seikel et al., 1997) of the external and internal intercostals forms a strong protective barrier for the lungs and heart, as well as an airtight

The accessory muscles include many that attach to the rib cage as well as muscles of the back, neck, and abdomen. They are recruited as necessary for deeper inspirations.

cavity that is essential for respiration. When contracted, the internal intercostals pull down on and lower the entire rib cage, thus decreasing the volume of the thoracic cavity.

Accessory Muscles of Respiration   Many other muscles that attach to the rib cage, as well as muscles of the back, neck, and abdomen, play changing roles in respiration, according to the needs of our bodies. The deeper we need to breathe, the more muscles we will call on to help elevate the rib cage and enlarge the volume of the thoracic cavity. Therefore, many of these muscles are known as **accessory muscles of respiration**. They are listed in Table 4.1.

The abdominal muscles are active during expiration by compressing the abdominal contents, which exerts upward pressure on the diaphragm and decreases the volume of the thoracic cavity.

Muscles of the Abdomen   The muscles of the abdomen play an important part in exhalation. As a group, four muscles of the abdomen work as a unit to compress the contents of the abdominal cavity, which helps in exhalation by exerting upward pressure on the diaphragm. When the abdominal muscles contract, the contents of the abdominal cavity are forced upward, thus forcing the roof of the cavity, the diaphragm, upward as well. This has the effect of decreasing the volume of the thoracic cavity.

■ TABLE 4.1

Accessory Muscles of the Neck, Thorax, and Abdomen and Their Possible Function in Respiration

MUSCLE	FUNCTION
Neck	
Scalenes	Elevate ribs 1 and 2
Sternocleidomastoid	Elevate rib cage
Thorax	
Costal levators	Elevate rib cage
Pectoralis major	Elevate rib cage
Pectoralis minor	Depress ribs 3 to 5
Serratus anterior	Elevate ribs 1 to 9
Serratus posterior inferior	Depress ribs 9 to 12
Serratus posterior superior	Elevate rib cage
Subclavius	Elevate rib cage
Subcostals	Lower rib cage
Transverse thoracic	Depress rib cage
Abdomen	
External oblique	Compress abdomen
Internal oblique	Compress abdomen
Rectus abdominis	Compress abdomen
Transverse abdominal	Compress abdomen

Pleural Linkage

For respiration to occur, the lungs have to increase and decrease their volume, and the only way they can do this is to expand and contract. However, the lungs contain very little muscle, so the only way that they can move is by some external force. This external force is generated through the structure and linkage of the lungs and thorax (see Figure 4.6).

Pleural linkage refers to the negative pressure within the pleural space between the visceral and parietal pleurae that attaches the lungs and thorax and forces them to operate as a unit.

Each lung is covered on the outside by a thin sheet of membrane, the **visceral pleura**. The inner surface of the thorax is lined with another layer of membrane, the **parietal pleura**. These two pleural layers are really one continuous membrane folded back on itself, rather than two separate membranes. Between these two pleurae (plural of pleura) is a very small potential space, the **pleural space**, containing a liquid, the **pleural fluid**. The visceral and parietal pleurae are separated only by this thin layer of liquid. Because of the chemical composition of the pleural fluid, the pleural space and pleural fluid are negative in pressure, with a value of about -6 cm H_2O (Seikel et al., 1997). When two structures are close together and the pressure between them is negative, the two

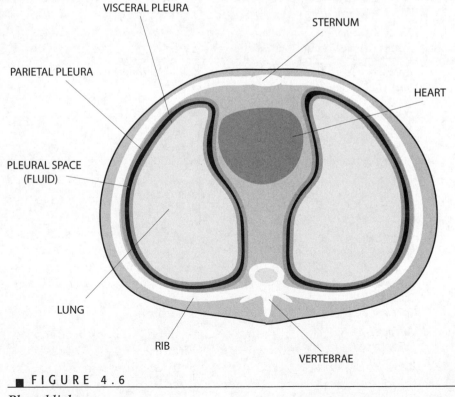

VISCERAL PLEURA
STERNUM
PARIETAL PLEURA
HEART
PLEURAL SPACE
(FLUID)
LUNG
RIB
VERTEBRAE

■ F I G U R E   4 . 6

Pleural linkage.

tend to be sucked closer together. Because the pressure in the pleural space is negative and never changes to positive, the lungs and thorax are permanently pulled close together and, in effect, function as one unit. Whatever the thorax does, or however the thorax moves, the lungs are drawn along as well. When the thorax expands due to muscular activity, the lungs expand as well. When the thorax decreases in volume, so do the lungs. Keep in mind that there are no structural attachments such as ligaments or tendons between the thorax and lungs; it is only the negative pressure in the pleural space that keeps them connected. Hence, the name of this attaching mechanism is **pleural linkage**.

This relationship is not completely one-sided, however, because the lungs also have an effect on the thorax. The lungs are connected to the thorax, so they prevent the thorax from expanding to its maximum capacity. Without the lungs, the thorax would be in a more expanded state. Without the thorax, the lungs would be in a more deflated state.

The pleurae not only play a crucial role in linking the lungs to the thoracic cavity, but they also have other functions. A second function of the pleurae is to provide a smooth, friction-free surface for the lungs and thorax to move against each other. If there were no fluid between the surfaces of the lungs and thorax, each cycle of respiration would bring the two directly into contact, creating friction and pain. The third function of the pleurae is a protective one. Each lung is encased in its own airtight visceral pleura. If one pleura is penetrated, for instance by a knife or gunshot wound, the lung will collapse, a condition known as **pneumothorax**. However, the other lung will remain intact and airtight, and survival is not at stake.

Moving Air Into and Out of the Lungs

We are now in a position to integrate concepts of how air behaves with the structure of the respiratory system in order to understand how we actually breathe. Basically, we move air into and out of the lungs by increasing and decreasing the air pressure inside the lungs. When air pressure inside the lungs, the **alveolar pressure** (P_{alv}) is negative, air from the atmosphere is forced to enter the respiratory system, because, as we learned in Chapter 2, air moves from an area of higher pressure to an area of lower pressure. This is inhalation, or inspiration. When P_{alv} is positive, air from inside the lungs is forced out of the respiratory system to the atmosphere. This is the process of exhalation, or expiration.

Inhalation   To bring air into the lungs, the P_{alv} must become negative so that air will be forced to flow into the respiratory system. To decrease P_{alv}, we must increase the volume of the thoracic cavity and lungs. We do this by contracting the diaphragm, which flattens out, increasing the vertical dimension of the thorax. Simultaneously, the external intercostal muscles contract, pulling the entire rib cage upward and slightly outward. This increases the back-to-front and side-to-side dimensions of the thorax. The lungs, attached by means of pleural linkage, are pulled in the same direction as the thoracic cavity and therefore increase in volume. As soon as the lungs begin to expand, the P_{alv} falls below P_{atmos}, reaching around -1 to -2 cm H_2O at the height of inspiration (Zemlin, 1998). As the P_{alv} decreases, air from the atmosphere is forced into the respiratory system through either the mouth or nose. The air travels throughout the bronchial tree, eventually reaching the alveoli in the lungs. There the fresh oxygen diffuses into the blood capillaries surrounding the alveoli and is carried by the circulatory system to every cell in the body.

Inhalation and exhalation are regulated by alveolar pressure (P_{alv}): When P_{alv} is negative, air is drawn into the lungs; when P_{alv} is positive, air is forced out of the lungs.

Exhalation   The reverse process occurs in exhalation. For air to exit the respiratory system, the P_{alv} must be higher than P_{atmos}, so the volume of the lungs must decrease. To achieve this, the diaphragm relaxes back to its dome-shaped position, decreasing the vertical dimension of the thorax. The external intercostal muscles relax, allowing the rib cage to return to its original position, which decreases the back-to-front dimensions of the thorax. The relaxation of the diaphragm and rib cage gives rise to elastic recoil forces. Correspondingly, the lungs also decrease their volume. As lung volume decreases, P_{alv} increases to about $+2$ cm H_2O relative to P_{atmos}. Air carrying carbon dioxide (CO_2), brought to the lungs by the circulatory system, is forced out of the lungs and respiratory system until the P_{alv} reaches atmospheric levels. At the end of each inhalation and each exhalation the P_{alv} equals the P_{atmos}, and for a brief instant air does not move either into or out of the system. The cycle of breathing in and out then begins again.

Rate of Breathing

These cycles of inhalation and exhalation start at the instant of birth and continue until the instant of death. The process occurs when we are awake and asleep, when we breathe vegetatively for life, and when we modify our breathing for speech. Table 4.2 shows how the rate of breathing changes from infancy to adulthood and how it also depends on level of activity.

Differences in breathing between children and adults occur because the structures and functions involved in respiration mature from infancy through childhood. Numerous anatomical and physiological changes occur during the first year of life, including the following: The alveoli increase in number and size; the alveolar ducts increase in number; the alveolar surface area increases; lung size and weight increase; the thoracic cavity enlarges and changes in shape; the angle of the ribs changes with upright posture; rib cage muscle bulk increases; and pleural pressure becomes more subatmospheric (Boliek, Hixon,

■ TABLE 4.2

Rates of Breathing in Breaths per Minute (BPM) according to Age, Gender (Male: M; Female: F; Not Specified: NS), and Activity

AGE	GENDER	ACTIVITY	BPM
Infants	NS	Awake	40–70
	NS	Asleep	24–116
5 years	NS		25
7 years	M + F		19
10 years	M		16
	F		18
15 years	NS		20
Adults	NS	Quiet breathing	12–18
Adults	M	Heavy activity	21
Adults	F	Heavy activity	30

Source: Data integrated from Seikel et al. (1997); Zemlin (1998); Hoit et al. (1990).

Watson, & Morgan, 1996). Maturation of the nervous system also contributes to the development of more mature breathing patterns with increasing age.

Lung Volumes and Capacities

Respiration deals with volumes and pressures of air. A system of classifying certain volumes of air in relation to respiration was established in 1950. These classifications are useful, because they allow both laboratory and clinical measurements to be made in various populations of individuals. Volumes can be compared in children and adults, or between normally developing children and children with cerebral palsy, or between young adults and elderly adults, and so on. Using these volumes also allows us to make comparisons of how breathing changes in different positions and with different tasks, including speech.

Lung volumes are single, nonoverlapping values; lung capacities include two or more lung volumes.

Respiratory volumes and capacities are measured with a **wet spirometer** (Figure 4.7). This instrument has a tube connected to a container that is open at the bottom. The tube goes right through the container. The open-bottomed container is situated within another container filled with water. When the individual breathes into the tube, the water is displaced and the amount of displacement is measured.

Lung volumes are single, nonoverlapping values, whereas lung capacities include two or more lung volumes. Both kinds of measurements are expressed in cubic centimeters (cc or cm^3), liters (l), or milliliters (ml). All three measurements are equivalent. Examples of lung volumes and capacities are given in Table 4.3.

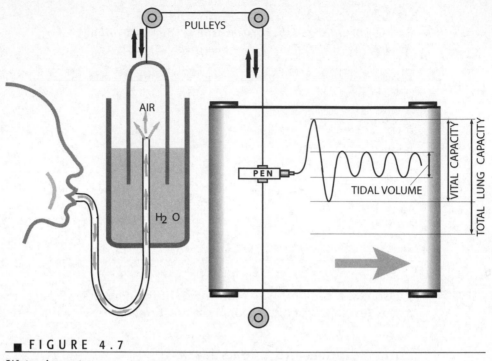

■ FIGURE 4.7

Wet spirometer.

Resting Expiratory Level **Resting expiratory level** (REL) is neither a volume nor a capacity, but refers to a state of equilibrium in the respiratory system. In this state, the natural tendency of the lungs to collapse is balanced by the natural tendency of the thorax to expand. If we could separate the lungs from the thorax, the lungs would deflate instantly. On the other hand, the thorax, separated from the lungs, would expand. The opposing forces of the lungs and thorax keep the lungs always slightly expanded and the thorax always slightly compressed in relation to each other. When P_{alv} equals P_{atmos}, these two opposing forces are in equilibrium, so air does not go into or out of the system. This state of affairs occurs very frequently; in fact, every time you complete a breath in or a breath out, the P_{alv} and P_{atmos} are in equilibrium for a brief instant before the next inhalation or exhalation begins again. Thus, the endpoint of a normal quiet exhalation is the resting expiratory level, which, because it occurs at the end of every exhalation, is also called the **end-expiratory level** (EEL). At this level there is still more air in the lungs that could be exhaled by using the expiratory muscles to pull down on the rib cage, compress the abdominal contents, and decrease lung volume even further.

Resting expiratory level refers to a state of equilibrium within the respiratory system in which air is neither entering nor exiting the system because alveolar pressure and atmospheric pressure are equal.

■ **TABLE 4.3**

Some Lung Volumes and Capacities

LUNG VOLUMES (SINGLE VOLUMES, NO OVERLAP)	
Tidal volume (TV)	Volume of air inhaled and exhaled during a cycle of respiration
Inspiratory reserve volume (IRV)	Volume of air that can be inhaled above tidal volume
Expiratory reserve volume (ERV)	Volume of air that can be exhaled below tidal volume
Residual volume (RV)	Volume of air remaining in the lungs after a maximum expiration and that cannot be voluntarily expelled
LUNG CAPACITIES (INCLUDE TWO OR MORE VOLUMES)	
Vital capacity (VC)	Volume of air that can be exhaled after a maximum inhalation (includes IRV + TV + ERV)
Functional residual capacity (FRC)	Volume of air remaining in the lungs and airways at the end-expiratory level (includes ERV + RV)
Total lung capacity (TLC)	Total amount of air the lungs can hold (includes TV + IRV + ERV + RV)

Lung Volumes

Lung volumes refer to the amount of air in the lungs at a given time and how much of that air is used for various purposes, including speech (Solomon & Charron, 1998). Lung volumes include tidal volume (TV), inspiratory reserve volume (IRV), expiratory reserve volume (ERV), and residual volume (RV). Figure 4.8 shows graphically the relationships among various lung volumes and capacities.

Tidal Volume   **Tidal volume** (TV) refers to the volume of air that we breathe in and out during a cycle of respiration. Tidal volume varies, depending on age, build, and degree of physical activity. Values for adult males during quiet breathing range from around 600 to 750 cc (600 to 750 ml; 0.6 to 0.75 l). A mild degree of physical exertion increases TV to approximately 1670 cc. Further increasing physical activity increases TV to about 2030 cc (Zemlin, 1998). In general, females inhale and exhale less air during each cycle of breathing than do males, about 450 cc for quiet breathing (Seikel et al., 1997).

> The amount of air breathed in and out during one cycle of respiration is called tidal volume (TV) and varies depending on age, gender, and level of physical exertion.

Children with their smaller lungs have a lower TV than adults, ranging from approximately 200 cc at age 7 to just under 400 cc at age 13. The gender difference in TV seen in adult males and females becomes more evident in children as they develop. Table 4.4 shows that at ages 7 and 10, boys and girls have similar values for TV. By age 13 boys have a larger TV, and by age 16 boys and girls have attained essentially adult values of 560 cc for boys and 410 cc for girls.

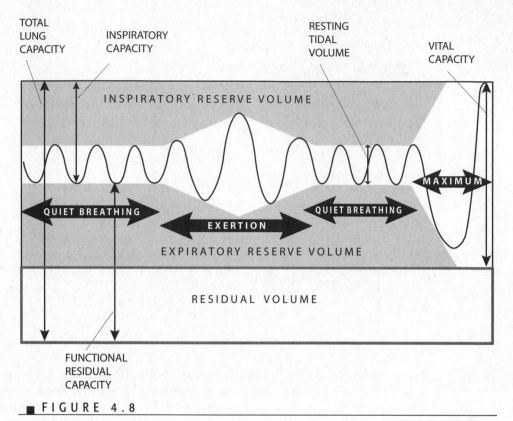

Lung volumes and capacities.

Inspiratory reserve volume (IRV) is the amount of air that can be inhaled above tidal volume.

Inspiratory Reserve Volume   **Inspiratory reserve volume** (IRV) refers to the amount of air that can be inhaled above TV. If you breathe in normally as you would for a quiet breath, you should find that you can still inhale considerably more air, instead of breathing it out right away. This extra amount of air is the IRV. The value for adults ranges from about 1500 to 2500 cc. The IRV can be used by speakers to obtain more air for a particularly long or particularly loud utterance.

The amount of air that can be exhaled below tidal volume is the expiratory reserve volume (ERV).

Expiratory Reserve Volume   **Expiratory reserve volume** (ERV) is the amount of air that can be exhaled below TV. Once you have breathed out a normal tidal breath, you should find that you can keep on exhaling for a while. You should also feel some muscle movement around your abdominal area as you breathe out below the tidal level. Figures for this volume in adults range from 1000 to 2000 cc. Values for children range from around 500 cc for 7-year-olds to 1180 cc for 13-year-old boys

■ TABLE 4.4

Lung Volumes and Capacities (cc) for Boys (B) and Girls (G) at Ages 7, 10, 13, and 16

	7		10		13		16	
	B	G	B	G	B	G	B	G
TLC	2120	2090	3140	2980	4330	3740	6200	4980
VC	1670	1580	2510	2340	3550	2990	5080	3780
IC	1140	1090	1740	1550	2370	2050	3260	2430
FRC	980	970	1400	1430	1970	1690	2940	2560
ERV	530	480	770	780	1180	940	1810	1350
RV	450	490	630	640	790	760	1120	1210
TV	200	190	260	280	390	350	560	410

Source: Adapted from Hoit et al. (1990).

and 940 cc for 13-year-old girls (Hoit et al., 1990). Singers might use a large portion of ERV to sustain a long phrase without replenishing the air.

Residual Volume   Lung tissue is always slightly stretched because of pleural linkage to the thorax. Therefore, in a healthy individual, the lungs can never be completely deflated and always contain some volume of air. Consequently, there must always be some corresponding air pressure in the lungs. The air that remains in the lungs even after a maximum exhalation is the **residual volume** (RV). This amount of air, around 1000 to 1500 cc in adults, can never be voluntarily expired. Newborns do not have this amount of RV. Infant lungs are much larger in relation to the thorax than are adult lungs. Thus, infant lungs are not expanded to the degree that adult lungs are, resulting in much less of an RV. As the child matures, the relationship between the lungs and thorax becomes increasingly adultlike, and the amount of RV increases. By age 7 the value is around 450 to 500 cc, by age 10 it is approximately 630 cc, by age 13 it has increased to almost 800 cc, and by 16 years the adult range is acquired.

> Residual volume (RV) refers to the amount of air that is always in the lungs and cannot be exhaled voluntarily.

Dead Air   A small amount of volume of air in the lungs and airways is known as **dead air**. This is about 150 cc worth of air that is not involved in oxygen–CO_2 exchange. This air, at any time, is in the upper respiratory passage and in the bronchial tree. It is the very last to be inhaled and is therefore the first to be exhaled during the next cycle of respiration (Zemlin, 1998). Correspondingly, the last 150 cc of air that is expired from the alveoli during exhalation remains in the dead air spaces and is the first to reenter the alveoli (even though it still has CO_2 in it).

Lung Capacities

Lung capacities combine various lung volumes, and include vital capacity (VC), functional residual capacity (FRC), and total lung capacity (TLC). One of the most important of these, in terms of speech production, is vital capacity.

Vital Capacity   **Vital capacity** (VC) is the combination of tidal volume, inspiratory reserve volume, and expiratory reserve volume. In other words, VC is the maximum amount of air that a person can exhale after having inhaled as deeply as possible. Vital capacity represents the total amount of air available for all purposes, including speech. It does not include residual volume, which is not under voluntary control. Like many of the lung volumes, VC depends on the age and size of the individual. Five-year-old girls and boys have a VC of about 1000 cc and 1250 cc, respectively (Zemlin, 1998). By age 7, VC is around 1500 to 1600 cc and increases to about 2000 cc by age 9. By 13 years of age the amount has increased by approximately 1000 cc for boys and 500 cc for girls. By age 17 years, boys have a VC of around 4500 cc, while the value for girls is about 3750 cc. The average value of 5000 cc is typically used for VC in adults. Vital capacity has been shown to decrease slightly with advancing age, which some researchers have linked to decreased voice production capabilities in older adults.

Vital capacity (VC) is the maximum amount of air a person can exhale after a maximum inhalation and is the total amount of air available for all purposes including quiet breathing, breathing during exertion, speaking, singing, etc.

Functional Residual Capacity   **Functional residual capacity** (FRC) is the amount of air remaining in the lungs and airways at the resting expiratory level, that is, at the end of a normal quiet exhalation. Thus, FRC combines the expiratory reserve volume and the residual volume and averages approximately 2500 to 3500 cc in young adults. In 7-year-olds, FRC is a little under 1000 cc and increases to the 1400 cc range at age 10 and to around 1700 to 2000 cc by 13 years. By age 16, adult levels are reached.

The amount of air remaining in the lungs and airways at the resting expiratory level is called the functional residual capacity (FRC).

Total Lung Capacity   **Total lung capacity** (TLC) refers to the total amount of air that the lungs are capable of holding, including tidal volume, inspiratory reserve volume, expiratory reserve volume, and residual volume. Like the other volumes and capacities, TLC is developmental, increasing with age, and influenced by gender. Values for 7-year-old boys and girls are in the 2000 cc range. Ten-year-olds have a TLC in the high 2000 and low 3000 cc range. By age 13 a gender difference emerges, with boys averaging around the mid 4000 cc range and girls around the 3700 cc range. By age 16 the difference is more pronounced, with males demonstrating values in the 6000 cc range and female values in the 5000 cc area.

Lung volumes and capacities can be expressed as a percentage of vital capacity—e.g., tidal volume for life breathing is approximately 10 percent VC, whereas speech breathing involves around 20 percent VC.

■ TABLE 4.5

Group Means of Three Age Groups of Subjects
for Some Lung Volumes and Capacities, in cc

	AGE: 25	50	75
TLC	6740	7050	6630
VC	5350	5090	4470
FRC	3120	3460	3440
ERV	1730	1500	1280

Source: Adapted from Hoit & Hixon (1987).

Development of Lung Volumes and Capacities   In general, lung volumes and capacities increase from infancy through puberty, and adult values are apparent by age 16, as can be seen in Table 4.4. Lung volumes and capacities seem to stay stable until the later adult years, when they start to decrease with advancing age. Hoit and Hixon (1987) have provided averages for some lung volumes and capacities for three age groups of adults: young adults (25-year-olds), middle-aged adults (50-year-olds), and elderly adults (75-year-olds). See Table 4.5, which shows that both vital capacity and expiratory reserve volume decrease somewhat with increasing age. This decrease may be implicated in some kinds of speech problems.

Lung volumes and capacities are often expressed as percentages of VC. The REL is around 35 to 40 percent VC. This means that we can inhale 60 to 65 percent more air above REL in order to fill the lungs to their maximum capacity. Conversely, at this point the lungs still hold 35 to 40 percent of air that could be breathed out. Below 35 to 40 percent VC, the individual is drawing on ERV. Figure 4.9 is a schematic representation of some lung volumes expressed as percentages of VC.

Differences between Breathing for Life and Breathing for Speech

Although it sounds like a simple enough process, breathing is actually an amazingly complex function that is integrated with other body functions, including metabolism, regulation of body temperature, fluid and acid–base balance, and others (Boliek et al., 1996). Furthermore, breathing for vegetative purposes (often called life breathing or quiet breathing) and breathing to generate a power supply for speech involve different motor strategies. Breathing for life is usually (although not always) an unconscious, automatic process, with the rate and extent of breathing determined by the needs of our bodies at a particular moment in time. We take in greater amounts of air when performing vigorous exercise than we do when sitting quietly and reading a book, for

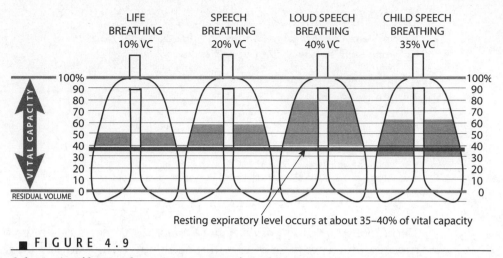

Resting expiratory level occurs at about 35–40% of vital capacity

■ **F I G U R E   4 . 9**

Schematic of lung volume as a percent of vital capacity.

example. These different levels of air intake are determined reflexively depending on the oxygen levels in our blood.

Breathing for speech complicates the process, because the need for appropriate gas exchange is integrated with linguistic considerations. These include, for example, the need to take breaths at linguistically appropriate places in order not to break the flow of speech, the need to take an appropriate amount of air for the utterance to be produced, and the need to generate an adequate length of exhalation to be able to say more than a few syllables in one breath. The respiratory system is also involved in the prosodic aspects of speech, such as variations in F_0 and intensity, syllable and word stress, and emphasis (Metz & Schiavetti, 1995). Human speech represents fine control and precise neural integration of the activity of seventy to eighty muscles from respiratory, laryngeal, pharyngeal, palatal, and facial muscle groups (Davis, Zhang, Winkworth, & Bandler, 1996). For speech breathing, the automatic nerve signals to the many different muscles involved in respiration and speech production must be replaced by voluntary nerve signals to the same muscles (Smith & Denny, 1990).

Based on linguistic and prosodic considerations of speech, four major changes occur when we switch from breathing for life to breathing for speech: the location of air intake, the ratio of time for inhalation versus exhalation, the volume of air inhaled per cycle, and the muscle activity for exhalation. See Table 4.6.

Location of Air Intake   The first change concerns the location of air intake. Both inhalation and exhalation in life breathing typically occur

Speech breathing is more complicated than quiet breathing because of the need to integrate ventilatory needs with linguistic considerations such as the appropriate place in the utterance to take a breath, appropriate amount of air for the upcoming utterance, and prosodic variations.

■ **TABLE 4.6**

Four Changes That Occur when Switching from Life Breathing to Speech Breathing

CHANGE	LIFE	SPEECH
Location of air intake	Nose	Mouth
Ratio of time for inhalation versus exhalation	Inhale: 40% Exhale: 60%	Inhale: 10% Exhale: 90%
Volume of air	500 cc 10% VC	Variable, depending on length and loudness of utterance, 20 to 25% VC
Muscle activity for exhalation	Passive: Muscles of thorax and diaphragm relax	Active: Thoracic and abdominal muscles contract to control recoil of rib cage and diaphragm

through the nose, unless the individual has some kind of blockage due to a cold, enlarged adenoids, deviated septum, or the like. Breathing through the nose is healthy for a number of reasons. First, tiny cilia are embedded in the mucous membrane lining the nasal cavities. Similar to the cilia in the trachea, the cilia in the nasal cavities help to filter the air entering the respiratory system by trapping particles of dust and pollution and preventing them from entering the rest of the respiratory system. Second, the mucous membrane lining of the nasal cavities acts to both moisten and warm the ingoing air. (If you have ever slept in a very dry room, you know firsthand the pain of breathing in very dry air.)

Breathing through the nose is healthier than breathing through the mouth because the air gets warmed, moistened, and filtered, but breathing through the mouth is more efficient for speech.

Inhaling and exhaling for speech, on the other hand, occur through the oral cavity. This is a much more efficient location for speech breathing because the air coming in through the mouth has less of a distance to travel to the lungs, and the air exiting the mouth is the source for most of the speech sounds we make.

Ratio of Time for Inhalation versus Exhalation   The second change involves the ratio of time for inhalation versus exhalation. In life breathing, the interval of time for inhalation is nearly the same as for exhalation, with inhalation consuming about 40 percent of the time and exhalation taking up about 60 percent of the time. Each breath in and breath out takes approximately 2 seconds (s), depending on age, bodily requirements, and other factors.

Inhalation and exhalation times are approximately equal for life breathing, whereas speech breathing requires a quick inhalation and a prolonged exhalation.

The ratio of inhalation time to exhalation time changes dramatically for speech breathing. Inhalation time shortens to about 10 percent of the total cycle, whereas exhalation time extends to about 90 percent of the cycle. Exhalation for speech can last up to 20 to 25 s, instead of the approximately 2 s duration in life breathing. This ratio is efficient for speech, which is produced on the expiratory phase of respiration. Speech would be very choppy if we had to pause every few seconds for an air refill and if each inhalation took 2 s. By shortening the inhalatory phase and lengthening the exhalation phase, we can generate a smooth stream of speech. This pattern of quick inspirations and more extended exhalations holds true even for infants and very young children.

Volume of Air Inhaled per Cycle   The third change involves the volume of air taken in per cycle. For each successive breath we take in around 500 cc (TV), breathe out the same amount, take in another 500 cc, breathe it out, and so on.

This 500 cc is about 10 percent of the average vital capacity of around 5000 cc. Thus, for life breathing we do not inhale as much air as our lungs are capable of holding, but only around 10 percent of that amount. For TV, an adult generally inhales up to around 50 percent of VC and exhales down to about 40 percent, that is, down to REL.

For speech breathing, the amount of air taken in and expired per cycle differs, depending on the utterance to be said. A short utterance ("Hi, how are you?") requires a lot less breath than a long utterance ("Have you read the latest psychological thriller that the great author— what's his name—just got out?"). In general, speaking is initiated at volumes above the REL and within volumes that are about twice as much as quiet, tidal breathing (Solomon & Charron, 1998).

In terms of the percentage of vital capacity for normal conversational speech, we tend to breathe in up to about 60 percent of VC per utterance and exhale during the utterance down to REL at 35 to 40 percent VC (Porter, Hogue, & Tobey, 1995). Thus, we use around 20 to 25 percent of vital capacity per utterance, compared to 10 percent for quiet breathing. For loud speech we use around 40 percent of VC, with inhalation being initiated at higher percentages of vital capacity (up to approximately 80%) and ending at REL. Children use a higher percentage of the VC for speech, generally beginning speech at around 65 percent VC and ending at about 30 percent. Children also breathe below REL for speech purposes much more than adults (Stathopoulos, 1997). Classically trained singers use much larger volumes during singing, sometimes even using the full vital capacity (Watson & Hixon, 1985; Watson, Hixon, Stathoupoulos, & Sullivan, 1990).

The volume of air inspired and expired for life breathing is around 500 mL on average. The volume for speech is approximately double.

Muscle Activity for Exhalation   The fourth change concerns the muscle activity for exhalation. For both life and speech breathing, inspiration is an active process requiring contraction of the diaphragm and external intercostal muscles to increase the volume of the thoracic cavity and lungs. For life breathing, exhalation is a passive process, relying solely on elastic recoil forces, whereas muscle activity plays a crucial role in controlling exhalation for speech. To understand the difference between exhaling for life compared to speech, we need to examine exhalation in more detail.

During exhalation the thoracic cavity and lungs must decrease in volume in order for the P_{alv} to increase and cause the outflow of air from the lungs. This decrease in volume is achieved by four forces that cause the thorax and lungs to recoil to their original positions. First, gravity acts to pull downward on the raised rib cage, thus forcing the thorax and lungs to decrease in volume. Second, the muscles that are contracting and lifting the rib cage relax, allowing the rib cage to return to its original position. The diaphragm also relaxes and resumes its dome shape, thus decreasing the vertical dimension of the thorax. Third, elasticity of the respiratory tissues and lungs returns the tissues that have been extended to their original positions. The fourth force involved in this recoil is the **torque** of the ribs. Torque refers to a twisting, rotary force. During inspiration, the cartilaginous portions of the ribs twist slightly. During exhalation, the ribs untwist as they return to their original positions, and this untwisting generates force. Together, these four restoring forces are called **recoil forces**. The more the thoracic cavity is enlarged during inspiration, the greater the recoil forces that are generated to return the rib cage to its original position during expiration.

The air pressures generated by these recoil forces are referred to as **relaxation pressures**. After you have inspired and increased your lung volume, recoil forces begin to return the structures to the rest position, generating a positive P_{alv}. At 100 percent VC, P_{alv} is around 60 cm H_2O. As lung volume decreases, the positive P_{alv} decreases as well. For speech, we inhale up to approximately 60 percent VC, yielding a P_{alv} of about 10 cm H_2O (Figure 4.10). Relaxation pressures can also be negative. The 0 point represents resting lung volume, the state of equilibrium during which $P_{alv} = P_{atmos}$. Resting lung volume occurs at 38

> Relaxation pressures are generated by recoil forces including gravity, muscle relaxation, tissue elasticity, and rib cage torque.

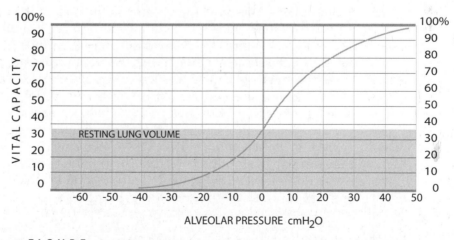

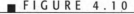

■ FIGURE 4.10

Relaxation pressures.

percent VC. When the lungs are compressed during forced expiration, the system tends to recoil in the opposite direction, that is, to expand to its rest position. In this case, P_{alv} is negative and air flows into the lungs. What the relaxation pressure curve shows is that at lung volumes above 38 percent VC the inspiratory process requires muscular force, and expiratory forces are passive. At lung volumes below 38 percent VC, the expiratory process requires muscular force, and the inspiratory process is passive (Zemlin, 1998).

The amount of positive pressure needed for speech is generally about 5 to 10 cm H_2O for normal conversation. For speech, there must be some way to control these pressures, and this leads us to the fourth difference between breathing for life and breathing for speech.

The exhalation portion of respiration for life is passive. For speech, on the other hand, exhalation is an active process, making use of muscle forces to control the necessary pressures. This control is achieved by a checking action of the inspiratory muscles, which regulates the rate at which the thoracic cavity and lungs return to their original positions after they have been displaced during inspiration. Various rib cage muscles are recruited to prevent the thoracic cavity and lungs from deflating too quickly, and abdominal muscles are used to continue exhalation below REL. That is, for pressures above REL, the muscles of inspiration continue to contract in order to provide a counteracting force to the deflating rib cage and lungs. Below REL, muscles of expiration (primarily the abdominal muscles) begin contracting in order to continue decreasing the volume of the thorax and lungs and thus prolong exhalation. The way that the abdominal muscles are involved is that they press inward on the abdominal contents (stomach, intestines, and so on), forcing the contents upward against the diaphragm. This upward pressure on the floor of the thoracic cavity further decreases the volume of the thorax and lungs. The internal intercostal muscles may also contract to depress the rib cage further.

> During exhalation for speech breathing the inspiratory muscles continue to contract, exerting a checking action that regulates the speed at which the thoracic cavity and lungs deflate.

This pattern of muscle activity for speech exhalation varies depending on factors such as the intensity of the utterance, emphasis on specific parts of the utterance, and linguistic stress on particular words and syllables. The pattern also varies depending on age. Children generate higher tracheal pressures for speech than do adults, and younger children use higher tracheal pressures than older children (Solomon & Charron, 1998). This may occur because children typically speak more loudly than adults, and louder speech is produced with higher pressure levels. The structure and function of children's respiratory systems probably also contribute to the higher pressures they produce.

Air Pressures and Flows in Respiration

A lot of recent research has been devoted to the measurement of various respiratory parameters in normal children and adults. These kinds of normative data form the basis of comparison for measurement of respiratory problems that can interfere with speech production. The analysis of respiratory parameters during either speech or nonspeech activities yields measures of air pressures, airflows, lung volumes, and chest and abdomen movement. For our discussion of these respiratory variables, we will use a framework developed by Hixon and his colleagues and described in depth by Solomon and Charron (1998). This framework focuses on four respiratory features important for speech production: pressure, volume, flow, and chest wall shape.

> Pressure, volume, airflow, and chest wall shape are important features of respiration for speech.

Pressure refers to the forces generated by the respiratory process, which form the power supply for speech. **Volume** refers to the amount of air in the lungs and airways. **Flow** refers to the change in volume of air over a certain period of time. **Chest-wall shape** refers to the positioning of the chest wall (rib cage, diaphragm, and abdominal muscles) for speech breathing activity. These four elements are closely related to each other. The positioning of the chest wall (and, due to pleural linkage, of the lungs) results in a particular volume of air in the lungs. The volume of air within the lungs directly influences the pressure in the lungs, and the volume change over time causes air to flow into and out of the respiratory system.

Because of the relationships among these respiratory parameters, it is possible to measure one parameter directly and then to make inferences about other parameters. For example, researchers and clinicians often measure chest wall shape and use this information to estimate lung volume changes. This kind of information is extremely useful in characterizing aspects of breathing in normal and disordered speech.

Air Pressures　　The pressures necessary for speech include pressure inside the lungs (P_{alv}), pressure below the vocal folds, called subglottal pressure or tracheal pressure (P_s or P_{trach}), and pressure inside the mouth, or oral pressure (P_{oral}). Air pressures are often measured with a **manometer** (Figure 4.11), a device with dials calibrated to show pressure changes in terms of cm H_2O. A person blows into an attached mouthpiece, generating pressure, which displaces the dials.

Because the dials on this instrument must be read, it is not suitable for measuring pressures that change rapidly, such as those during speech. Rather, static pressures can be measured, so we can determine how much pressure a person can generate and sustain for a period of time. This kind of measure is useful for evaluating how much pressure can be built up by an individual with some kind of problem, such as a neurological problem or a cleft palate (Decker, 1990).

For pressures within the oral and nasal cavities that change very rapidly during speech, it is necessary to convert pressure changes into electrical signals, which are then processed and read by an appropriate instrument, such as

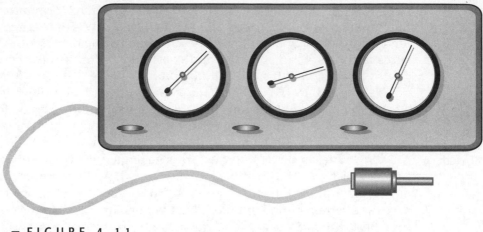

■ FIGURE 4.11

Manometer.

an FM recorder or a computer. This change is made by means of a pressure transducer fitted into a tube that can be placed in the oral cavity or mounted in masks placed over the mouth and face (Decker, 1990). With this technique, the pressure variations recorded can be stored for later viewing and analysis.

The pressures used in speech are typically measured and expressed in units of cm H_2O. The pressure needed for conversational speech is low, somewhere around 5 to 10 cm H_2O. This is a small proportion of the total pressure that a person can generate. For instance, most 5-year-old children can generate 35 to 50 cm H_2O when blowing as hard as possible. Adults can generate 60 cm H_2O or more. For normal conversational speech, although the pressures needed are low, they have to be sustained for different amounts of time, which means that the muscles of the chest wall must produce carefully graded forces (Solomon & Charron, 1998). Within the overall pressures needed for speech, the pressures also vary instant by instant, depending on the emphasis on a syllable or word, the changes in vocal amplitude, and so on. In general, children talk at higher tracheal pressures than adults (Stathopoulos & Sapienza, 1997). For louder speech, both children and adults generate greater tracheal pressures to increase intensity (Stathopoulos & Sapienza, 1993). For instance, to increase vocal intensity by 8 to 9 dB, a person would have to double P_{trach} (Titze, 1994).

Tracheal and alveolar pressures are not usually measured directly because, although it is possible to make direct measurements, the procedure involves inserting a needle into the trachea, which is a highly invasive procedure. Fortunately, P_{trach} is easy to measure indirectly by measuring P_{oral}. A small tube connected to a pressure transducer is placed inside the mouth just past the lips,

The pressure needed for conversational speech is around 5 to 10 cm H_2O.

and the pressure inside the mouth during the closure portion of a stop consonant is measured (Smitheran & Hixon, 1981). The strongest oral pressures generated during the closed portion of a voiceless stop consonant (e.g., /p/) are almost identical to P_{alv} and P_{trach}. Why should this be? For the /p/ sound, we close our lips, raise the velum to close the velopharyngeal passage and prevent air escaping into the nose, and open the vocal folds. We are still exhaling, however. Thus, the pressures throughout the system (i.e., P_{alv}, P_{trach}, and P_{oral}) are essentially the same at this moment. So, if we measure P_{oral} at this instant, we can say with some confidence that the P_{oral} is equal to P_{trach} and to P_{alv}. Using this indirect method, pressures have been compared in normally speaking children and adults and between individuals with and without speech disorders.

Airflow   Airflow (or volume velocity) is a measure of a volume of air moving in a certain direction at a particular location per unit of time. For instance, airflow can be measured in milliliters per second (ml/s) or liters per minute (l/min). Airflow through the speech production system is strongly related to the structures above the trachea that open and close to valve the airway (Solomon & Charron, 1998). These structures include the larynx and the articulators. Air flows into and out of the lungs due to muscular and recoil forces.

The outward flow of air through the system is modified by the various resistances to this flow created as the larynx and other articulators open and close. If the larynx allows too much air to flow through the glottis during vocalization, the voice will be heard as breathy. If too little air is permitted through the glottis because the vocal folds are closed too tightly, the voice may be perceived as tense and strained. Resonance of the voice is also affected by airflow and the resistance to flow. If the soft palate does not offer enough resistance to the airflow, too much air flows into the nasal cavities, resulting in hypernasality and nasal emission. On the other hand, if some kind of blockage, such as enlarged adenoids, causes too much resistance to the flow of air through the nose, the person sounds hyponasal.

Airflow for speech is related to the resistence to flow exerted by the valving action of the larynx and articulators.

The device usually used to measure airflow is called a **pneumotachograph** This instrument includes a mask (like an anesthesia mask) that fits over the face. The air being exhaled from the mouth exits through a channel that is hooked into a pressure sensor. Flow from the mouth and nose can also be measured separately using a divided face mask and separate pressure sensors for the nose and mouth. The output of the pneumotachograph can be stored on an instrument such as an FM tape recorder or computer and then displayed for analysis. Flow can be measured over the duration of an utterance and calculated in milliliters per syllable or milliliters per second. Alternatively, peak flow (i.e., greatest flow) can be measured per second during the production of stops and fricatives. In terms of syllables, Boliek, Hixon, Watson, and Morgan (1997) found that toddlers used about 100 ml per syllable. However, the

■ TABLE 4.7

Average Flow Rates (in ml/s) for 7-Year-Old Children and Adult Men and Women for Sustained /a/

BOYS	GIRLS	MEN	WOMEN
95.9	71.6	112.4	93.7

Source: Baken, 1996.

amount of flow per syllable appears to depend on age, as younger children use more flow, which decreases as they mature. Hoit, Banzett, Brown, and Lorring, (1990) reported that children aged 7 to 16 years used approximately 35 to 60 ml/syllable.

Flow rates in millilieters per second (ml/s) have been calculated for children and adults. Table 4.7 provides flow rate information based on data reported in the literature and provided by Baken (1996).

In terms of peak flow, Borden et al. (1994) noted that a speech sound produced with a rather high pressure and flow, such as /s/, might show a pressure of 7 cm H_2O and a flow of around 500 ml/s. Peak airflow during the release of stop sounds is high, approximately 600 ml/s for children and 900 ml/s for adults (Stathopoulos & Weismer, 1985; Subtelny, Worth, & Sakuds, 1966; Trullinger & Emanuel, 1983). The lower peak flows shown by children may be due to a combination of physical and physiological factors, such as children's smaller vocal tracts, greater vocal tract resistances, and lower elastic recoil of the lungs (Solomon & Charron, 1998).

Individuals who have greater than normal airflows during speech may valve the airstream inefficiently, allowing too much air to escape. This is often seen in people with neurological diseases. However, it is important to keep in mind that abnormalities of airflow during speech cannot be attributed only to the respiratory system, because the larynx and other articulators contribute to airflow measures (Solomon & Charron, 1998).

Lung Volume and Chest-Wall Shape   Volume refers to the amount of air in the lungs and is measured either in liters (l), milliliters (ml), cubic centimeters (cc or cm^3) or as a percentage of vital capacity (%VC). Lung volume can be measured directly with a spirometer or estimated from rib cage (RC) and abdominal movement. Spirometers are useful in determining volumes such as vital capacity and tidal volume, but cannot be used to measure lung volumes during speaking. In speaking situations, **respiratory kinematic analysis** is used, in which lung volumes are estimated from RC and abdominal movement. The rationale for this kind of analysis is that the RC and abdomen displace volume as they expand

Respiratory kinematic analysis is used to estimate lung volumes from movements of the rib cage and abdomen.

and contract during inhalation and exhalation. The movements of these structures therefore reflect the changing volumes of the thorax and abdomen.

Movements of the rib cage and abdomen can be measured with either a **plethysmograph** or with **linearized magnetometers** A plethysmograph consists of an elastic band covering a coil of wire. One elastic band fits around the chest and one around the abdomen. As the person's chest and abdominal walls expand and contract, the changes in their cross-sectional areas are measured. These changes are sent to an amplifier and recorder, or computer. This method allows the degree of movement of the RC and abdomen to be assessed independently, and the movements can also be combined to calculate lung volume.

Movements of the chest wall and abdomen can also be measured by a magnetometer. A magnetometer is composed of two coils of wire. An electric current is passed through one coil and generates an electromagnetic field. This electromagnetic field in turn induces an electric current in the other coil. The strength of the voltage induced by the electromagnetic field depends on the distance separating the coils. If one coil is placed on a person's back and the other directly opposite on a point along his or her thorax or abdomen, the changes in the diameters of the rib cage or abdomen can be calculated in relation to the changing strength of the current.

Measures generated with these types of kinematic analyses typically include lung, RC, and abdominal volume intiations and terminations. In other words, the volume of the lungs, RC, or abdomen is measured at the beginning and end of an utterance. The volume of air expended equals the initiation value minus the termination value.

Breathing Patterns for Speech

Measurements of pressure, flow, volume, and chest wall shape have been used to establish patterns of breathing for speech. It has been found, for example, that during speech the abdomen is smaller and the rib cage is larger than in their respective relaxation positions. This positioning is efficient for speech, because when the abdominal wall moves inward, it pushes the diaphragm upward and expands the lower rib cage. This allows the diaphragm to make quick, strong contractions, which facilitates the quick inspirations and the constantly changing pressures needed for speech (Hixon, Goldman, & Mead, 1973). During speech, the rib cage and abdomen move continuously to generate the necessary changes in lung volume. Most lung movement is accomplished through rib cage adjustments, because a greater portion of the surface of the lung is adjacent to the rib cage than to the diaphragm. Therefore, the rib cage is more efficient than the abdominal wall at moving air from the lungs (Solomon & Charron, 1998). Research using kinematic analysis has shown that just before a person starts to speak he or she automatically positions the chest wall in such a way as to quickly and efficiently generate the necessary pressures (Baken & Cavallo,

1981). These chest wall movements (known as **prephonatory chest wall movements**) are influenced by the speaking task, such as the length of the upcoming utterance. Prephonatory chest wall movements also depend on the person's lung volume when speech is initiated. At high lung volumes, the respiratory structures can passively generate P_{alv} of around 5 to 8 cm H_2O, which is more than enough for normal speech. Therefore, at high lung volumes, the chest wall might not need much setting up for speech. At lower lung volumes that do not produce enough P_{alv} for speech, the chest wall may need to quickly make muscular adjustments immediately before beginning to speak (McFarland & Smith, 1992).

Kinematic analysis has also provided information about the lung volumes used for speech. For instance, speech is produced in the midrange of VC (Manifold & Murdoch, 1993; Mitchell, Hoit, & Watson, 1996). However, lung volumes differ both between individuals and within individuals producing different utterances. Individuals use lung volumes during speech that are not much greater than quiet breathing, suggesting that normal conversational speech is a very efficient procedure. Kinematic analysis has also shown that lung volumes, pressures, and flows are influenced by linguistic considerations, such as clause boundaries and the number of clauses in a sentence (Winkworth, Davis, Adams, & Ellis, 1995). People tend to time their inspirations with naturally occurring breaks in the linguistic message, which enhances the overall fluency of speech. Pauses for breath that do not occur at grammatical junctures disrupt the flow of speech and result in the perception of disfluent speech. In fact, individuals who stutter tend to pause at linguistically inappropriate places in a sentence, which contributes to the perception of stuttering (Eisen & Ferrand, 1995).

> An efficient chest-wall posture for speech involves a smaller abdominal position and a larger rib cage position relative to relaxation.

Another speech breathing pattern relates to the complexity of the speaking activity. More complex speaking tasks seem to result in a smaller number of syllables per breath group, slower speaking rate, and greater average volume of air expended per syllable (Mitchell et al., 1996). The amount of air breathed in is strongly influenced by the loudness of the intended utterance. When speaking very loudly, we inhale a greater volume of air in a shorter amount of time in order to preserve speech fluency while meeting the normal bodily demands of gas exchange (Russell, Cerny, & Stathopoulos, 1998). On the other hand, during very soft speech, individuals typically begin utterances at a much lower lung volume.

> Lung volumes, pressures, and flows are influenced by linguistic considerations such as clause boundaries and the number of clauses in a sentence.

The type of phoneme being said also influences respiration. Voiceless stops and fricatives need a high flow, while voiced stops and fricatives need a lower flow (Russell & Stathopoulos, 1988). Differences also exist in respiratory function between regular conversational speech and whispering. During whispering, individuals tend to terminate breath groups at lower lung volumes, use fewer syllables per breath group, and expend more air per syllable. Also, P_{trach} is lower

■ TABLE 4.8

Patterns of Speech Breathing

CHEST WALL SHAPE

Abdomen smaller, rib cage larger than during relaxation

VOLUME

Midrange of VC

Approximately twice the volume of quiet tidal breathing

LINGUISTIC INFLUENCES

Inspirations timed with naturally occurring breaks in the linguistic message

Complexity of speaking task

Intended loudness

Type of phoneme

Whispering

when a person whispers than during normal conversational speech (Stathopoulos et al., 1991). Table 4.8 lists the typical patterns of speech breathing.

Changes in Speech Breathing over the Lifespan

Like many other functions involved in speech production, breathing for speech undergoes developmental change throughout the lifespan. Children have smaller lungs and thoracic cavities than adults, resulting in smaller vital capacities. Lung width, lung length, and total capacity continue to increase until 14 to 16 years of age (Stathopoulos & Sapienza, 1997). Children produce speech using a higher percentage of their lung capacity and also use lower lung volumes to end their utterances than adults (Stathopoulos & Sapienza, 1997). Children seem to use more effort and are less efficient in producing speech. However, these respiratory variables in children are related to how fluent the child is. Children who use many voiced fillers ("um," "er," "uh," etc.) and many pauses and hesitations in their speech generally show fewer syllables per breath and use more lung volume for each syllable (Hoit et al., 1990). Therefore, speech fluency is very important to take into account when making clinical judgments of speech breathing. A client whose speech or reading is slow and halting, with many fillers and hesitations, would be expected to produce fewer syllables per breath and expend more air per syllable than another client of the same age who is more fluent.

Changes also occur in older adults' respiratory patterns for speech, resulting from changes in anatomy and physiology over the span of years. For instance, the costal cartilages ossify and calcify; thoracic shape changes; the force

With aging, changes occur to the respiratory system, including ossification of the costal cartilages, loss of alveolar surface tension, and reductions in the force and rate of muscle contraction.

and rate of respiratory muscle contraction decreases; there is a progressive loss of alveolar surface tension and pulmonary capillary blood volume; and overall lung size decreases (Sperry & Klich, 1992). These changes affect the recoil pressures of the lungs, resulting in decreases in vital capacity, expiratory reserve volume, and inspiratory reserve volume and increases in residual volume. Sperry and Klich (1992) compared younger and older women's speech breathing. The groups were found to differ in lung volumes and also in speech breathing patterns. For example, the younger group had an average VC of 3356 cc, and the older group had an average VC of 2456 cc. The older adults did not start to phonate immediately after inhaling and wasted two to three times more air than did the younger speakers.

Research has also shown that older individuals inhale more deeply to higher lung volume levels and use more air per syllable than younger speakers. Older persons also tend to inhale more often than younger individuals, perhaps because they waste more air than younger people. However, despite these changes, older adults' speech is usually as intelligible as younger adults'. Older adults may adjust to these kinds of anatomical and physiological changes in order to maintain adequate respiratory support for clear speech. For instance, older adults may compensate by talking more slowly in order to maintain intelligibility. These aging effects seem to be fairly uniform until around 60 to 70 years, after which the effects become more variable among individuals.

s u m m a r y

- The respiratory system consists of the pulmonary system (lungs and airways) and the chest-wall system (rib cage, abdomen, and diaphragm).
- Inhalation and exhalation occur when P_{alv} decreases and increases, forcing air into and out of the system.
- Lung volumes and capacities refer to different amounts of air in the lungs at a given time; these amounts change over the lifespan.
- Four important changes occur when breathing for speech rather than for life:

location of air intake, ratio of inhalatory to exhalatory time, volume of air per cycle, and muscle activity for exhalation.
- Breathing patterns for speech are influenced by linguistic considerations, including speaking task complexity, clause boundaries, and loudness of the intended utterance.
- Speech breathing changes over the lifespan, due to changes in the structure and function of the respiratory system.

1. Draw a diagram of the pulmonary system, and describe each of the components.
2. Explain how the lungs are able to expand and contract even though they contain very little muscle.
3. Describe how the respiratory system changes over the lifespan in terms of rate of breathing, lung volumes and capacities, and speech breathing.
4. Identify and describe the four differences between breathing for life and breathing for speech. For each difference, explain why a person with spastic cerebral palsy might have difficulty in making the switch.
5. Explain the concept of resting expiratory level and discuss its role in the measurement of lung volumes and capacities.

chapter 5

Clinical Application
Respiratory Breakdowns That Affect Speech Production

chapter objectives   *After reading this chapter, you will*

1. Be aware of the general principles of clinical management of speech breathing problems.

2. Understand the problems in respiratory function in Parkinson's disease.

3. Be able to describe differences in lung volumes and capacities in cerebellar disease and cervical spinal cord injury.

4. Be able to explain the parameters of respiratory function in cerebral palsy.

5. Understand how speech breathing is affected in patients who are mechanically ventilated.

6. Appreciate the role of respiratory function in voice disorders and hearing impairment.

Numerous different types of structural or neurological problems can affect the respiratory system and the structures of the system, or the function of any part of the system, or both. If a person has a compromised respiratory system, not only will breathing for life be more effortful, but breathing for speech will also be affected. The difficulty may be with the respiratory muscles themselves or with the nervous supply to the respiratory muscles, or it may be due to a generalized weakness that hinders the individual from sitting or standing properly, thus interfering with breath support for speech. Postural problems are particularly evident in neurological disorders, such as Parkinson's disease, cerebellar problems, spinal cord injury, and cerebral palsy. Breathing for speech may also be affected in individuals who are mechanically ventilated (i.e., who have life support for breathing), in people with voice disorders, and in hearing-impaired individuals. See Table 5.1.

It is important to appreciate two general principles that apply to the clinical management of speech breathing problems. First, the amount of air needed to produce speech is not very much greater than that required for normal breathing activities at rest (Dworkin, 1991), around 20 percent of VC. However, this amount of air must be managed efficiently for speaking purposes. Some clinical researchers have suggested that if a patient can generate a steady stream of P_s of 5 cm H_2O for 5 seconds or longer, the respiratory system may be sufficient to support speech (Netsell & Hixon, 1992). However, although some patients with neuromuscular respiratory difficulties may be able to perform this static kind of task, they may not be able to coordinate the more

■ TABLE 5.1

Some Diseases and Disorders in Which Parameters of the Respiratory System May Be Affected

CONDITION	RESPIRATORY PARAMETERS
Parkinson's disease	Changes in chest-wall shape, reduced rib cage movement, and increased displacement of abdomen Reduced VC Reduced P_{oral}
Cerebellar disease	Reduced VC Abrupt changes in motions of the chest wall Utterances initiated below normal lung volumes
Cervical spinal cord injury	Reduced VC, IRV, and ERV Larger than normal lung volumes at beginning and ending of speech exhalation Larger abdominal volumes than normal Fewer than normal syllables per breath
Cerebral palsy	Reduced VC Difficulty accessing IRV and ERV Weakness and deformities of chest wall Abnormally high airflows during speech
Mechanical ventilation	Higher than normal P_{trach} Excessively high TV
Voice problems	Clavicular breathing Higher than normal P_{trach} Higher lung volume initiation and lower lung termination for speech
Hearing problems	Exhaling for speech at low lung volumes Excessive air expenditure per syllable

dynamic and complex respiratory maneuvers that are required for speech breathing. Thus, in a clinical situation, it is critical to measure the patient's static and dynamic respiratory skills.

The second principle is that treatment needs to be tailored to the patient's specific respiratory difficulty. For example, patients with too much muscular tone may need treatments that will help them to relax their muscles. Patients with posture problems may benefit from braces or girdles for abdominal support. Patients with cerebellar problems often need treatment to improve their balance and sense of position. Patients with too little muscular tone require exercises that increase the strength of the muscles used for inhalation and exhalation.

Keeping these two principles in mind, we will examine speech breathing as it relates to some medical and clinical conditions.

Conditions That Affect Speech Breathing

Parkinson's Disease

Parkinson's disease (PD) is a progressive neurological disease characterized by a rigidity of muscles that restricts the range of movement of the affected structures. If the respiratory and/or other structures involved in speech production are affected, speech will be affected as well. In fact, PD is typically associated with speech that is monotonous, distorted in terms of articulation, breathy, and weak. The weakness and low vocal intensity, which are very typical, are important factors in communication, because they decrease the clarity and intelligibility of the person's speech (Ramig, 1992). The breathy, weak voice is probably due in part to decreased respiratory support (Ramig, Countryman, Thompson, & Horii, 1995). Research has shown that, when breathing for speech, patients with PD often have a different chest wall shape than normal. Normally, in the upright body position, the rib cage moves more easily than the abdomen, above resting expiratory level. Therefore, when the diaphragm contracts, the rib cage moves more than the abdomen. In individuals with PD,

Patients with Parkinson's disease often show reduced movement of the rib cage and greater displacement of the abdomen during speech breathing, which is opposite to the normal pattern.

the rigidity of chest wall muscles results in reduced movement of the rib cage and more displacement of the abdomen (Solomon & Hixon, 1993). Because of the limited rib cage movement, patients may show a reduced vital capacity. However, despite the different chest wall shape, some individuals with PD can probably generate adequate P_{trach} for speech. Individuals who cannot generate enough pressure may not be able to produce speech of normal intensity.

Even if patients with PD can generate enough P_{trach}, they often cannot build up as much P_{oral} as normal speakers. This suggests that the individual with PD probably loses pressure through the lips or through the velopharynx (Solomon & Hixon, 1993). It seems that some of these speakers are able to produce enough respiratory driving pressures for speech, but may have difficulty with controlling the airstream using the articulators. In addition, the lower than normal P_{oral} seen in some speakers with PD may contribute to their lack of intelligibility because of inadequate pressure buildup in the mouth necessary for sounds such as stops and fricatives.

Because the breathing system has been reported to be one of the first speech production subsystems affected in PD, strategies to improve breathing function are often targeted in treatment programs. These strategies should be based on the patient's breathing physiology. For example, teaching patients to speak in short phrases may be more successful than trying to get them to increase their lung volume, because of the rigidity of the chest wall. One main complaint in PD is reduced vocal intensity. Increasing intensity is often targeted in treatment and is accomplished by increasing P_{trach}, as well as by increasing the strength of the vocal fold closure. Strategies include increasing respiratory effort through tasks such as breathing in and out as much and as forcefully as possible; sustaining voiceless sounds, such as /s/ and /f/, for as long as possible; taking deep breaths frequently; speaking at the beginning of the exhalation without wasting breath; and sustaining vowels for as long as possible (Ramig et al., 1995).

> Treatment strategies for increasing intensity in Parkinson's disease often focus on increasing respiratory support.

Cerebellar Disease

Respiratory function has also been studied in speakers with cerebellar disease. The cerebellum is important in the coordination of voluntary movement, because it regulates the speed of movement, direction of movement, force of movement, and so on. If the cerebellum is injured by disease or trauma, this smooth coordination is lost, and movements tend to become jerky and uncoordinated. The person looks like he or she is intoxicated, with an unsteady, lurching gait. If the speech production system is affected, the person's voice may fluctuate unpredictably in pitch and loudness, and the individual loses the ability to make the fine adjustments to F_0 and intensity that are necessary for stress and emphasis. Speech therefore becomes slow, and syllables tend to be produced with excess and equal stress, giving an almost robotic sound to the speech. This type of speech is called *scanning* speech. It is possible that an underlying respiratory disorder contributes to these speech problems, because the respiratory system provides the energy for speech production and is involved in the regulation of loudness, pitch, and stress. This is important to know, because treatment could then be focused on the underlying problem of speech breathing.

Research has shown that some subjects with cerebellar disease have total lung capacities within normal limits, but have vital capacities below normal limits (Murdoch, Chenery, Stokes, & Hardcastle, 1991). The reduction in VC is probably the result of the breakdown in the coordinated action of the components of the chest wall, such as abrupt changes in the motions of the rib cage and abdomen and motion jerks. Some patients in the study by Murdoch et al. (1991) even breathed in during exhalation for speech, a pattern termed by the authors "inspiratory gasps." These gasps seem to be caused by momentary breakdown in the control of the outgoing airflow for speech. Another abnormality in speakers with cerebellar disease was the lung volume level at which they initiated speech. Typically, normal individuals begin to speak at about twice their resting tidal end-expiratory levels, and they end the utterance either at or just above functional residual capacity (FRC). The majority of the patients with cerebellar problems initiated utterances below normal lung levels. Many began their utterances at a lung volume just barely higher than their resting tidal end-expiratory levels, and two speakers actually initiated utterances below REL.

Patients with cerebellar disease sometimes show a reduced vital capacity resulting from the breakdown in the coordination of chest-wall activity.

Understanding these kinds of details about respiratory patterns has important clinical applications. For example, it might be helpful to teach patients with these kinds of breathing characteristics to begin each utterance at a higher lung volume.

Cervical Spinal Cord Injury

Individuals who have suffered cervical spinal cord injury (CSCI) often have respiratory problems. Injury to the part of the spinal cord that supplies nerve impulses to the muscles of respiration can result in weakness or paralysis. If the diaphragm is affected, the person may not be able to breathe at all and will need mechanical ventilation. Even when the diaphragm is not affected and the individual is able to breathe by himself or herself, speech may be affected if the person has difficulty in generating adequate pressures and flows. This could result in reduced loudness, imprecise consonant production (because of the problem in generating the P_{oral} necessary for stops and fricatives), abnormally short breath groups, and slow inspirations (Hoit et al., 1990).

Individuals who have suffered a cervical spinal cord injury may have an abnormally small vital capacity, inspiratory capacity, and expiratory reserve volume, but normal resting tidal volume and breathing rate.

Patients with CSCI have been reported to have much smaller than normal VC, inspiratory capacity (IC), and expiratory reserve volume (ERV). Resting tidal volume and breathing rate, however, may be normal. Hoit et al. (1990) found that most patients with CSCI in their study began and ended their exhalations for speech at larger lung volumes than normal. Also, the injured individuals had larger abdominal volumes, whereas healthy speakers kept the abdomen at smaller volumes during speech breathing. Most speakers with spinal cord injuries produced fewer than normal syllables per breath. However, similar to that of healthy individuals, average flow per syllable ranged from about 35 to 80 cc. Apparently, what some of the patients did was to compensate for their muscular impairment by taking in larger amounts of air. This increased the resulting recoil pressure so that they would not have to rely on the muscles of exhalation to speak. The downside of this compensatory strategy was that the number of syllables produced per breath was reduced. Despite this minor disadvantage, this kind of strategy could be very useful as a clinical tool. Individuals with CSCI can be taught to take in larger amounts of air, to help them increase loudness and project their voices better.

Massery (1991) provided an excellent example of the importance of clinical management of speech breathing in patients with CSCI problems. He described a child of not quite 4 years of age with a CSCI. During the initial evaluation the child could only produce two syllables per breath. Treatment focused on chest wall development, such as body positioning, muscle strengthening, and coordination exercises. After two months the child was able to produce eight syllables per breath and spoke in full sentences.

Cerebral Palsy

Many children and adults with cerebral palsy (CP) face problems with respiratory function that affect their speech production to lesser or greater degrees. Different forms of CP may affect respiratory function in different ways. *Spastic* CP is a condition in which the affected structures are hypertonic and weak. When the chest-wall muscles are involved, the person's inhalations tend to be shallow, and expirations are forced and uncontrolled (Massery, 1991). *Athetoid* CP is characterized by the presence of involuntary movements that interfere with normal voluntary movements. This condition is more likely to result in irregular and uncontrolled breathing, with involuntary bursts of air during inhalation and/or exhalation. These sudden movements are probably due to abnormal involuntary movements of the chest wall (Solomon & Charron, 1998). With *ataxic* CP, the person lacks coordination, resulting in irregular rate, rhythm, and depth of tidal breathing.

> Children with cerebral palsy typically have reduced vital capacities and find it difficult to access their inspiratory and expiratory reserve volumes because of their weak and/or spastic muscles.

All the parameters of respiratory function (pressure, flow, volume, and chest-wall shape) may be affected in children (and adults) with CP. Pressures and volumes may be lower than normal. In fact, children with CP have smaller than normal vital capacities. Also, because such children have weak muscles, they have difficulty in using their respiratory muscles to access ERV (that portion of the lung volume below REL). Use of this air requires activation of the expiratory muscles. Often these speakers have difficulty going above TV into the IRV because of difficulty in using the inspiratory muscles. Thus, these children are not able to pull air into or force air out of the lungs voluntarily as well or as much as able-bodied children (Solomon & Charron, 1998). Another by-product of this weakness is that these children often have to use a much larger proportion of their already reduced VCs for speech. In addition, children with CP may valve the airstream inefficiently at any location of the vocal tract, including the larynx, velopharynx, or other articulators. This wastes air, so airflows are typically abnormally high during speech.

The shape of the chest wall is an extremely important variable in treating children with CP. The most efficient position of the chest wall for speech is one in which the abdomen is smaller and the rib cage larger than during relaxation. Deformities of the chest wall are common in children with CP (Davis, 1987). This is likely due to hypertonic and/or weak muscles, as well as to postural problems. For instance, children with spastic CP spend a lot of time in a flexed position. This causes breathing that actually gets worse as they develop, along with deterioration in vocal quality and loudness (Workinger & Kent, 1991). The child's attempts to compensate for the abnormal tone might also contribute to the increasing difficulty in breathing for speech. On the other hand, children with athetoid CP become more posturally stable as they mature, and their speech may become more intelligible.

Strengthening the muscles of the chest wall may improve a child's ability to generate greater P_{trach} and a correspondingly louder voice (Solomon & Charron, 1998). Strengthening the respiratory muscles can also help to increase VC and to improve endurance for breathing. The child may then be able to produce more syllables on one breath and to talk for longer periods of time. This was demonstrated by Cerny, Panzarella, and Stathopoulos (1997), who used a muscle-conditioning protocol in which children with low muscle tone wore a face mask that provided resistance against the outgoing breath stream. They wore the mask for 15 minutes each day, 5 days a week, for 6 weeks. Even though speech itself was never targeted during training, the children showed increases in P_{trach} and vocal loudness during both normal and loud speech, demonstrating the efficiency of working on the underlying respiratory difficulty.

Treating respiratory function in children with cerebral palsy involves strengthening the respiratory muscles and improving postural support.

Other respiratory exercises are designed to improve speech breathing coordination. A child can be taught to inspire quickly and deeply and to exhale in a slow and controlled manner while speaking. This technique is called inspiratory checking, because the deep inhalation results in increased lung volume and greater pressures available for speech. To control the expiration, the child must use his or her inspiratory muscles to counteract the passive recoil forces at high volumes (Netsell & Hixon, 1992). Other techniques are used to focus only on inspiration or on expiration (e.g., sniffing and blowing exercises) or on switching voluntarily between the two (Solomon & Charron, 1998).

Improving postural support can be very helpful in treating respiratory function. When children with CP have an individually adjusted seating system that changes the positioning of their body in ways that improve posture, VC can be increased and children can exhale for longer amounts of time. Boliek (1997) described the respiratory function of Katie, a preschooler who was born prematurely and who had spastic CP and respiratory problems. When she was unsupported, Katie began phonation below REL and her voice sounded breathy and strained. With appropriate support, she began speaking at higher lung volumes and ended her utterances at or above REL, which is more similar to able-bodied children. Thus, proper support can maximize respiratory capacity for speech.

Another important way of improving posture and respiration for speech is by abdominal trussing. Corsets, braces, wraps, and belts can be used to push the individual's abdomen inward, forcing the diaphragm upward and lifting the rib cage. This makes exhalation more efficient, so lung volume, maximum inspiratory and expiratory pressures, maximum flow, and maximum phonation time all increase, according to Watson (1997). Watson also found an added advantage in that, because individuals could speak for a longer time with trussing, they were able to pause at more linguistically appropriate places, thus increasing the fluency of their speech.

Mechanical Ventilation

Problems with speaking while mechanically ventilated include inability to control the timing of ventilator cycles and dealing with abnormally high tracheal pressures.

Understanding respiratory patterns in speech production has become important in the treatment of individuals who, because of various disorders, such as CP, cervical spinal cord injury, asthma, emphysema, and head or neck cancer, are dependent on a mechanical respirator to breathe. The person is attached to a ventilator by a tube called a *cannula* that fits tightly into a *stoma* (hole) in his or her neck, leading to the trachea. The ventilator has an inspiratory phase, during which air is pumped into the person's respiratory system. In this phase, P_{trach} increases because of the increase in the density of the air within the trachea. Exhalation occurs as the individual's thorax and lungs recoil, forcing the pumped air out of the system. P_{trach} decreases during exhalation.

In some cases, if the patient's ventilatory function is greatly compromised, no air is allowed to flow into the upper airway, but is directed fully into the trachea. However, some individuals are able to speak using the air from the ventilator. In this case, a small portion of the air that is pumped into the trachea is allowed to flow upward through the larynx and vocal tract so that it can be used to power speech.

Although some people who are mechanically ventilated are able to speak, they often have difficulties in doing so. Several problems exist. First, the individual may be unable to control the timing of ventilator cycles. Second, the tracheal pressures generated by the ventilator are abnormally high and change rapidly. Third, these individuals must balance the aeromechanical requirements of speech production with the body's air exchange needs (Hoit, Shea, & Banzett, 1994).

Differences in speech breathing behavior have been found between normal speech and ventilator-dependent speech. For example, Hoit et al. (1994) reported that the tidal volumes of most ventilator-dependent subjects were as much as three times larger than those of normal subjects. Normal TV is around 500 cc. The subjects studied by Hoit et al. (1994) had TVs ranging from 700 to 1470 cc. Marvin, however, reported that ventilator TV is typically closer to normal values in subacute care ventilator patients (2000, personal communication). Hoit et al. (1994) also found differences in P_{trach}, which for these ventilator-dependent patients ranged from 13.9 to 26 cm H_2O, whereas the P_{trach} needed for speech in healthy subjects is around 5 to 10 cm H_2O. Another difference was that, rather than producing speech on an exhalation, the ventilator-dependent patients began to speak as P_{trach} rose during inspiration and stopped as P_{trach} fell during expiration. These patients usually began speaking 0.3 to 0.7 second(s) after the onset of inspiration and stopped speaking around 0.7 to 1.1 s after the inspiratory flow ceased. Hoit, Hixon, Watson, and Morgan (1990) found that the time at which the individual stopped speaking was usually influenced by the linguistic structure of the utterance. However, sometimes these patients stopped speaking when P_{trach} dropped below about 2 cm H_2O. For the most part, individuals did not take advantage of the full speaking time available to them. Average speaking duration ranged from 59 to 81 percent of the patient's potential speaking time. Therefore, speakers produced a smaller than normal number of syllables per breath.

Based on these findings, the authors suggested that a promising strategy for maximizing speech duration is to encourage the patient to continue speaking as far into the expiratory portion of the cycle as possible, until voicing begins to fade with the falling P_{trach}. However, although this strategy can increase speaking time, it might also result in frequent linguistically inappropriate breaks in the speaker's discourse. Hoit et al. (1990) suggested that these breaks may actually be beneficial, because they signal the listener that the speaker plans to continue talking.

Patients with certain disorders, such as cervical spinal cord injury, who require mechanical ventilation are often good candidates for placement of a speaking valve, such as the Passy-Muir valve. This is a one-way valve that fits into the stoma in the patient's neck. When the patient wants to speak, the valve can be closed using positive pressure generated in the trachea. The air is therefore prevented from exiting the trachea and consequently is exhaled through the larynx. This allows the patient to use the larynx to generate voice.

Voice Disorders

Much less information is available about respiratory function in voice disorders than in neurological disorders. Nevertheless, respiratory parameters are often the focus of treatment for various voice disorders. For example, by focusing on

---

Tracheal pressures reported for mechanically ventilated individuals range from around 14 to 26 cm H_2O.

Ventilator-dependent patients have been found to begin speech during the inspiratory cycle and stop speaking during the expiratory cycle.

breathing, tensions that are generalized throughout the chest, as well as the larynx and vocal tract, can be reduced (Colton & Casper, 1996). The systems involved in speech are closely intertwined, and tensions in one system affect the other systems. Colton and Casper (1996) suggested that reducing tension in the respiratory muscles helps to assure continuous airflow from inspiration through expiration, and this in turn helps to reduce laryngeal tension.

Stemple (1997) proposed that voice therapy should take a holistic approach to integrating respiration and phonation. He noted that many techniques used commonly in voice therapy are based on modifying air pressures and flows. For instance, the *pushing technique* is often used to help patients with a paralyzed vocal fold to close the vocal folds more strongly and thereby to prevent too much air from flowing through the larynx and being wasted. The *yawn-sigh technique,* on the other hand, is designed to help individuals who use a hyperfunctional voice and close their vocal folds too tightly to generate an easier flow of air. Other procedures are designed to eliminate *clavicular* breathing, in which the person raises his or her shoulders on inspiration, which produces strain in the neck and laryngeal areas.

> Many techniques used to treat patients with voice disorders, such as the pushing technique and the yawn-sigh technique, are based on modifying air pressures and airflows.

Hyperfunctional voice production is often associated with higher P_{trach}, indicating increased respiratory effort. Hyperfunctional voice disorders have been described as being associated with shallow breathing, poor coordination of expiration and phonation, and a clavicular breathing pattern, as well as disrupted inspiratory and expiratory cycles of tidal volume breathing. Some patients with hyperfunctional voice disorders complain of a loss of breath and respiratory fatigue during voice production, according to Sapienza and Stathopoulos (1995). They reported that children with nodules used greater amounts of air for speech than children with normal voice, as demonstrated by the higher lung volume initiation and lower lung volume termination for utterances. This may have been a compensatory response to the nodules, because nodules prevent the vocal folds from closing properly, allowing air to leak out. Therefore, the individual needs more volume in order to maintain enough pressure during speech. Clinically, it would be more efficient for the person to initiate the speech utterance at a higher percentage of the lung capacity, and he or she could then also end the utterance above REL, which would lessen the strain on the respiratory and laryngeal muscles (Sapienza, Stathopoulos, & Brown, 1997).

Hearing Impairment

People who are deaf or hard of hearing often seem to have trouble in controlling the airstream for speech. The respiratory system itself does not appear to be deviant, but coordinating the breath stream with articulation and voicing

People who are deaf or hard of hearing sometimes have difficulty coordinating the expiratory airflow for speech with articulation and voicing.

poses a problem. For instance, deaf speakers have been shown to begin exhaling for speech at volumes well below normal. Also, deaf subjects often expend too much air. For example, some deaf speakers use 180 cc per syllable, and end their utterances around 500 cc below FRC (Whitehead, 1983). Speakers who take in too little air, use too low an operating point in the dynamic range of respiration, and waste air in breathy voice are forced to pause more often for breath, often at syntactically inappropriate places (Lane, Perkell, Suirsky, & Webster, 1991).

Recent advances in hearing technology, such as cochlear implants, have helped children and adults to increase their sensitivity to auditory stimuli. Interestingly, once auditory sensitivity is heightened, coordinating respiration with the other speech systems seems to improve. For example, Lane et al. (1991) examined speech breathing in three adults before and after each had a cochlear implant. Once the speakers received auditory input from the implant, in every case they modified their speech breathing in a more normal direction. The authors reported, for example, changes in average airflow, in the volume of air expended per syllable, and in speech termination levels. Table 5.1 summarizes the respiratory parameters that may be affected in different disorders.

Clinical Study

Background

Mr. Stevens is a 78-year-old man who was diagnosed with Parkinson's disease five years ago. He was referred by his neurologist to your outpatient rehabilitation center for a speech evaluation and possible treatment. Family members, including Mrs. Stevens and their three adult children, have complained about difficulty in understanding him. Mrs. Stevens reports that his voice is extremely soft, that he sounds "breathless," and that he "mumbles." The children all live out of state and communicate mostly with their parents through phone calls, since their parents do not own a computer. Of late, Mrs. Stevens is finding it more and more difficult to get her husband to talk to the children on the phone. She's hoping that speech therapy will improve his ability to communicate.

Clinical Observations

Upon meeting Mr. Stevens, you are struck by his stooped posture, and you note that his head hangs forward, both when standing and sitting. As his wife indicated, his speech intelligibility is reduced due to low intensity, lack of normal prosody, and slurred speech.

Acoustic Measures

Using a handheld spirometer, you obtain Mr. Stevens's vital capacity both in his typical stooped posture and with postural support that helps to improve the alignment between his head and chest. In addition, you have Mr. Stevens sustain the /a/ vowel for as long as possible, in order to determine his maximum phonation time, which is a measure of available breath support for speech purposes. This activity is also done under the two conditions of his stooped and improved posture. Spirometric measurements under the stooped postural condition indicate a VC of 2800 ml, compared to the norm of 4470 ml for his age group. When provided with postural support, his VC improved to 3500 ml. Maximum phonation time also improved from 3.5 seconds with extremely breathy voice to 9 seconds with a stronger voice quality.

Clinical Questions

1. How can this diagnostic information be used to set treatment goals for this patient?
2. What other respiratory measurements might be helpful in the diagnosis and treatment of this patient?
3. Suggest two treatment goals that would be appropriate for Mr. Stevens, based on the above information.

summary

- Two general principles apply in the clinical management of respiratory function: First, the patient's static and dynamic respiratory ability must be measured; second, the treatment must be tailored to the patient's specific breathing difficulty.
- Patients with Parkinson's disease may have a different chest wall shape than normal because of the rigidity of the chest wall muscles.
- Patients with cervical spinal cord injury may not be able to breathe on their own and may need mechanical ventilation; if the person can breathe, he or she may have difficulty generating adequate pressures and flows for speech.
- Many children and adults with cerebral palsy face problems with respiratory function affecting pressure, flow, volume, and shape.
- Several problems exist in speaking on a mechanical ventilator, including the abnormally high tracheal pressures generated and rapidly changing pressures.
- Subtle problems in respiratory function may occur in some voice disorders and in hearing impairment.

1. Do you agree or disagree with the suggestion that, if a patient can sustain a steady stream of subglottal air pressure of 5 cm H_2O for 5 seconds, the respiratory system may be sufficient to support speech? Provide a detailed rationale for your answer.

2. How does the rigidity that is a hallmark of Parkinson's disease affect respiratory and speech production?

3. Make a table of similarities and differences in respiratory function in patients with cerebellar disease and in those with cervical spinal cord injury.

4. Compare respiratory function in spastic, athetoid, and ataxic cerebral palsy.

5. Identify two problems in respiratory and speech function in individuals who are mechanically ventilated.

6. Explain why some behavioral techniques used in voice therapy are based on modifying respiratory function.

The Phonatory System

After reading this chapter, you will

1. Be familiar with the structures of the larynx and the myoelastic-aerodynamic theory of phonation.
2. Understand the complex, nearly periodic sound wave of the human voice.
3. Be able to explain the sources and measurement of jitter and shimmer.
4. Appreciate the physiologic and acoustic bases of vocal registers.
5. Be able to describe differences between normal and abnormal voice qualities.
6. Become acquainted with measures of voice quality such as harmonics-to-noise ratio and electroglottography.

The phonatory system is comprised of the larynx. This small organ is the means by which air provided by the respiratory system is converted into sound through an extraordinarily complex process. The process involves air pressures and flows and the muscular and elastic properties of the vocal folds that are housed in the larynx. To gain an appreciation of the process of the air-to-sound conversion, it is imperative to be familiar with the structure of the larynx and vocal folds and the way in which the structures operate.

The Vocal Mechanism

The vocal mechanism includes the laryngeal skeleton plus joints, three pairs of folds, and extrinsic and intrinsic muscles.

Laryngeal Skeleton

The laryngeal skeleton is made up of one bone and nine cartilages. Three of the cartilages are unpaired and six are paired. The unpaired cartilages are the thyroid, cricoid, and epiglottis; the paired cartilages include arytenoids, corniculates, and cuneiforms. The cartilaginous framework of the larynx is suspended from the hyoid bone (Figure 6.1).

Bones and Cartilages   The **hyoid bone** is a small U-shaped bone that forms the attachment for the tongue. The larynx is suspended from this bone by a sheet of membrane, the **hyothyroid membrane**. The hyoid bone consists of the body in the front and the major horns forming the long sides of the U. Projecting slightly upward from each major horn is a small protrusion, the minor horn.

The larynx is suspended from the hyoid bone by the hyothyroid membrane.

Inferior to the hyoid bone is the **thyroid cartilage**, which is the largest cartilage of the larynx. This structure is formed by two laminae, or plates of cartilage, that are fused in the front. The fusion of these plates occurs at an angle, which is more acute in men than in women. This protrusion is known as the Adam's apple and, because of the different angles, it is generally more prominent in men than in women. A small, V-shaped notch, the *thyroid notch*, is apparent at the top surface of the laryngeal protrusion. Two long projections, the *superior horns*, one at either side of the thyroid, extend upward and connect by means of ligaments to the hyoid bone. Two shorter projections, the *inferior horns*, extend downward and articulate with the sides of the cricoid cartilage. The posterior portion of the thyroid is open. The vocal folds are attached to the inner surface of the thyroid, just below the thyroid notch, at a fibrous structure, the **anterior commissure**.

The anterior commissure of the thyroid cartilage forms the anterior attachment for the vocal folds.

The second unpaired cartilage, the **cricoid** (Latin for *signet ring*) is so called because of its shape, being narrow in the front (the arch) and flaring to a larger, squarish plate in the back. The shape of this posterior plate explains its name, the *quadrate lamina*. The cricoid is a complete ring of cartilage located inferior to the thyroid, just above the first ring of the trachea. A sheet of membrane, the **cricotracheal membrane**, runs between the inferior margin of the cricoid and the superior margin of the first tracheal ring.

The third unpaired cartilage, the **epiglottis**, is a broad cartilage shaped rather like an oak leaf. It is attached to the inner surface of the thyroid cartilage, just below the thyroid notch, by the *thyroepiglottic ligament* and attaches to the

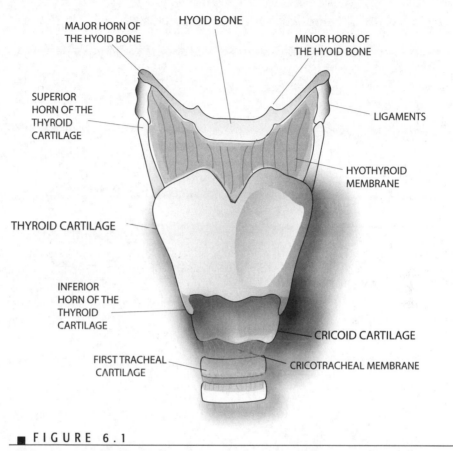

MAJOR HORN OF
THE HYOID BONE

HYOID BONE

MINOR HORN OF
THE HYOID BONE

SUPERIOR
HORN OF THE
THYROID
CARTILAGE

LIGAMENTS

HYOTHYROID
MEMBRANE

THYROID CARTILAGE

INFERIOR
HORN OF THE
THYROID
CARTILAGE

CRICOID CARTILAGE

FIRST TRACHEAL
CARTILAGE

CRICOTRACHEAL MEMBRANE

■ F I G U R E   6 . 1

Anterior view of the larynx and trachea.

body of the hyoid bone by way of the *hyoepiglottic ligament*. The epiglottis performs an important function during swallowing by folding downward over the entrance to the larynx and acting as a bridge to direct food and liquids to the esophagus. It is less important, however, in the production of voice.

The paired **arytenoid cartilages** are small structures located on the superior surface of the quadrate lamina of the cricoid. They are pyramidal in shape, being broad and flattish at their base and extending upward to more of a point at their apex. Two projections extend from their base. The first, the elastic **vocal process**, projects anteriorly toward the thyroid cartilage. The second projection, the **muscular process**, projects laterally and posteriorly. The arytenoids play a crucial role in phonation, because the vocal folds are attached to the vocal processes. Various muscles of the larynx attach to the muscular processes and move the arytenoids, allowing the attached vocal folds to be opened and closed.

Figures 6.2 through 6.4 show various views of the cartilages of the larynx.

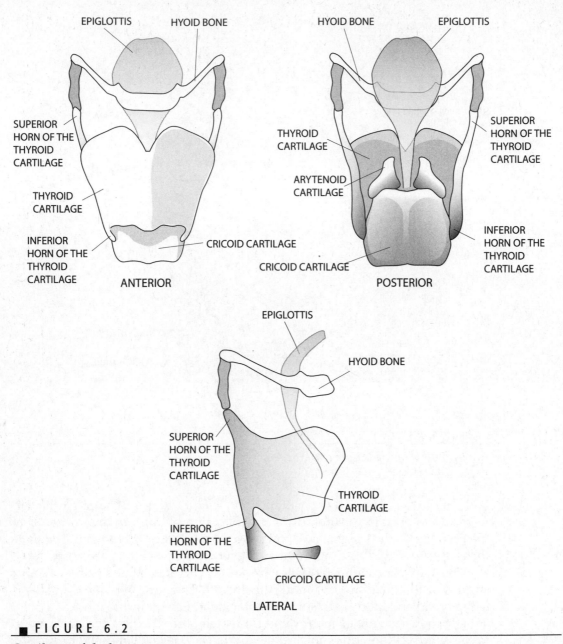

■ FIGURE 6.2

Cartilages of the larynx.

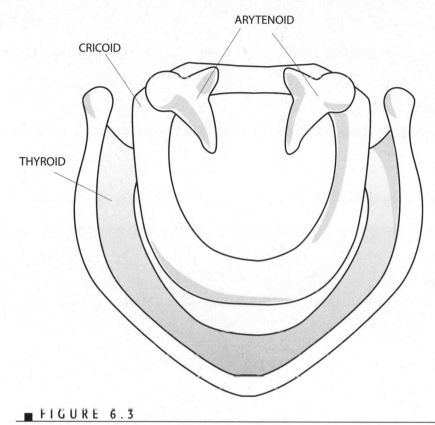

CRICOID

ARYTENOID

THYROID

■ FIGURE 6.3

Superior view of laryngeal cartilages.

There are several cartilages that do not appear to play an important role in voice production. The paired **corniculate cartilages** are located at the apex of the arytenoids, but may not be present in all individuals. The paired **cuneiform cartilages** are small, elastic rods of cartilage, embedded within the **aryepiglottic folds**. Their primary function may be to stiffen these folds. The structures of the laryngeal skeleton are described in Table 6.1.

Joints of the Larynx   There are two pairs of joints in the larynx, both of which are crucial in the production of a normal voice. The **cricoarytenoid joints** are formed by the articulation between the base of each arytenoid and the superior surface of the quadrate lamina of the cricoid. The joints are *diarthrodial*, allowing a wide range of motion of the arytenoids, which can glide medially and laterally, as well

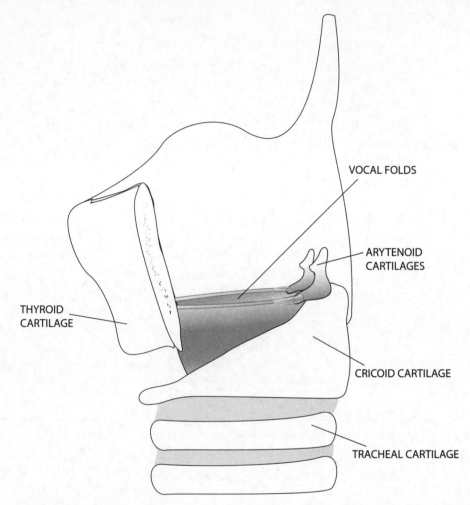

VOCAL FOLDS

ARYTENOID
CARTILAGES

THYROID
CARTILAGE

CRICOID CARTILAGE

TRACHEAL CARTILAGE

■ FIGURE 6.4

Cutaway of thyroid cartilage showing vocal folds and relationship between tracheal, arytenoid, and cricoid cartilages.

as move backward and forward in a rocking motion. Since the vocal folds are connected to the vocal processes of the arytenoids, any movement of the arytenoids affects the positioning of the vocal folds. When certain laryngeal muscles that are attached to the muscular processes contract, the muscular processes move anterolaterally, bringing the vocal processes to the midline. The attached vocal folds are therefore closed (adducted). Conversely, when the muscular processes are pulled posteriorly, the vocal processes and the attached vocal folds are separated (abducted). Thus, the cricoarytenoid joints are instrumental in vocal fold opening and closing.

The posterior portion of the vocal folds attach to the vocal processes of the arytenoid cartilages.

■ TABLE 6.1

Structures of the Laryngeal Skeleton

BONE	
Hyoid	Attachment for tongue; larynx suspended from it by means of the hyothyroid membrane.

UNPAIRED CARTILAGES	
Cricoid	Complete ring of cartilage; most inferior portion of larynx; connects to trachea by cricotracheal membrane.
Epiglottis	Elastic, leaf-shaped cartilage attached to hyoid and thyroid; folds downward to close entrance to larynx.
Thyroid	Largest cartilage; articulates with cricoid; vocal folds attach to anterior commissure.

PAIRED CARTILAGES	
Arytenoids	Located on superior aspect of quadrate lamina of cricoid; vocal folds attach to vocal processes; laryngeal muscles attach to muscular processes.
Corniculates	Located at apex of arytenoids.
Cuneiforms	Elastic rods of cartilage embedded within the aryepiglottic folds.

JOINTS	
Cricoarytenoid	Between base of arytenoids and superior surface of quadrate lamina; involved in adduction and abduction of vocal folds.
Cricothyroid	Between inferior horns of thyroid and lateral aspect of cricoid; involved in F_0 regulation by elongating and shortening vocal folds.

The **cricothyroid joints** are located between each inferior horn of the thyroid and the sides of the cricoid cartilage. These joints allow the thyroid cartilage to tilt downward toward the arch of the cricoid or the cricoid cartilage to tilt upward so that the arch comes closer to the thyroid. When either the cricoid or thyroid moves in this way, the distance between the arytenoid cartilages in the back and the thyroid cartilage in front increases. Because the vocal folds are attached to the vocal processes of the arytenoids posteriorly and to the anterior commissure of the thyroid anteriorly, increasing the distance between these two points has the effect of stretching the vocal folds, making them more tense and thin. When the vocal folds are elongated, stretched, and tense, they vibrate more rapidly, resulting in a higher F_0 and in the perception of a higher pitch. The cricothyroid joints, then, are the main agents of F_0 regulation in the human voice.

> The cricoarytenoid and cricothyroid joints permit the vocal folds to be opened, closed, tensed, and relaxed.

Valves within the Larynx

The larynx is essentially a hollow tube with three sets of valves inside it that open and close to perform various functions. The valves are made of bundles of connective tissues and muscle fibers called folds and are arranged from superior to inferior within the larynx. They include the *aryepiglottic folds*, the **false** (or ventricular) **vocal folds**, and the **true vocal folds**. Figure 6.5 shows the positions of the false and true vocal folds.

Aryepiglottic Folds   The most superior of the folds, the aryepiglottic folds, run from the sides of the epiglottis to the apex of each arytenoid cartilage. They are sheets of connective tissue and some muscle fibers that contract in a circular or sphincteric action to pull the epiglottis backward and to close the entrance of the larynx during swallowing.

The larynx contains three sets of folds located from superior to inferior: the aryepiglottic, the ventricular (false), and the true vocal folds.

False Vocal Folds   The false or ventricular folds lie inferior to the aryepiglottic folds and just superior and parallel to the true vocal folds. They are not as richly supplied with muscles as are the true folds and are only capable of limited movement. They close during swallowing, during effortful activities such as lifting heavy objects, and during natural functions such as excretion or childbirth. They normally remain

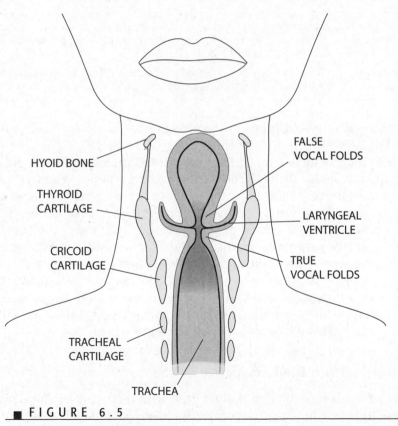

HYOID BONE

THYROID
CARTILAGE

CRICOID
CARTILAGE

TRACHEAL
CARTILAGE

TRACHEA

FALSE
VOCAL FOLDS

LARYNGEAL
VENTRICLE

TRUE
VOCAL FOLDS

■ F I G U R E   6 . 5

Coronal view of the larynx.

open during phonation, closing only under pathological conditions. Separating the false from the true vocal folds is a small space, the **laryngeal ventricle**. This space contains glands that secrete mucus, keeping the larynx moist and lubricated.

True Vocal Folds   The true vocal folds are the most complex of the laryngeal valves. Only within the past two decades have the extraordinary nature and degree of their complexity been determined, thanks primarily to the work of a Japanese otolaryngologist and voice scientist, M. Hirano, and his colleagues. The vocal folds consist of five layers, including the thyroarytenoid muscle, three layers of mucous membrane surrounding the muscle, and a layer of epithelium covering the mucous membrane. Hirano and others' research using highly sophisticated technology such as electron microscopy has revealed the differing cellular compositions and the different mechanical properties of these layers. The outermost layer of the vocal folds is the epithelium, an extremely thin but tough layer of tissue. A basement membrane connects the epithelium to the underlying layer. Deep to the epithelium and basement membrane is the mucous membrane, called the **lamina propria**, which itself is composed of three layers. The superficial layer of the lamina propria, also known as Reinke's space, is made mostly of elastic fibers, giving it a high degree of pliability. The intermediate layer of the lamina propria is also composed of elastic fibers, but is more dense and less flexible than the superficial layer. The third layer of the lamina propria, the deep layer, is made up chiefly of collagen fibers and is less flexible than the intermediate layer. The final structure that makes up the vocal folds is the **thyroarytenoid muscle**. This is the main mass of the vocal folds and is considerably thicker and denser than the other layers. Figure 6.6 provides a cross-sectional view of the vocal folds.

The true vocal folds consist of five layers: the epithelium, the three-layered lamina propria (superficial, intermediate, deep), and the vocalis muscle

Cover-Body Model   The five layers of the vocal folds have been classified by Hirano and his colleagues on the basis of the differing degrees of stiffness of the layers. **Stiffness** refers to the resistance of a structure to being displaced. The opposite of stiffness is **compliance**, which refers to the ease with which a body can be displaced. Hirano's model of the vocal folds is known as the **cover-body model**. The *cover* consists of the epithelium and the superficial layer of the lamina propria. The transition, or **vocal ligament**, encompasses the intermediate and deep layers of the lamina propria. The thyroarytenoid muscle forms the *body* of the vocal folds. Each layer has its own mode of vibration, depending on its structural composition and stiffness properties. Clearly, the vocal folds are a multilayered and extremely complex vibrator. This structural complexity gives rise to a sound wave that is acoustically complex and that results, in turn, in a rich and resonant human voice.

The cover-body model groups the vocal folds into three layers based on degree of stiffness: The cover is the least stiff, the vocal ligament is more stiff, and the body has the greatest degree of stiffness.

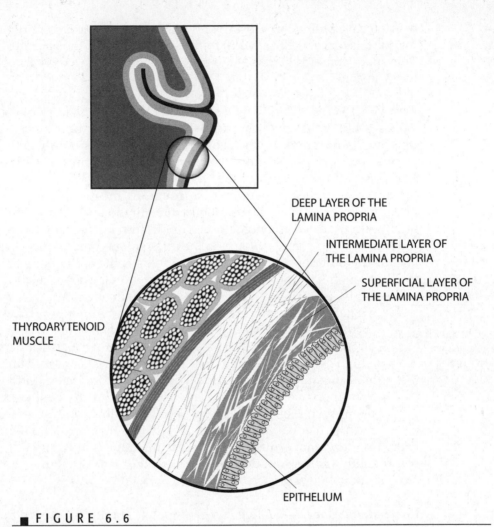

DEEP LAYER OF THE
LAMINA PROPRIA

INTERMEDIATE LAYER OF
THE LAMINA PROPRIA

SUPERFICIAL LAYER OF
THE LAMINA PROPRIA

THYROARYTENOID
MUSCLE

EPITHELIUM

■ **F I G U R E 6 . 6**

Cross-sectional view of layers of the vocal folds.

The membranous
glottis is bounded by
the vocal ligament and
forms the anterior three-
fifths of the entire
glottis; the cartilaginous
glottis is bounded by
the vocal processes
and accounts for the
posterior two-fifths.

Glottis   The space between the true vocal folds is the **glottis**, divided
into the **membranous glottis** and the **cartilaginous glottis**. The membranous glottis, which forms the anterior three-fifths of the entire length
of the glottis, is bounded by the vocal ligament on either side. The vocal
processes form the lateral edges of the cartilaginous glottis, which accounts for the posterior two-fifths of the glottis. The membranous glottis is around 15 mm in adult males and 12 mm in adult females. The
cartilaginous glottis varies from about 4 to 8 mm in length, depending
on the person's sex, age, and build. Children's vocal folds are much

shorter. The shape of the glottis varies, depending on the positioning of the vocal folds.

For quiet breathing, the glottis is open, but not to its greatest extent. The vocal folds are in a paramedian position. The glottis opens more widely when one needs to inhale greater amounts of air, for example, during vigorous exercise. This position is known as forced abduction. For phonation the glottis is closed, with the vocal folds in the median position. Whispering is produced with the membranous glottis closed and the cartilaginous glottis open. See Figure 6.7.

Muscles of the Larynx

The muscles of the larynx are divided into extrinsic and intrinsic groups.

Extrinsic Muscles   The **extrinsic muscles**, also known as the *strap muscles*, are those that have one point of attachment to the larynx, either at the hyoid bone

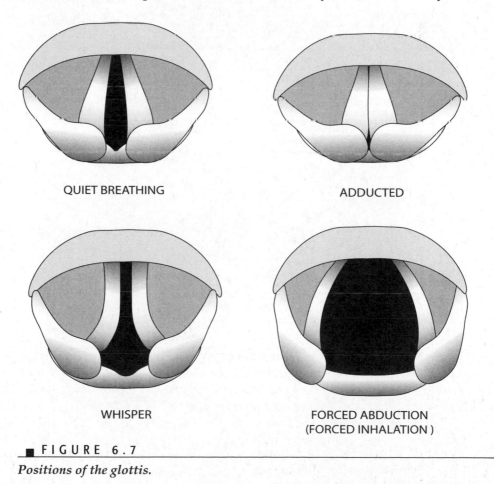

QUIET BREATHING   ADDUCTED

WHISPER   FORCED ABDUCTION (FORCED INHALATION)

■ FIGURE 6.7

Positions of the glottis.

The extrinsic laryngeal muscles are divided into infrahyoid and suprahyoid groups and anchor the larynx in the neck.

or another laryngeal cartilage, and the other point of attachment to a structure outside the larynx, such as the sternum or the cranium. The extrinsic muscles form a network that surrounds the larynx and anchors it in position. The extrinsic muscles, in turn, are subdivided into the **infrahyoid** and the **suprahyoid muscles**.

The infrahyoids have their external point of attachment at structures below the hyoid bone, including the sternum and scapula; the suprahyoids have one point of attachment to structures located above the hyoid bone, including the mandible and temporal bone. The infrahyoids, when they contract, pull the entire larynx downward. Contraction of the suprahyoids pulls the entire larynx upward in the neck. These large up and down movements of the larynx occur mainly during swallowing. Figure 6.8

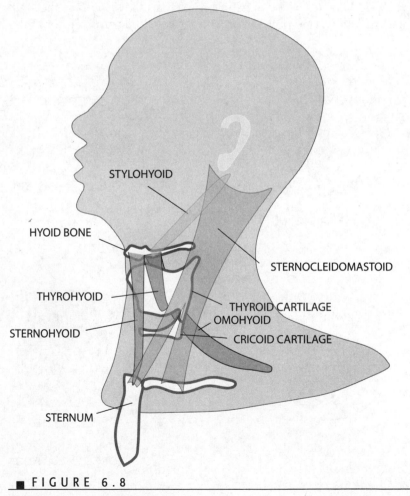

■ **F I G U R E   6 . 8**

Extrinsic muscles of the larynx.

■ TABLE 6.2

Extrinsic Muscles of the Larynx

SUPRAHYOIDS	INFRAHYOIDS
Anterior and posterior digastric	Sternohyoid
Stylohyoid	Omohyoid
Mylohyoid	Sternothyroid
Geniohyoid	Thyrohyoid
Hyoglossus	

shows some of the extrinsic muscles of the larynx. The muscles are listed in Table 6.2.

Intrinsic Muscles   There are five intrinsic muscles of the larynx. These muscles have both their origin and insertion within the larynx itself. Two of the five muscles function to adduct the vocal folds, one muscle is the vocal fold abductor, one elongates and tenses the folds, and one forms the main body of the vocal folds. The intrinsic muscles of the larynx are shown in Figure 6.9.

The first adductor is a paired muscle, the **lateral cricoarytenoid** (LCA). This muscle arises from the lateral border of the cricoid and inserts into the muscular process of the arytenoids. When it contracts, it pulls the muscular process in an anterior and medial direction. This has the effect of pulling the vocal processes toward each other in an inward and downward movement. The vocal folds, attached to the vocal processes, are also brought toward each other, closing the membranous glottis.

> The lateral cricoarytenoid muscle is one of two vocal fold adductors and closes the membranous glottis.

The **interarytenoid** (IA) **muscle** is the second adductor. This is an unpaired muscle consisting of two bundles of muscle fibers: the *transverse* portion, which runs horizontally across the posterior portions of the two arytenoid cartilages, and the *oblique* portion, whose fibers run from the base of one arytenoid to the apex of the other arytenoid, and vice versa. This arrangement of fibers forms a cross between the posterior surface of the arytenoids. When the interarytenoid muscle contracts, it glides the arytenoid cartilages medially toward each other, closing the posterior portion of the glottis.

> The interarytenoid muscle consists of the transverse and oblique portions and acts to close the cartilaginous glottis.

The paired **posterior cricoarytenoid** (PCA) **muscle** is the only one that opens the vocal folds. The PCA is a large, fan-shaped muscle that originates on the posterior aspect of the cricoid cartilage and inserts into the muscular process of each arytenoid cartilage. Upon contraction, the muscular processes are rotated posteriorly, which has the effect of pulling the vocal processes away from each other and opening the vocal folds.

> The posterior cricoarytenoid muscle is the only vocal fold abductor.

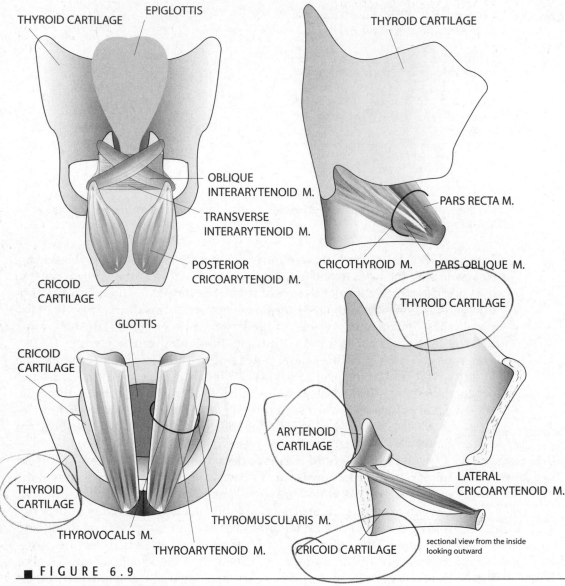

■ FIGURE 6.9

Intrinsic muscles of the larynx.

The paired **cricothyroid** (CT) **muscle** is also composed of two sets of muscle fibers. The *pars recta* portion originates at the lateral surface of the cricoid cartilage. Its fibers run at an almost upright angle to insert into the inferior border of the thyroid cartilage. The *pars oblique* portion originates at the same place as the pars recta, but its fibers run in a more angled direction and insert at the anterior surface of the inferior horn of the thyroid cartilage. This muscle

The cricothyroid muscle includes the pars recta and pars oblique and regulates vocal pitch; the thyroarytenoid muscle or vocalis forms the main body of the vocal folds.

functions as a pitch changer. When it contracts, the thyroid cartilage is tilted downward toward the cricoid, thus increasing the distance between the anterior commissure of the thyroid and the arytenoid cartilages. Because the vocal folds are attached anteriorly at the anterior commissure and posteriorly at the arytenoids, increasing the distance between these points stretches and elongates the vocal folds, decreasing their mass per unit of area and increasing the longitudinal tension placed on them. This increases their rate of vibration, resulting in a higher frequency (which may be perceived as a higher pitch).

The fifth muscle, the thyroarytenoid (TA), forms the main mass of the true vocal folds. This part of the vocal folds comprises the body in the cover-body model. The TA is a paired muscle, coursing from the anterior commissure to the arytenoids. The more lateral fibers, sometimes known as the *thyromuscularis,* insert into the muscular process of each arytenoid. The more medial fibers, sometimes referred to as the thyrovocalis, insert into each vocal process. However, this is not truly a two-part muscle like the interarytenoid, and the entire muscle, including both lateral and medial fibers, is often termed the *vocalis.* The TA is opened, closed, tensed, and relaxed by the contractions of the other intrinsic muscles. It also, however, can exert internal tension that stiffens it and helps to increase the rate of vibration of the vocal folds. The intrinsic muscles of the larynx are listed in Table 6.3.

■ **TABLE 6.3**

Intrinsic Muscles of the Larynx

MUSCLE	ATTACHMENTS	FUNCTION
Lateral cricoarytenoid	Lateral cricoid to muscular process of arytenoid	Adduct vocal folds
Interarytenoid		
Transverse	Lateral margin of one arytenoid to lateral margin of other arytenoid posteriorly	Adduct vocal folds
Oblique	Base of one arytenoid to apex of other arytenoid posteriorly	Adduct vocal folds
Posterior cricoarytenoid	Posterior cricoid to muscular process of arytenoid	Abduct vocal folds
Cricothyroid		
Pars recta	Anterior cricoid to inferior border of thyroid	Elongate and tense vocal folds
Pars oblique	Anterior cricoid to anterior surface of inferior horn of thyroid	Elongate and tense vocal folds
Thyroarytenoid		
Muscularis	Anterior commissure to muscular process	Body of vocal folds; shorten and relax folds
Vocalis	Anterior commissure to vocal process	Body of vocal folds; tenses folds

Myoelastic-Aerodynamic Theory of Phonation

The vocal folds act as a sound generator by vibrating the air coming through the larynx from the lungs, thus setting up a sound wave in the vocal tract. The **myoelastic-aerodynamic theory of phonation**, proposed in the 1950s, is the most widely accepted model of voice production. This model describes voice production as a combination of muscle force (*myo*), tissue elasticity (*elastic*), and air pressures and flows (*aerodynamic*).

To initiate vocal fold vibration, the vocal folds must close. This is achieved by the LCA and IA muscles, which exert a force called **medial compression**. When medial compression holds the vocal folds closed at the midline, the pressure of the air beneath the folds (subglottal pressure, P_s, or tracheal pressure, P_{trach}) begins to increase. When the P_s is strong enough, it overcomes the resistance of the closed vocal folds and forces them apart. A puff of air escapes into the vocal tract, setting the air within the tract into vibration, in much the same way as the tuning fork in Chapter 2. This sound wave is then transmitted through the vocal tract, where various vocal tract valves modify the sound. Meanwhile, the vocal folds have begun to close again due to the interaction of two forces. First, once the folds have been forced apart, they begin to recoil back to the midline, due to their natural elasticity. As they begin to close, they form a narrow channel. Second, the air passing through this constriction formed by the closing vocal folds becomes negative in pressure due to the effect of the **Bernoulli principle**. According to this principle, air passing through a narrow channel increases in velocity and decreases in pressure. The decrease in pressure between the folds further helps to close them completely by pulling them toward each other. Once again, P_s begins to build up and the whole process repeats itself. One such opening and closing of the folds constitutes one cycle of vocal fold vibration. During speech, of course, the vocal folds vibrate hundreds of times per second. Note that for phonation to occur the vocal folds do not have to be completely closed, but cannot be farther apart than around 3 mm.

Medial compression is the muscular force exerted by the lateral cricoarytenoid and interarytenoid muscles to close the vocal folds.

Vertical and Longitudinal Phase Differences during Vibration Because of their layered structure, the vocal folds vibrate in an extremely complex fashion. Rather than opening and closing as a whole, the folds open from bottom to top and close from bottom to top in an undulating way. This complex vibration is due to timing differences in the way that the vocal folds open and close along both their vertical and horizontal dimensions. Vertically, as the inferior edges of the folds are beginning to close, the superior margins are still open. As the air flows upward through the glottis, creating negative pressure, the closing movement also progresses upward. While the superior margins of the folds are closing and then closed, the inferior edges are already beginning to open again as P_s

The mucosal wave is created by the slight differences in the timing of opening and closing between the top and bottom margins of the vocal folds.

builds up and forces them apart. This slight time lag between the opening and closing of the inferior and superior portions of the vocal folds is known as the **vertical phase difference**.

There is a similar timing lag between the opening and closing of the vocal folds from back to front. They open from their posterior attachment at the vocal processes to the anterior portion at the anterior commissure. They close, however, in an anterior to posterior direction. This lag in closure is called the **longitudinal phase difference**.

These timing differences give the vibration of the vocal folds an undulating, wavelike motion, which is particularly evident in the loose and pliable cover layer of the folds; this has been termed the **mucosal wave**. Figure 6.10 provides schematic representations of the opening and closing of the vocal folds.

The complex vibration of the vocal folds generates a periodic, complex sound wave, consisting, as do all such waves, of a fundamental frequency (F_0) and harmonics. The F_0 is the rate at which the vocal folds vibrate and corresponds to the perceived pitch of the voice. The undulating vibration is crucial for the production of a normal voice. Disturbance or disruption of the mucosal wave interferes with voice production and results in various types of vocal

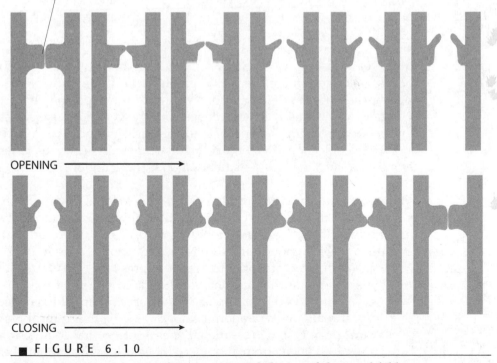

VOCAL FOLDS

OPENING ⟶

CLOSING ⟶

■ FIGURE 6.10

Schematic representation of the opening and closing of the vocal folds.

problems. The vocal folds vibrate for as long as the individual is producing a voiced sound. For a voiceless sound or to inhale, the vocal folds are opened by the PCA.

Voice Fundamental Frequency   As with any vibrator, the rate of vibration of the vocal folds depends on their length, mass and tension. The greater the length and mass and the less the tension and stiffness, the slower the vocal folds will vibrate and the lower the person's pitch, and vice versa. Vocal F_0 is determined primarily by the tension of the vocal fold cover, rather than by the actual length of the vocal folds (Kent, 1997a). We change vocal F_0 continuously during speech, depending on whether the utterance is a question or statement, on which particular words and syllables are emphasized, and so on. Children, with their small and thin vocal folds, tend to have a high frequency of vibration (around 250 to 300 Hz for boys and girls prior to puberty). Adult females have an average F_0 of 180 to 250 Hz, and adult males, with their generally longer and more massive vocal folds, range in F_0 between approximately 80 and 150 Hz.

> Vocal fundamental frequency is determined primarily by the tension of the vocal fold cover.

Voice Intensity   Intensity is controlled by regulating subglottal pressure, primarily through increasing and decreasing medial compression. When medial compression is increased, the vocal folds press together more tightly and for a longer period of time, causing the P_s to build up more strongly. Therefore, when the folds are blown apart by the P_s, they are blown apart more forcefully. Due to their elastic recoil, the vocal folds also come together again more forcefully, creating a stronger excitation of the air in the vocal tract. The sound wave that is generated, therefore, has a greater amplitude and intensity. During speech, the vocal folds continuously modify their tension characteristics to change F_0 and intensity in accordance with the verbal message. These continuously varying changes give rise to the prosody (melody) of speech, the rising and falling inflections that signal linguistic meaning (such as whether an utterance is a question or a statement), mood, and emotion.

Pressures Involved in Phonation   For the vocal folds to vibrate, the pressure below the vocal folds must be higher than that above so that air will flow through the glottis. The relative difference between the subglottal (tracheal) pressure and supraglottal pressure is the driving pressure forcing air to flow through the glottis, the **transglottal pressure**. This transglottal difference in pressure forces the vocal folds to vibrate if they are in an appropriate closed position. The minimum amount of P_s needed to set the vocal folds into vibration is known as the **phonation threshold pressure** (P_{th}). For conversational speech at normal loudness levels, this pressure ranges from about 3 cm H_2O at low fundamental frequencies to around 6 cm H_2O at high fundamental frequencies (Kent, 1997a). At

> Phonation threshold pressure refers to the minimum subglottal pressure needed to set the vocal folds into vibration.

higher F_0 the vocal folds are thinner and stiffer, so more pressure is needed to set them into vibration. For a low F_0, a P_{th} of around 3 to 4 cm H_2O corresponds to a voice amplitude level of around 45 to 65 dB SPL (Kent, 1997a). Higher pressures are needed for louder speech. Pressure for a loud yell, for example, needs to be around 50 cm H_2O.

The Complex Sound Wave of the Human Voice

The vocal folds, because of their layered structure and varying levels of stiffness, vibrate in an extremely complex and undulating manner, unlike the more rigid vibration of a tuning fork. Because the sound produced by the larynx is complex, it must share the characteristics of other complex sounds. In other words, the laryngeal tone has a fundamental frequency and harmonics, just like other periodic complex sounds. The F_0 corresponds to the perceived pitch of the voice, while the harmonics contribute to the **quality** of the voice. In acoustic terminology, quality refers to the relationship between the frequencies in a complex tone and their amplitudes. Perceptually, the term quality relates to the unique timbre or tone of a sound. People's voices can usually be distinguished by quality. For example, if you and a friend both say /a/ with the same F_0, others will still be able to distinguish between your voices. Your voices sound different, even when the pitch is perceived as the same, because the amplitudes of the harmonics in your voices are different. The same is true with musical instruments. Middle C on a piano and middle C on a violin have the same F_0. However, unless you are totally tone deaf (which very few people are), you can easily tell the difference between the two instruments; each has a uniqueness of tone, which is related to the acoustic quality of the instrument.

The relationship between the frequencies and amplitudes in a complex sound determines the quality of the sound.

Glottal Spectrum   The F_0 and harmonics of the human voice can be well visualized on a line spectrum. The spectrum of the human voice is known as the **glottal spectrum** (see Figure 6.11).

The glottal spectrum does not represent the sound of the voice you actually hear, because the sound is modified as it travels through the vocal tract and out the mouth or nose. Rather, the glottal spectrum represents the sound that you would hear if you could somehow place a microphone at the larynx, before the sound travels through the rest of the vocal tract. The glottal spectrum shows that the F_0 is the lowest frequency and has the greatest amplitude. As the harmonic frequencies increase, their amplitudes decrease in a systematic way at a rate of 12 dB per octave (an octave refers to a doubling or halving of frequency). Thus, the glottal spectrum shows a loss of 12 dB from 100 to 200 Hz, another loss of 12 dB from 200 to 400 Hz, another loss of 12 dB from 400 to 800 Hz, and so on. Because of this decrease of acoustic energy as frequency increases,

The glottal spectrum depicts the laryngeal tone, in which the fundamental frequency has the greatest amplitude and successive harmonics have decreasing amplitude levels.

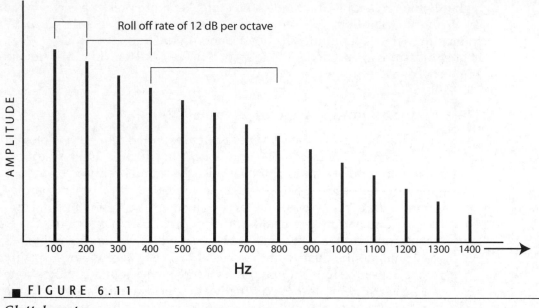

Glottal spectrum.

there is more acoustic energy in the lower frequencies of the voice and less in the higher frequencies. At the very highest frequencies, acoustic energy is miniscule. There are about 40 harmonics in the human voice that have at least some acoustic energy. Acoustic energy in the human voice has been shown to be significant up to around 4000 or 5000 Hz.

Harmonic Spacing   When we alter the pitch of our voice in conversational speech, it is the F_0 that we are manipulating by adjusting the rate of vocal fold vibration. We also change the **harmonic spacing**, which refers to the distance between the harmonic frequencies in a complex sound (see Figure 6.12). You can see why harmonic spacing changes with different F_0 if you recall that harmonics are whole-number multiples of the F_0.

If an individual has an F_0 of 100 Hz, the harmonics would be 200, 300, and 400 Hz, and so on, up to around 4000 or 5000 Hz. If this individual raises his or her pitch by increasing F_0 to, say, 200 Hz, the harmonics are now 400, 600, and 800 Hz, and so on, up to around 4000 or 5000 Hz. The spacing between the harmonic frequencies has increased from 100 to 200 Hz, and there are now fewer harmonics in the person's voice. Thus, at an F_0 of 200 Hz not only does the person's pitch sound higher, but the complexity of his or her voice has also changed. The higher the person's F_0, the wider the harmonic spacing is. This helps to explain why children's voices sound so different from adults' voices. Prepubertal children have an F_0 that is considerably higher than adults'

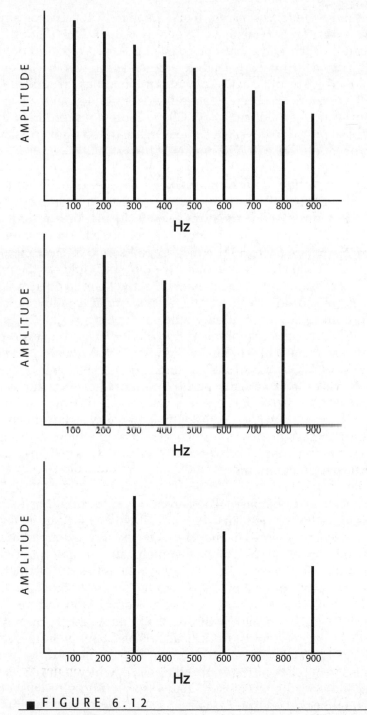

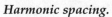 FIGURE 6.12

Harmonic spacing.

(around 300 Hz, compared to approximately 100 Hz for adult males and 200 Hz for adult females). Not only is their pitch much higher, but, because of the wider harmonic spacing, their voices do not have the rich, resonant quality of adult voices. The fewer harmonics in the child's voice result in a quality that is thinner than an adult's. This quality has historically been an advantage for child singers in church and concert choirs, such as the Vienna Boys Choir. In previous centuries, this purity of voice was so prized in boys that some were castrated (known as castrati) in order to prevent the voice from changing at puberty.

Nearly Periodic Nature of the Human Voice   Because of their tissue and mechanical characteristics, the vocal folds do not vibrate in a completely even, periodic manner. There are always small fluctuations in frequency and amplitude, resulting in an almost but not quite periodic sound. For example, you are trying to produce an /a/ sound as steadily as possible at an F_0 of 200 Hz. You are holding your vocal folds at the precise degree of tension and stiffness that will allow them to open and close 200 times per second. If your vocal folds vibrate in a totally periodic manner, each cycle of vibration would take exactly 1/200 second(s). Because the vocal folds vibrate nearly periodically, however, one cycle may last 1/200 s, the following cycle may last 1/199 s, the next cycle may last 1/203 s, and so on. This timing variability between cycles of vibration is called **frequency perturbation** or, more commonly, **jitter**.

A similar variability between cycles is also true of amplitude. If you say /a/ and try to keep your loudness level as steady as possible, despite your best intentions your vocal folds will vibrate with slightly different amplitudes for each cycle. This variability is known as **amplitude perturbation** or **shimmer**.

Sources of Jitter and Shimmer   These cycle-to-cycle variations in frequency and amplitude have been shown to be caused by many factors, including neurologic, biomechanic, aerodynamic, and acoustic. For example, the left and right vocal folds may not be exactly symmetrical, but may differ slightly in their mass and tension. Or there may be more mucus on one fold than another, causing one to have slightly more mass than the other. Variations in lung pressure can also cause perturbations in vocal fold amplitude and frequency, because P_s fluctuates slightly during the buildup and release of pressure through the vocal folds. The articulators also have an influence on vocal fold vibration. Whenever the tongue moves forward, for example, it pulls the hyoid bone forward and upward, which in turn raises the larynx. Raising the larynx can change the stiffness of the vocal folds, thereby perturbing the F_0 (Titze, 1994). Aerodynamic events can also produce fluctuations in vocal fold cycles of vibration. As the air is

---

The distance between the harmonic frequencies in a complex sound is referred to as harmonic spacing.

The human voice is not completely periodic, but has minute cycle-to-cycle changes in frequency and amplitude, called frequency and amplitude perturbation, respectively.

Frequency perturbation is often called jitter; shimmer is another name for amplitude perturbation.

Factors that contribute to jitter and shimmer include neurologic, biomechanic, aerodynamic, and acoustic.

forced through the glottis, it can become unstable and turbulent, resulting in rapid pressure fluctuations in the vocal output (Titze, 1994).

Measurement of Jitter and Shimmer   To evaluate jitter and shimmer, it is necessary to measure the period of each cycle of vocal fold vibration. Current computer technology allows what used to be an incredibly complex mathematical procedure to be achieved at the push of a button (or a click of the mouse). Many commercially available instruments and software packages measure jitter and shimmer, including the Visi-Pitch and the Computerized Speech Lab by Kay Elemetrics, a program called CSpeech developed by Milenkovic, and others.

A disadvantage is that many of these programs use different mathematical algorithms to calculate jitter and shimmer, making it difficult to compare results from different instruments. Also, the units of measurement of jitter and shimmer differ between programs. Some programs measure jitter in percentages and some use milliseconds. Some measure shimmer in percentages and some use decibels.

Problems exist with jitter measurement because cycle-to-cycle frequency variability is affected by F_0, with higher F_0 being more difficult to measure. Some algorithms that are used to calculate jitter take this factor into account and some do not. In addition, because the measurement of jitter depends on a precise determination of the period of the voice signal, it may not be valid to calculate jitter for a voice that is aperiodic.

Despite these disadvantages in jitter measurement, much has been learned about vocal function using this technique. For instance, the slight degree of cycle-to-cycle variability in vocal fold vibration is such a natural part of human voice production that too little jitter and shimmer in the voice result in a perception of unnaturalness. The work of many researchers has shown that jitter levels of around 1 percent or less are normal in the human voice.

Titze (1991b) worked out a mathematical model of jitter, manipulating various aspects of the neuromuscular function of the vocal folds, and found that the very lowest level of jitter in the human voice is around 0.2 percent. These figures accord well with much research showing that jitter values in normal voices range from around 0.2 to 1 percent. Jitter values above this level indicate that the vocal folds are vibrating in a way that is not as periodic as it should be.

Jitter values in normal voices range from around 0.2 to 1.0 percent, while shimmer values below around 0.5 dB have been estimated to be normal.

High jitter levels suggest that something is interfering with normal vocal fold vibration and the mucosal wave. On the other hand, normal speakers can actually decrease the level of jitter in their voices with practice. For example, Ferrand (1995) showed that normally speaking women decreased their jitter levels from around 0.6 percent to around 0.4 percent with practice. Jitter has also been used as an index of vocal maturation in children and as an index of vocal aging. Children have been shown to have higher jitter values than adults; elderly adults demonstrate higher jitter values than younger adults.

Shimmer has not been as thoroughly explored as has jitter, but researchers estimate that shimmer values below 0.5 dB are normal in the human voice.

Jitter and shimmer reflect, as Titze (1994) put it, the internal noises of the human body. Titze commented that if we could shrink to microscopic dimensions and travel through the human body we would see that much of the physical plant (the hydraulic, electrical, and chemical systems) exhibits complex back and forth motions. These micromovements impose fluctuations on what would otherwise be smooth and steady activity. The larynx is especially susceptible to small fluctuations in neural, vascular, respiratory, lymphatic, and other transport systems. Since most of the major lifelines of the human body pass through the neck, in close proximity to the larynx, the fluctuations leave small "footprints" in their path that become detectable in the vibratory patterns of the vocal folds.

Measuring cycle-to-cycle variability of vibration can allow us to detect changes in neuromuscular function or changes in the layers of the vocal folds that result in changes in the acoustic output, that is, the sound wave. The muscles controlling vocal fold vibration need to exert a certain degree of force to maintain a certain frequency and amplitude level. This force is generated and controlled by the nerves supplying the larynx. The more steadily these muscles can control vocal fold vibration, the more steady and periodic the acoustic signal generated, and the lower the jitter and shimmer. Problems in neuromuscular control can result in the vocal folds vibrating in a less stable manner, reflected in higher jitter and shimmer levels. Similarly, if vocal fold mass is increased, perhaps by a nodule or a cyst on the folds, not only is F_0 likely to decrease, but vibration will become less periodic and jitter and shimmer levels will increase.

Vocal Registers and Vocal Quality

Having examined the basics of how voice is produced, we are now in a position to fine-tune the discussion to encompass the different ways in which the vocal folds vibrate and the different qualities of sound that can be produced by the larynx. We all know intuitively that when we raise our pitches very high something feels different in the way that we use our vocal mechanism, and the same is true when we lower our pitch to the very bottom of our range. In fact, there are many different ways in which we can vibrate our vocal folds to create different qualities of sounds and different F_0. These qualities and the F_0 are related to vocal registers.

Vocal Registers

You may be familiar with the term **register** if you sing or play an instrument. Musically, a register refers to a particular part of the range of pitches of a voice

Vocal registers refer to a specific range of fundamental frequencies characterized by a particular mode of vocal fold vibration resulting in a particular quality.

The three most common registers in speech production are falsetto (loft), modal, and pulse (glottal fry).

or instrument. The entire range of F_0 in the human voice is enormous, from under 60 Hz in the basso voice to over 1568 Hz in the soprano voice (Zemlin, 1998). In singing, registers have been assigned particular names; thus *chest register* indicates a midrange of pitches, while *falsetto* refers to a much higher range of pitches. *Head register* is sometimes described as a mixture between chest and falsetto (Titze, 1994).

In terms of voice production, the range of F_0 is usually divided into three registers: **pulse**, **modal**, and *falsetto*. These are perceptually distinct regions of vocal quality that can be maintained over some ranges of F_0 and intensity. Pulse register refers to a range of very low F_0, which perceptually creates a creaky, popping sort of sound. Pulse is also called *vocal fry*, *glottal fry*, or *creaky voice*. Falsetto refers to a very high range of F_0, and is sometimes called *loft register*. Modal is the register most commonly used in normal conversational speech. This register is characterized by the kind of vibration described earlier in the chapter.

In modal register the vocal folds are somewhat shorter in length compared to their nonvibrating position, the cover is slack, and the body is fully involved in vibration (Titze, 1994). Table 6.4 shows some F_0 ranges associated with different registers.

A key characteristic that distinguishes registers is that each is produced by a different manner of vocal fold vibration. A particular pattern of vibration is usually confined to a certain F_0 range and, as the speaker goes beyond this range (either higher or lower), the vocal folds change their mode of vibration. This change in vibration results in a corresponding change in voice quality. Typically, this change in voice quality is abrupt and noticeable to the speaker

■ TABLE 6.4

Average Speaking Ranges for Males and Females at Five Different Registers

	MALES (Hz)	FEMALES (Hz)
Deepest range (pulse)	43–82[a]	87–165[a]
	25–80[b]	25–45[b]
Chest (modal)	98–147[a]	175–294[a]
	75–450[b]	130–520[b]
Midvoice	196–294[a]	349–587[a]
Falsetto	349–494[a]	659–988[a]
	275–620[b]	490–1130[b]
Whistle	523–698[a]	988–2093[a]

(Adapted from Baken, 1996, and Zemlin, 1998.)
Source: [a]Zemlin (1998).
　　　[b]Baken (1996).

and to his or her listeners. In fact, voice specialists and singing teachers seem to agree that a primary task in training for singing is to blend the registers by smoothing the transitions between them to the point where they are not detectable. In normal conversational speech, when the speaker reaches the upper limits of the modal range, the manner of vocal fold vibration suddenly changes and the sound shifts to the falsetto or loft register. Similarly, at the lower limits of the modal range, these adjustments in vocal fold vibration result in glottal fry or pulse register.

Physiologic and Acoustic Bases of Pulse and Falsetto Registers

High-speed photography has been used to study how the vocal folds vibrate in the pulse and falsetto (loft) registers.

Pulse   Using this technology, Zemlin (1998) showed that during pulse register the folds are tightly closed. However, their free borders seem to be lax, and subglottal air, as Zemlin (1998) put it, simply bubbles up between them. The vocal folds vibrate at a rate ranging from about 30 to 80 Hz, with an average of approximately 60 Hz. The vocal folds are closed for a much longer period during each cycle of vibration than they are in modal register. In modal register, the ratio of time that the vocal folds are closed compared to the time that they are opening and closing is approximately equal, with the closed portion lasting for about half the cycle. In pulse register the folds are closed for around 90 percent of the cycle, and opening and closing movements together account for only about 10 percent of the cycle.

> Pulse is characterized by a very low range of fundamental frequencies and a long closed phase, as well as biphasic or multiphasic closure.

Not only are the vocal folds closed for most of the cycle, but they also vibrate in a very different manner from the modal register. They go through **biphasic closure** or **multiphasic closure** in each cycle. That is, instead of just opening and closing, they open, close slightly but not all the way to the midline, open again, and then close all the way and stay closed for 90 percent of the cycle. Pulse register also differs from modal in terms of the air pressure needed to set the vocal folds into vibration. The P_s needed in modal register is approximately 5 to 10 cm H_2O, whereas that needed for pulse is only about 2 cm H_2O (Zemlin, 1998).

Acoustically, the waveform of an utterance produced in pulse register looks like what Titze (1994) called a series of wave packets. After each vocal fold closing, there is a burst of acoustic energy. This energy dies out, leaving a temporary interval during which there is no acoustic energy. This interval has been dubbed by Titze the **temporal gap**. Below about 70 Hz, the human ear seems to be able to detect these bursts of acoustic energy, followed by gaps of silence, within each glottal cycle. This is what is heard as the creaky, popping sound of pulse register. Above 70 Hz or so, a continuous sound is perceived, rather than the individual acoustic pulses and temporal gaps.

Pulse is a perfectly normal register and is used by many people at the ends of phrases and sentences. This register is an extension of the lower limits of the modal pitch range. Clinically, though, the use of pulse register becomes a problem when it is used habitually, instead of just at the very end of sentences.

Falsetto   High-speed photography has also been used to examine vocal fold vibration in falsetto. In this register the folds appear very long and stiff, very thin along the edges, and often somewhat bow shaped. This elongated shape suggests that the vocal folds are very tense, due to the extreme degree of longitudinal tension exerted by the cricothyroid muscle. The glottis is tight and narrow. The cover of the folds is lax, and the vocal ligament is tensed (Titze, 1994). The edges of the glottis vibrate during phonation, and often the vocal folds do not meet at the midline because of the extreme tension placed on them. The vocal ligament and body of the folds do not vibrate as fully as they do in modal and pulse registers, resulting in a less complex vibration.

> Falsetto is characterized by a very high range of fundamental frequencies, extremely tense vocal folds, and a less complex mode of vibration resulting in a thin quality.

Because of both the high speed of vibration and the less complex manner of vibration of the vocal folds during falsetto, the quality of the tone is almost flutelike (Zemlin, 1998). When the F_0 is very high, the harmonics are widely spaced, giving the sound a thinner quality, compared to the richer quality of a lower pitched sound. Another factor that contributes to the distinctive quality of falsetto voice is the slightly breathy component that results from the vocal folds never quite closing during vibration.

Spectral Characteristics of Pulse and Falsetto   Spectrally, the different registers have different shapes, much like different musical instruments. For instance, a brass instrument such as a trumpet has many harmonics, giving it a shallow spectral slope. A woodwind instrument like a flute, on the other hand, has fewer harmonics, resulting in a steep spectral slope. Similarly, the voice in pulse register, with its low F_0 and many harmonics, has a shallow spectral slope. The spectral slope is steeper for the high-pitched voice of falsetto, with its high F_0 and few harmonics. Using the qualities of musical instruments as an analogy, the sound of the voice changes from "brassy" to "fluty" as one goes from pulse to falsetto register.

Use of Different Registers in Singing and Speaking   Even though modal and falsetto registers are characterized by different vibratory patterns, there is actually a considerable amount of overlap between the upper limits of the modal range and the lower limits of the falsetto range. Most trained singers can produce a high note that is perceived as being within the modal register and can produce a note with exactly the same F_0 that is heard as the lower portion of the falsetto register. Also, some trained singers can push the modal register up

Modal is the most typically used register in normal conversational speech.

to very high limits, around 500 Hz (Titze, 1994). Abrupt changes in register are used in some kinds of singing, such as yodeling, country western, folk singing, soul, and gospel. In electronically amplified singing, the falsetto register is becoming more and more the acceptable register for high pitches. However, in classical Western styles of singing, such as opera, art song, and oratorio, noticeable register changes are generally unacceptable. Singers of these styles spend much time and effort learning to switch smoothly between registers, with no perceivable changes in quality.

For speech purposes, modal is the most typically used register, although it is common for individuals to drop to pulse register at the ends of phrases and sentences. Use of falsetto in conversational speech is less common. However, all three registers are normal modes of vocal fold vibration. In fact, switching between registers is sometimes necessary for linguistic, esthetic, or physiologic reasons. For instance, some African and Asian languages use abrupt changes in register to distinguish between phonemes (Titze, 1994). However, if a speaker uses primarily pulse or primarily falsetto for conversational speech, rather than primarily modal register, this is considered by speech–language pathologists to be a voice problem requiring therapy.

Voice Quality

Although an enormous amount of research has been devoted to investigating vocal quality, there is as yet no generally accepted definition of the term. One reason for this is that the concept of vocal quality has been used in different contexts. For example, a phonetician might use quality to distinguish between phonemes; a singer might refer to the quality of different registers; and quality might be used to describe voice types such as breathy, hoarse, and harsh (Childers, 1991).

Another reason is that voice quality is a multidimensional entity and is linked to numerous aspects of voice production, including F_0 and intensity. The quality of a person's voice is determined by how their vocal folds vibrate, as well as by the shape and configuration of their vocal tract (including length, degree of arching of the hard palate, size of the oral cavity in relation to size of the pharynx, and so on). For example, women have slightly different vocal tract configurations than men, so even if men and women produce a sound with the same F_0, we can still usually recognize the voice as male or female by its quality.

Hyperadducted vocal folds create a voice that sounds tense and harsh; hypoadducted vocal folds result in a breathy and weak voice.

The way that the vocal folds close during vibration plays an important role in shaping an individual's voice quality. Vocal folds that are adducted too tightly, with too much medial compression, are said to be **hyperadducted**. This can be caused by many different types of problems, ranging from vocal abuse to neurological diseases such as spasmodic dysphonia. When the folds are hyperadducted, the balance between muscular tension and P_s is upset. With the folds adducted too tightly, it takes more P_s to overcome the resistance of the folds. The resulting voice is perceived as tense, with what Colton and Casper (1996) termed a "hard edge" to the voice.

On the other hand, vocal folds that do not adduct as tightly as they should are said to be **hypoadducted**. This condition, too, can be caused by numerous factors, ranging from inappropriate usage to neurological problems such as vocal fold paralysis. As with hyperadduction, the balance between muscular and aerodynamic forces is upset. In this case, there is too little muscle force, so the vocal folds do not offer enough resistance to the flow of air. Air thus escapes between the vocal folds without being converted into acoustic energy. This loss of air creates turbulence as it passes through the vocal folds and adds a noisy, breathy quality to the vocal tone.

The quality of an individual's voice is usually easy to recognize, even without seeing the person. You probably all have friends who call you and don't bother to identify themselves, assuming that you will know who it is. And usually you do. However, although it is not difficult to perceive even small differences in people's voice quality, describing and measuring voice quality objectively is another matter altogether.

Probably hundreds of adjectives have been used to describe voice quality. Just a few are pleasant, strident, rough, raspy, shrill, clear, unpleasant, harsh, hoarse, tinny, and strained. This abundance of terminology, while it may be colorful, is a problem in the clinical management of voice disorders, because these terms are highly subjective. What is rough to me may be hoarse or strident to you. Professionals using these terms have no standard frame of reference for voice quality, which makes communication between them difficult.

Another problem with these subjective terms is that they do not indicate how the vocal folds are actually vibrating. There is no agreed on physiological basis for most of these terms. In other words, what is missing is an agreed on relationship between the perceptual aspect of how the person's voice is heard and the physiological and acoustic bases that are contributing to the perception of the voice in question.

Normal Voice Quality

It has proved to be very difficult to define voice quality. In fact, normal voice quality is often defined by default, as the absence of a problem. Colton and Casper (1996) brilliantly pinpointed the problem of defining normal voice:

> An accepted definition of normal voice does not exist. There are no established standards, and no boundaries of accepted norms have been set. Attempting to set such standards might be likened to defining what

Normal vocal quality encompasses many dimensions related to physical, physiological, acoustic, emotional, and social factors.

constitutes normal appearance. Voice, like appearance, comes in so many varieties. Cultural, environmental, and individual factors contribute to the determination of what is designated normal. And voice, again like appearance, does not remain constant. It changes throughout the lifespan; it changes in reaction to emotion; it changes in response to environment; it reflects the state of health of the body and of the mind. It would be extremely difficult, if not impossible, to have a single definition that would encompass all of the ways that a normal voice could sound. Normal is not a single state, but rather exists on a continuum. . . . The lack of a definition of normal voice creates problems in setting therapeutic goals and in describing abnormality and its degree of severity. There is no complete and objective template against which to measure and compare it. . . . If a voice improves, how can we measure that improvement? What can we compare it to? Which of the vocal attributes have contributed to its improvement? How much better is it? Is it normal?

Recently, however, voice experts have begun to determine voice quality in a way that has its basis in the actual functioning of the laryngeal mechanism. Despite the inherent difficulties in defining normal voice, researchers and clinicians have tried to specify various acoustic and physiological bases that form the foundation of normal voice.

Zemlin described six acoustic features of normal voice, including maximum frequency range, average fundamental frequency, maximum phonation time, minimum-maximum intensity, jitter, and noise.

Zemlin (1998) provided six specifiable parameters of voice production that contribute to a normal, clear vocal quality. These six parameters clearly demonstrate the multidimensional nature of voice quality and the interdependence of F_0, intensity, and quality.

The first is maximum frequency range. The normal voice is flexible in pitch during conversation. Speech that lacks this flexibility sounds very monotonous. Adults have a frequency range of around two to three octaves.

The second parameter is the average rate of vocal fold vibration during conversation, that is, SFF, or habitual pitch. We saw in Chapter 2 that children, adult women, and adult men demonstrate fairly typical F_0 levels during speech. F_0 levels that are much higher or lower than expected for a person's age and sex do not sound normal.

The third factor is air cost, or maximum phonation time, and refers to the longest period of time that an individual can sustain a vowel in one breath. An adult speaker should be able to sustain comfortable phonation for about 15 to 25 seconds (s). Children are expected to be able to sustain phonation for at least 10 s. A lack of ability to sustain phonation for the expected amount of time indicates a problem in adequately valving the airstream for speech.

Fourth is minimum-maximum intensity at various F_0 levels. We saw earlier, when discussing voice range profiles, that at a person's midrange of frequency a minimum-maximum SPL of 20 to 30 dB is normal. Zemlin (1998) suggested that an even wider range of 50 dB is within normal limits. At high and low F_0, we can only vary intensity by a few decibels. A person who shows a restricted range of decibel variation may have a voice problem.

The fifth parameter refers to the periodicity of vocal fold vibration, reflected acoustically in jitter. With mass, length, tension, and P_s held constant, normal vocal fold vibration will still be nearly, and not completely, periodic. However, more aperiodic vibration often results in a rough or hoarse-sounding voice.

Finally, Zemlin (1998) identified noise as the sixth parameter of quality. Noise results from turbulent airflow, with a random distribution of acoustic energy. Turbulent airflow is generated when an obstacle interferes with vocal fold vibration, causing air to flow in a less regular manner through the glottis. In a normal voice, the harmonic energy generated by the nearly periodic vibration should be much higher than any noise energy. Noise in the voice can be heard as breathiness, hoarseness, roughness, or any combination of these perceptual attributes. A small amount of noise in the glottal source may produce what Baken (1998) called a "fuzzy softness" or "velvety quality" to the sound. More turbulence might be heard as breathiness or huskiness, whereas a lot of turbulence is usually perceived as a hoarse voice.

Table 6.5 lists the six parameters of normal voice quality.

The normal voice has a steep spectral slope, so it should not have much energy at the higher frequencies. A spectrum that shows increased energy at higher harmonics may indicate that there is noise in the signal contributing to the increased energy. Noise in the signal, or **additive noise**, may be perceived as some form of dysphonia. Some noise in the spectrum, though, seems to be normal, particularly in women's voices, which lends a breathier quality to women's voices (Klatt & Klatt, 1990; Mendoza, Valencia, Munot, & Trujillo, 1996; Sodersten & Lindestad, 1990).

Abnormal Voice Qualities

Abnormal voice qualities, generically referred to as **dysphonia**, describe voices that sound deviant in terms of tone, pitch, and/or loudness. It is important to

---

■ **TABLE 6.5**

Parameters of Normal Vocal Quality

Maximum frequency range
Speaking F_0
Maximum phonation time
Minimum-maximum intensity at various F_0 levels
Periodicity of vibration
Noise generated by turbulent airflow

Source: Zemlin (1998).

Additive or spectral noise refers to excess noise in the voice spectrum, perceived as some form of dysphonia.

keep in mind that voice quality is multidimensional, so perceived problems in pitch and loudness often contribute to the perception of dysphonia, and vice versa. For example, research by Wolfe and Ratusnik (1988) has shown that moderately to severely dysphonic vowels are perceived by listeners to be significantly lower in pitch than clear or mildly dysphonic vowels. These authors reported that listeners matched dysphonic vowels with a perceived pitch that was on the average six semitones lower than the actual F_0 of the vowel. Thus, the relationship between the perception of pitch and the actual vocal F_0 seems to vary depending on voice quality. Conversely, the lower the pitch of the voice and the louder the voice, the greater is the likelihood of the voice being rated more severely dysphonic (Kempster, Kistler, & Hillenbrand, 1991).

Although professionals use many different terms to describe different voice qualities, the most currently accepted terms are **breathiness**, **roughness**, and **hoarseness**. A breathy quality refers to a vocal tone that sounds aspirated. You can actually hear the air escape during phonation. Roughness refers to a raspy sound in the voice, with the perception of a low pitch. Hoarseness refers to a combination of breathy and rough qualities in the voice (Eskenazi,

Breathiness, roughness, and hoarseness are the most commonly used terms to describe abnormal voice qualities.

Childers, & Hicks, 1990). Other professionals may use the same terminology in somewhat different ways. For instance, Colton and Casper (1996) do not distinguish between hoarse and rough vocal qualities. On the other hand, they describe many different kinds of voice qualities, including tense voice and strain-struggle voice.

In general, the terms breathiness, roughness, and hoarseness have become popular because these are the vocal qualities that are the most amenable to acoustic analysis. Researchers have therefore tried to measure these qualities acoustically in many different ways in order to generate some kind of objective method of relating the perception of abnormal voice to the relevant acoustic factors in the vocal signal. Numerous different acoustic measurements have been made on both normal and disordered voices in an attempt to find a cluster of measures that successfully separates normal from disordered voice. To date, this quest has not been completely successful.

Acoustic Characteristics of Breathy and Rough or Hoarse Voice

Some researchers have tried to characterize a voice as breathy or rough, depending on where in the glottal spectrum the additive, or **spectral noise**, occurs.

Breathy Voice When the vocal folds do not close properly, the result is a continuous flow of air during the entire vibratory cycle. The air leaking out generates a hissy kind of friction noise along with the tone generated by the vibrating vocal folds (Zemlin, 1998). The vocal folds are close enough to be vibrated, but the sound of air being continuously released accompanies the sound wave (Borden et al., 1994). The turbulent airflow pattern results in a less periodic acoustic signal. Because the periodic component of the voice source is weaker in the middle and high frequencies, noise tends to be especially noticeable above about 2 to 3 kilohertz (kHz) (Hillebrand & Houde, 1996). A breathy voice signal has more high-frequency energy than a nonbreathy signal. Some researchers found breathiness to be associated with a relative loss of acoustic energy between 2 and 5 kHz and with an increase in noise at frequencies higher than 5 kHz (Rihkanen, Leinonen, Hiltunen, & Kangas, 1994).

Breathy voice is associated with increased high-frequency energy.

Breathiness is an inefficient form of phonation, which usually results in a very limited intensity range, because less subglottal pressure builds up when the vocal folds do not close properly. In addition, the person with a breathy voice often uses three to four times the normal amount of air per second. Breathy voice is not always abnormal, however. Breathy or aspirated voice serves to distinguish between some phonemes in several languages. Zulu, for example, is a Bantu language spoken in South Africa that differentiates between aspirated and unaspirated voiceless stops such as /k/ and /kʰ/. In Zulu, these would be heard as two distinct phonemes, based on the degree of breathiness accompanying each. On the other hand, breathiness is also a very common symptom of both organic and functional voice disorders (e.g., vocal fold paralysis), and increased breathiness may be associated with aging.

Rough or Hoarse Voice   A rough or hoarse voice is a very common symptom of most laryngeal disorders. It can be the first indication of some kind of voice problem, ranging from a minor bout of laryngitis to a life-threatening cancerous tumor. Similar to the acoustic basis of breathy voice, hoarseness also seems to be partially determined by the amount of spectral noise, resulting from the flow of turbulent air through the glottis, in relation to the harmonic energy. However, hoarseness is also related to how periodically the vocal folds are vibrating. For instance, when the vocal folds are irritated or swollen, they vibrate in a less periodic fashion, because the inflammation prevents the cover of the vocal folds from vibrating as freely as normal, which interferes with the mucosal wave. Since aperiodic sound is noise, the more aperiodic the vibration is, the more noise that is imposed on the vocal sound. The noise that results in the perception of a hoarse voice tends to be more prevalent at lower frequencies, between 100 and 2600 Hz.

Hoarseness tends to be associated with increased noise at lower frequencies.

In sum, breathiness and roughness are both characterized by additive noise, but in breathiness the noise is located at the higher frequencies, and in roughness the noise occurs at the lower frequencies. A combination of these factors is also possible and does indeed occur frequently.

Ways of Measuring Registers and Quality

Over the past few decades, several ways have been developed to analyze various acoustic and physiological aspects of voice quality. Many of the instruments that perform these analyses are commercially available, relatively inexpensive, and safe and noninvasive.

One such analysis measures the **harmonics-to-noise ratio (HNR)**, which is a measure of the proportion of harmonic sound to noise in the voice measured in decibels. HNR quantifies the relative amount of additive noise in the voice signal (Awan & Frenkel, 1994). The higher the HNR is, the more the harmonic components of the voice predominate over the noise. The lower the HNR is, the more noise that exists in the voice. HNRs show a high correlation with perceptual judgments of voice quality, so this measure can be useful for making objective, quantitative assessments of breathiness, roughness, or hoarseness of a person's voice. Normal HNRs have been reported by various researchers for adult speakers, as shown in Table 6.6. HNRs for children and for elderly adults have been reported to be lower than for young and middle-aged adults (Ferrand, 1999, 2000).

Harmonics-to-noise ratio (or noise-to-harmonics ratio) quantifies the spectral noise in a voice signal by measuring the proportion of harmonic to inharmonic components.

A patient who obtains a lower than normal HNR is demonstrating additive noise in the voice. For example, if a person has some kind of problem in vibrating the vocal folds, due to a growth (e.g., a polyp or nodule), paralysis of one or both vocal folds, or other kind of laryngeal problem, a larger amount of air than normal escapes during vibration, creating turbulent noise (Pabon & Plomp, 1988). Aperiodic vocal fold vibration also creates additive noise, contributing to the low HNR and to the resulting perception of dysphonia.

Electroglottography   **Electroglottography**, also sometimes called **laryngography**, or, more simply, **EGG**, has become a popular method of evaluating vocal fold function noninvasively. Originally developed in the 1950s and re-

■ **T A B L E   6 . 6**

Average Adult Values for HNR Reported for Normally Speaking Adults

AUTHOR(S)	HNR (dB)
Awan & Frenkel (1994)	15.63 (males)
	15.38 (females)
Bertino et al. (1996)	7.23
Horii & Fuller (1990)	17.3 (males)
	19.1 (females)
Yumoto et al. (1982)	7.3

Electroglottography generates a waveform that reflects the opening and closing of the vocal folds.

fined in the 1970s by Adrian Fourcin, EGG works on the principles of conduction of electricity. Human tissues are good conductors of electricity, whereas air is a poor conductor. The EGG was developed to take advantage of this difference in conductivity between tissue and air.

A high-frequency signal of very low current is generated and passed through two surface electrodes held in place with a Velcro band at either side of the person's thyroid cartilage. The individual feels nothing, and the procedure is completely safe. Because tissue conducts electricity well, but air does not, when the vocal folds are closed, the current passes easily from one electrode to the other (in electrical terminology, the resistance is low). However, when the vocal folds are open, there is a relatively large body of air between them, and thus there is more resistance to the flow of current from one electrode to the other. This changing of resistance as the vocal folds open and close is displayed on a screen as a waveform, with time along the horizontal axis and relative amplitude of electrical voltage along the vertical axis.

This waveform is called the **Lx wave**; it reflects the surface area of contact of the vocal folds (see Figure 6.13). As the vocal folds close during vibration, the resistance to the electrical current decreases and the amplitude of the waveform increases. As the vocal folds separate during vibration, the resistance to the electrical current increases and the amplitude of the waveform decreases. Thus, the Lx waveform produces a record of vocal fold vibration during phonation. For voiceless sounds, there is no Lx waveform, because voiceless sounds are not produced with vocal fold vibration.

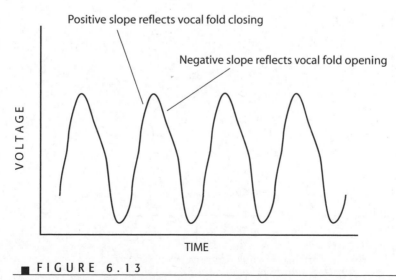

■ FIGURE 6.13

Lx wave of modal vibration.

The duty cycle refers to all the phases involved in a cycle of vocal fold vibration, including closing, closed, opening, and open.

The Lx waveform looks similar to acoustic waveforms, but what is being measured is very different. An acoustic waveform represents increases and decreases in air pressure. The Lx waveform shows increases and decreases of electrical activity, which corresponds to the opening and closing of the vocal folds. The Lx waveform reflects what is called the **duty cycle** of vocal fold vibration. The duty cycle refers to the phases of a vocal fold vibratory cycle, including the interval during which the vocal folds begin to close, the interval during which they are maximally closed, the interval during which they begin to open, and the interval during which they are completely open.

Baken (1992) provided a detailed interpretation of points along the Lx waveform and how they correspond to vocal fold vibration. See Figure 6.14. At point a the inferior margins of the vocal folds make their initial contact, signaling the start of the closing phase. Between points a and b, the lower margins continue to close. At point b the superior margins of the folds make initial contact. Between points b and c the superior margins continue to close. At point c, maximal contact between the vocal folds is achieved, signaling the end of the closing phase and the beginning of the closed phase. The interval between points c and d reflects the closed phase of the cycle. At point d the inferior margins of the vocal folds begin to separate, initiating the opening phase. The inferior margins continue to separate between points d and e. At point e the separation of the inferior margins is complete, and the superior edges begin to open. This point, with its abrupt change in slope, is referred to as a *knee* in the opening phase. During the interval between points e and f, the superior mar-

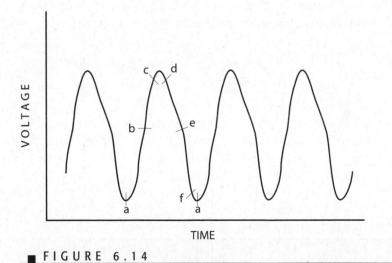

TIME

■ FIGURE 6.14

Points of vibration shown on the Lx wave.

gins of the vocal folds continue to open. At point f, contact between the vocal folds reaches its minimum, and during the interval between points f and a, the width of the glottis is at its greatest. The cycle then begins again.

It is important to keep in mind that the EGG represents relative contact area. The maximum peak on the Lx waveform does not necessarily mean that there is complete glottal closure. It is possible during vocal fold vibration for complete glottal closure to not occur at all. The vocal folds may be as much as 3 mm apart and vibration will still occur. In falsetto register, for instance, the glottis may not completely close during vibration. Just by looking at the Lx waveform, we would not be able to tell whether complete closure was occurring. We could tell that the peak represented maximum closure, but how close that actually is cannot be determined. It is also not possible to specify the precise time at which glottal opening or closing is initially achieved.

Electroglottography can indicate various voice qualities based on the shape of the waveform.

By counting the peaks in a specific interval of time in the Lx waveform, we can determine the person's F_0. A greater number of cycles per second can indicate that the person is using falsetto. A reduced number of cycles per second can indicate pulse register. Also, by evaluating the shape of the waveform, we can make judgments about the way in which the vocal folds are opening and closing. For instance, a longer than normal separation time between the folds may indicate a greater volume of air passing through the glottis, giving the person's voice a breathy quality. A longer than normal closed time between the folds may indicate that the person is using too much medial compression, giving the voice a hyperfunctional, pressed quality. An even, regular pattern of the cycles in the waveform reflects periodic opening and closing of the folds, whereas an irregular pattern shows less periodic vibration, which may sound perceptually like hoarseness. Sample Lx waves are given in Figure 6.15.

EGG and Register Because the Lx signal matches the vocal F_0, it is rather easy to assess register with the EGG. Each register is associated with a characteristic Lx wave. Modal register is characterized by Baken's (1992) description of the phases described previously. Note that the closing phase in modal register has a steeper slope than the opening phase. This reflects the fact that vocal fold closing is quick and abrupt, whereas vocal fold opening is slower and more gradual. The difference occurs because with the vocal folds closed P_s has to build up to the point at which it is stronger than medial compression, a relatively gradual process. On the other hand, once the vocal folds are open, their elastic recoil and the increasing P_{neg} between them act very quickly to close the folds.

Different registers can be assessed by electroglottography.

Lx waveforms of pulse register often show more than one peak per cycle, reflecting the biphasic or multiphasic closure pattern (Blomgren, Chen, Ng, & Gilbert, 1997). Pulse is characterized by a wave that has sharp, short pulses

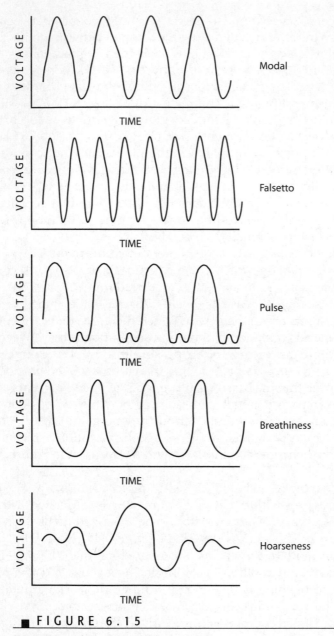

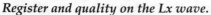

■ FIGURE 6.15

Register and quality on the Lx wave.

followed by a long closed glottal interval (Childers, 1991). The opening phase of vibration in pulse register may have one, two, or three minor openings and closings before the vocal folds close completely. Also, as you would expect, there are fewer cycles per second in pulse than in modal register.

In falsetto, the number of Lx cycles is greatly increased. The waveform also looks more nearly sinusoidal (almost like a pure tone), reflecting the extreme longitudinal tension and possible incomplete closure of the folds during vibration (Childers, 1991). Because of incomplete closure, the waveform does not show the less steep gradual opening and the steeper closing pattern typical of modal register. This shape typically indicates that the closed phase is absent, with the motion of the vocal folds remaining periodic, but alternating between a more and a less open glottis (Nair, 1999).

EGG Slope Quotients   Other ways of utilizing the EGG waveform have been developed that do not rely on visual inspection and subjective interpretation, but that are quantitative in nature. These measures are based on the duty cycle and the various proportions of time that each phase takes to complete. These types of EGG slope quotients are indications of vocal fold behavior during vocal fold contact (Fisher, Scherer, Guo, & Owen, 1996). EGG slope quotients have been obtained from normal voices and have also been applied to various types of disorders. In this kind of analysis, various phases of the duty cycle are measured in terms of their durations, and quotients are obtained by dividing certain durations into other durations. For example, the **closed quotient** (CQ) compares the duration of the closed phase to the time of the entire vibratory cycle. Because it reflects the proportion of time that the vocal folds are in contact with each other, it is related to the degree of medial compression being exerted. CQs in modal register typically range from around 0.50 to 0.60 (Nair, 1999). A higher CQ indicates a longer duration of closure, and a lower CQ reflects a shorter closure duration. For example, a CQ of 0.67 indicates a longer closed phase than one of 0.52. A louder voice shows a higher CQ than a softer one, and a "pressed" or tense voice generates a higher CQ than a soft or breathy voice. CQs for falsetto tend to be much lower because of the absence of a definitive closed phase. Thus, this measure may provide an "objective yardstick" of vocal hyperfunction or hypofunction (Orlikoff, 1991).

Another measure called the **contact index** (CI) is based on the ratio of the difference in time between the closing and opening phases, divided by the duration of the closed phase. The CI measure is apparently very sensitive to the mucosal wave of the vocal fold cover, so it can provide information about the way in which the vocal folds are vibrating in a particular register. A similar measure is the **closed-to-open ratio** (C/O ratio), which gives information about the relative durations of the closed and open phases of the duty cycle. From this information about how long the vocal folds are closed compared to how long they are open, the degree of hyper- or hypofunction of a person's voice can be determined. A longer closed phase results in a higher C/O ratio, whereas a lower C/O ratio indicates a shorter closed phase. Examples of EGG quotients are shown in Figure 6.16.

> Quantitative electroglottographic measures are based on the duty cycle and include the closed quotient, the contact index, and the closed-to-open ratio.

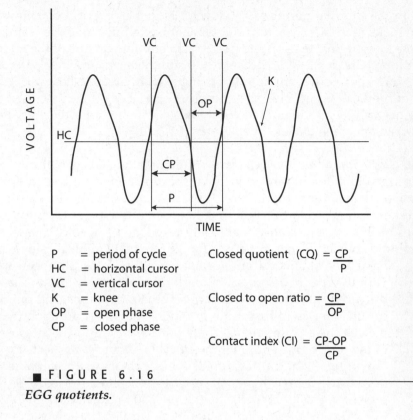

P = period of cycle	Closed quotient (CQ) = $\dfrac{CP}{P}$
HC = horizontal cursor	
VC = vertical cursor	
K = knee	Closed to open ratio = $\dfrac{CP}{OP}$
OP = open phase	
CP = closed phase	
	Contact index (CI) = $\dfrac{CP-OP}{CP}$

■ FIGURE 6.16

EGG quotients.

summary

- The larynx comprises one bone, nine cartilages, two pairs of joints, three sets of folds, and extrinsic and intrinsic muscles and is connected by membranes and ligaments.
- The myoelastic-aerodynamic theory of phonation describes one cycle of vocal fold vibration in terms of muscular, elastic recoil, and aerodynamic forces.
- The sound generated by the larynx is complex and nearly periodic and is characterized by a certain amount of jitter and shimmer.

- The vocal folds vibrate differently in different frequency ranges, giving rise to modal, pulse, and falsetto registers.
- Voice quality is a multidimensional entity that is influenced by the degree of adduction of the vocal folds during vibration, by F_0 and intensity, and by the vocal tract structures above the larynx.
- Breathiness and hoarseness can be characterized acoustically as additive noise in different areas of the voice spectrum.
- Some ways of measuring vocal quality acoustically include harmonics-to-noise ratio and electroglottography.

review exercises

1. Explain how the vocal folds adduct and abduct, describing all the relevant structures involved (cartilages, joints, muscles).

2. Discuss all the structures involved in the regulation of vocal F_0 and intensity.

3. Explain the relationship between voice quality and vocal registers, including a discussion of the physiological and acoustic parameters.

4. Compare jitter, shimmer, and harmonics-to-noise ratio in terms of the types of information that each provides.

5. Explain the relationship between EGG shape, EGG slope quotients, and vocal fold vibration.

chapter **7**

Clinical Application
Measures of Jitter, Shimmer, and Quality

chapter objectives   *After reading this chapter, you will*

1. Understand the clinical applications of jitter and shimmer measures.
2. Appreciate the relationship between jitter and normal aging of the laryngeal system.
3. Be able to describe the measurement of jitter in neurological disease.
4. Know how jitter levels are used as an indicator of laryngeal response to surgical, medical, and behavioral treatment.
5. Be familiar with the use of electroglottography as an indicator of vocal change.

Jitter and Shimmer Measures

The fact that normal jitter and shimmer can be quantified is very useful for making comparisons between normal and disordered voice production. Analyzing a speaker's vocal output to estimate the condition of his or her vocal mechanism is particularly attractive, because information about an individual's condition may be carried in vocal parameters such as F_0, intensity, jitter, and shimmer (Doherty & Shipp, 1988). These acoustic measurements have been used quite extensively to evaluate the effectiveness of behavioral, medical, and surgical treatments for various laryngeal disorders. Jitter measures have also been used to compare vocal motor control in different groups of speakers, such as children and adults who stutter and individuals with various vocal pathologies.

Laver, Hiller, and Beck (1992) identified four major clinical applications of acoustic analyses such as jitter and shimmer. First, because these methods are quick and easy, they can be a valuable tool in screening programs in schools and hospitals to identify people who are at risk for laryngeal pathology, such as children who yell a lot or people who use their voices professionally. The second application is the assessment of patients visiting the family doctor with complaints of harshness or hoarseness. In the current climate of managed care and cost control, the use of an automatic acoustic system could justify referring a patient for a laryngeal examination by an ear, nose, and throat specialist. Third, such acoustic analysis has been shown to be useful in supplementing diagnostic evaluation of vocal problems. With acoustic analysis, it is often possible to detect early changes in speech and voice that cannot be perceived by ear (Silbergleit et al., 1997). Fourth, acoustic analysis of jitter and shimmer has become an accepted way of monitoring voice changes over time of patients receiving surgery, radiotherapy, chemotherapy, or speech therapy, or of tracking deterioration or remission of voice function in progressive diseases.

In addition to screening and assessment, jitter measures have been used to study normal aspects of vocal development across the lifespan. It has been found, for example, that normal age-related changes in the tissues of the vocal folds may cause irregularities in their vibratory pattern (Orlikoff, 1990).

Major clinical applications of acoustic analyses include screening programs to identify people at risk for vocal pathologies, comprehensive diagnostic evaluation of vocal problems, and monitoring vocal changes over time.

These changes can have adverse effects on the quality of phonation, such as increased hoarseness or roughness. However, physiological health is an extremely important variable in aging of the voice. Many authors have shown that elderly individuals in good health tend to have younger-sounding voices than younger individuals in poor health. Orlikoff (1990) highlighted this important point by comparing jitter values between young healthy men, old healthy men, and old men with hypertension (high blood pressure). The values for all three groups fell within normal limits (less than 1%). However, the elderly subjects with hypertension fell much closer to the upper limits, while the young subjects' values fell closer to the lower limits. The elderly healthy subjects' values fell in between lower and upper limits. Thus, it seems that subtle aspects of vocal motor control may decline somewhat in the later years, particularly in the face of poor health.

Jitter and Shimmer Measures in Communication Disorders

Jitter and shimmer measures have been used extensively to document vocal function in patients with various types of communication disorders. These include neurological diseases such as amyotrophic lateral sclerosis and

Parkinson's disease; mechanical problems such as damage from endotracheal intubation; laryngeal cancer, functional voice problems, and stuttering.

Amyotrophic Lateral Sclerosis   Amyotrophic lateral sclerosis (ALS) is a progressive neurological disease in which all the motor functions of the body deteriorate due to damage to the motor nerves that supply all the voluntary muscles of the body, including those involved in speech production. Jitter and shimmer tend to be greater in women with ALS than in healthy women. This is a clinically important factor: Even women who are able to speak fairly clearly often demonstrate deviations in F_0, jitter, and shimmer. These differences show that there seems to be degeneration in the speech muscles before this degeneration is actually heard as impaired speech. Acoustic analysis may therefore provide a means by which early oral-facial and laryngeal signs of the disease can be detected. The findings of Silbergleit et al. (1997) corroborate this notion. They compared jitter and shimmer in patients who had ALS, but who had perceptually normal voices, and in healthy individuals. The ALS patients showed greater jitter levels. The authors suggested that the increased jitter resulted from changes in the laryngeal musculature. However, patients with motor disorders also have difficulties in getting rid of mucous secretions, so it is possible that the increased jitter was due to increased accumulations of mucus on the vocal folds. Whatever the reason or reasons, the higher jitter scores may indicate the beginning of an overall disruption in laryngeal function. The fact that acoustic analysis can detect differences in vocal characteristics before the human ear picks them up can help in making important treatment decisions, such as when to begin implementing treatment and the most functional types of treatment for individual patients.

Parkinson's Disease   Jitter and shimmer measures have also been used to evaluate the outcome of new or different types of treatment for voice problems. In Parkinson's disease (PD), for instance, the underlying pathophysiology is the reduction in the neurotransmittor **dopamine**. Patients with PD often suffer from voice difficulties, including hoarseness, reduced loudness, and reductions in pitch range. Acoustically, these individuals have shown higher F_0, higher jitter, lower intensity, decreased phonational range, and decreased dynamic range (Gamboa et al., 1997). A new treatment for PD is **fetal cell transplantion** (FCT), in which suitable fetal cells are transplanted into the appropriate site in the patient's brain. The aim of this procedure is to replenish the missing dopamine and thus alleviate the symptoms.

Measures of jitter and shimmer have been used to evaluate the outcome of new or different types of treatments for voice problems.

One investigation has found that, although FCT surgery was effective in improving overall motor performance of the patients studied, the acoustic results, including jitter and shimmer values, showed that the surgery did not systematically improve the patients' phonation or articulation capacities (Baker, Ramig, Johnson, & Freed, 1997). The patients involved were only mildly affected with PD, so it is important to know that voice symptoms in mild PD may not benefit from this type of surgery.

Endotracheal Intubation   Other medical and clinical uses of jitter and shimmer have also been reported. One very practical outcome that has resulted from jitter and shimmer analysis is changes in the administration of general anesthesia. Whenever a person has a general anesthetic, a breathing tube is inserted into their trachea through the larynx. This is called **endotracheal intubation**. Taking the tube out is referred to as *extubation.*

Endotracheal intubation often produces various degrees of temporary and sometimes permanent damage to the laryngeal mechanism. The damage can be mild, such as microscopic alterations of the mucosal tissues, or more severe, such as gross tissue damage to the mucosa, connective tissues, and muscles. Laryngeal cartilages may be dislocated, requiring corrective surgery (Horii & Fuller, 1990). More severe damage may result in complete loss of voice, called **aphonia**, and less severe damage can produce varying degrees of dysphonia.

> Objective documentation of the effects of intubation on the larynx has led to the development of less damaging tubes for endotracheal intubation.

Horii and Fuller (1990) made voice recordings of adults on the evening preceding surgery (not laryngeal surgery) and again within 24 hours following extubation. Greater jitter and shimmer levels were evident in the patient's voices even after this short-term intubation, which ranged from 1.5 to 23.5 hours. This kind of objective documentation of the effects of intubation on the vocal mechanism has led to the development of less damaging kinds of tubes for endotracheal intubation.

Laryngeal Cancer   Another example of the effectiveness of jitter measurement in a medical context was provided by Orlikoff et al. (1997). They used jitter levels to document the extent of laryngeal impairment in advanced laryngeal cancer and to investigate the effectiveness of nonsurgical treatment. Orlikoff et al. (1997) reported that since 1983 Memorial Sloan-Kettering Cancer Center in New York has instituted a larynx preservation protocol (LPP) for the treatment of certain kinds of cancer of the larynx and throat. This treatment is based on a combination of chemotherapy followed by radiation therapy (RT). Patients are monitored for their response to this therapy. If they do not respond within a certain amount of time, they are referred for a **laryngectomy**, in which part or all of the larynx is removed.

The authors studied men with advanced squamous cell carcinoma of the larynx involving one or both vocal folds. They obtained voice-frequency data before each cycle of the patients' chemotherapy. Orlikoff et al. (1997) found a dramatic reduction in jitter across chemotherapy cycles. The average jitter value fell from 4.34 percent before the first chemotherapy treatment to 1.52 percent, measured before the last administration of chemotherapy. Although 1.52 percent is still above the levels of normal adult males without pathology, it is clearly closer to the normal range. Patients who did not respond to the chemotherapy and RT did not show this marked drop in jitter levels. The authors concluded that the significant reduction or elimination of a laryngeal tumor is associated with increased vocal stability, as reflected in the reduced jitter levels.

Functional Voice Problems   Jitter analysis has also been used to justify certain types of behavioral voice therapy for functional voice problems, which are problems that are not caused by disease, growths, trauma, or other neurological or organic problems. Many patients referred for voice therapy have these functional problems, often related to improper use or overuse of the voice. Although numerous techniques are used to treat these functional disorders, there is very little objective evidence that they actually work. Many voice therapies, including manual circumlaryngeal therapy (a form of laryngeal massage therapy), yawn-sigh, accent method, and progressive relaxation, aim to reduce or to eliminate excess muscle tension in the laryngeal area.

The effectiveness of specific vocal techniques such as manual circumlaryngeal therapy has been documented using acoustic measures such as jitter and shimmer.

Roy et al. (1997) measured the effects of manual circumlaryngeal therapy in adult female patients with voice disturbances. In addition to perceptual measures (i.e., a judgment regarding the severity of the sound of the voice), they obtained acoustic measurements of F_0, jitter, and shimmer of voice pre- and posttherapy. Perceptually, there was a significant reduction in average severity of the voice disturbance after therapy. Acoustically, there were significant reductions in jitter and shimmer. More of these kinds of studies need to be done to document objectively the improvement of voice due to treatment.

Stuttering   In addition to these different kinds of voice problems, jitter and shimmer have also been used to differentiate between the speech of children who stutter and normally fluent peers. This is important, particularly at the initial stages of stuttering, because it is often difficult to distinguish between normal disfluency and stuttering. Subtle acoustic markers have been sought that can help to make these fine distinctions, which are often difficult to make on the basis of perceptual characteristics of the child's speech.

As children mature, they exhibit greater laryngeal control and more stable vocal fold vibration, with correspondingly less jitter and shimmer (Glaze, Bless, Milenkovic, & Susser, 1988; Hall & Yairi, 1992). Hall and Yairi (1992) suggested that measures of jitter and shimmer may help to detect subtle problems in laryngeal function that may exist even in the fluent speech of young children who may be beginning to stutter. These researchers found that although jitter values were similar between the young stutterers and nonstutterers who participated in their study, shimmer values were substantially higher for the children who stuttered than for the nonstuttering children. Importantly, these higher shimmer levels were identified in the speech of 3- to 4-year-old children who had just recently begun to stutter. This may indicate that subtle differences in laryngeal functioning or in the complex interaction among the laryngeal, respiratory, and vocal tract systems are present at very early stages of the disorder. Jitter and shimmer measures, therefore, may help to distinguish between those children who stutter or who are at risk for stuttering and those children who are going through a period of normal nonfluency.

Measures of Voice Quality

Deviations from normal voice quality are apparent in a large diversity of communication disorders, including voice disorders caused by benign and malignant tumors; neurological disorders, such as Parkinson's disease and ALS; strokes and head trauma; and hearing impairment. Aging also affects vocal motor control and voice quality, and this has important clinical implications.

Need for Objective Measures of Voice Quality   In the past ten or so years, many new surgical techniques have been developed to treat vocal disorders, with the express purpose of restoring or maintaining as normal a vocal quality as possible. This has generated a heightened interest in exploring methods and techniques for measuring and quantifying vocal quality. With more objective measures of voice quality, such as those provided by acoustic and EGG measures, evaluation of the problem can be more precise so that the most appropriate treatment for the patient can be determined. Equally important is the ability to objectively assess and quantify the outcome of treatment in order to satisfy not only the patient and therapist, but also the insurance companies and

Objective measures of voice quality are critical in clinical situations because of the multidimensional nature of voice quality.

HMOs who, typically, are paying for the treatment. It is much easier to justify the cost of treatment when you can provide numbers that show differences in vocal function and quality before and after treatment, rather than having to persuade skeptical finance officers based on subjective opinions. No insurance company is going to hand out hundreds or thousands of dollars when you say, "Treatment worked. Mr. B's voice sounds much clearer and less breathy." A much stronger case for the effectiveness of the treatment is made when data are available showing decreases in jitter and shimmer after treatment, as well as increases in HNR, normalized EGG quotients, expanded phonational and intensity ranges, and so on.

Objective measures are also critical in the clinic, because voice quality is a multidimensional entity that includes aspects of F_0, intensity, rate of speech, and other parameters. Clinically, it is important to sort out which aspects are involved in a patient's vocal problem in order to target the relevant dimensions for therapy. For instance, a low-pitched, hoarse voice can be associated with many voice problems, including nodules or other tumors on the vocal folds, vocal fold paralysis, and so on. A traditional method of treatment has been to teach the patient to raise his or her pitch, in the expectation that the raised pitch will increase the clarity of the individual's tone. This therapy is based on the notion of **optimum pitch**. That is, every individual has a certain range of pitches that is the most efficient, vocally speaking, for him or her to produce. It is thought that a person who habitually uses a pitch range that is either below or above the optimum is placing strain on the vocal mechanism, which in turn results in hoarseness.

Recently, with the more widespread use of objective measures of F_0 and quality, researchers and clinicians have found that often, although the patient's pitch sounds very low, his or her F_0 is actually within normal limits. Thus, the treatment procedure of teaching the patient to use a higher pitch range may not be physiologically appropriate and, in fact, could do more harm than good to the patient. A study by Wolfe and Ratusnik (1988) illustrates this point. They reported on a male speaker with a very rough voice who was diagnosed as having thickened vocal folds with a small area of leukoplakia (white patches) on one vocal fold. They noted that the initial impression of this individual's voice quality was that of severe hoarseness. Perceptually, the patient's pitch was judged to be appropriate for his age and sex. Instrumental analysis, however, revealed that his average F_0 was 213 Hz, which is much higher than the modal range for a male. The fact that this patient was actually using falsetto was overlooked at first, because the roughness of his voice made the pitch sound much lower than than the actual F_0. After treatment the patient was able to produce a clearer voice in the modal register well within the average male range.

Aging   EGG quotient data have shown that elderly men have less complete vocal fold closure than younger men (Higgins & Saxman, 1991). This is consistent with physiological evidence of laryngeal degeneration in aging men, including degeneration of the vocal ligament and mucosa, ossification of the laryngeal cartilages, and bowing of the vocal folds due to muscle atrophy. However, the elderly women in Higgins and Saxman's (1991) study did not show a similar lack of complete closure, according to the EGG data. Again, this is consistent with laryngeal physiology. It has been well established that laryngeal degeneration in women starts later and is less than that of men. These findings demonstrate the importance of accounting for the variable of age when assessing vocal pathology. Otherwise, the effects of normal aging on laryngeal behaviors could be mistaken for those of laryngeal pathology.

These EGG data are corroborated by HNR measures, which have demonstrated acoustically that laryngeal function changes with aging. For instance,

> Acoustic and electroglottographic information has been used to identify vocal changes that occur with normal aging.

Ferrand (1999) compared three age groups of normally speaking women: young adults, middle-aged adults, and elderly adults. The young and middle-aged women obtained similar HNRs, but the elderly women's HNRs were much lower. Therefore, both EGG and HNR measures demonstrate that it is not clinically appropriate to compare data of elderly speakers with data from young speakers to diagnose or treat vocal pathology.

EGG and Vocal Disorders   Numerous studies have used EGG measures to document vocal changes resulting from behavioral voice therapy or surgery. For example, Motta, Cesari, Iengo, and Motta (1990) evaluated a large group of individuals with a variety of voice problems, including functional hypokinetic dysphonia (i.e., breathy voice with no apparent vocal fold pathology), functional hyperkinetic dysphonia (excessive vocal fold adduction, but no pathology), nodules, polyps, and Reinke's edema (overall swelling of the cover of the vocal folds). Patients underwent EGG before and after surgery or speech therapy. The authors reported that the Lx wave always became more normal in those patients with functional dysphonias after speech therapy; 45 percent of individuals with nodules, polyps, or Reinke's edema showed complete normalization of the Lx wave after surgery. Fifty-five percent of the patients presented a different Lx wave than normal after surgery, but after speech therapy this 55 percent also normalized.

EGG and Spasmodic Dysphonia   EGG has been used to investigate the effects of Botox treatment in **adductor spasmodic dysphonia** (ADSD). ADSD is a neurological voice disorder in which the individual has spasms of the vocal folds. During these **laryngospasms**, the folds adduct so tightly that they are very difficult to set into vibration. The medial compression is so great that the P_s cannot force the vocal folds apart. The voice quality of individuals with this disorder is often so strained and tense that it has a strangled sound to it. This kind of quality is, in fact, called *strained-strangled.* Over the past ten or so years, a procedure known as **Botox injection** has been used to alleviate these laryngospasms in some patients with ADSD. Botox is the trade name for botulinum toxin, which is the toxin found in improperly canned food. If ingested from an affected can, this toxin can make a person very sick and even die. However, when used properly under medical treatment, miniscule amounts of the toxin can be very helpful in relieving certain kinds of muscle spasms. The toxin is injected into the affected muscle, which in the case of ADSD is usually the thyroarytenoid muscles, and the toxin temporarily weakens or even paralyzes the muscle. Therefore, during vibration the vocal folds are unable to close with too much medial compression, allowing for much easier phonation. Often, though, the patient's voice after Botox injection is rather breathy and weak, especially for the first week or two.

Electroglottography is useful in cases of adductor spasmodic dysphonia because the measure quantifies vocal fold contact area.

However, the effects of the injection are not permanent, and the patient's voice starts to lose the breathy quality and become more strained as time goes on. The person is typically reinjected every three to six months, depending on how long the effects last.

Because EGG measures quantify vocal fold contact area, such measures are very helpful in voice disorders in which hyper- or hypofunction is the major problem. This is particularly useful in ADSD, because the laryngospasms typically obscure the vocal folds during direct viewing with videostroboscopy or endoscopy. Fisher et al. (1996) have used EGG to investigate whether laryngeal function changes before and after Botox injection in patients with ADSD. They argued that it is important to obtain measures that quantify voice characteristics during the postinjection period as a way of identifying, for example, dose levels that result in voice improvement with minimal adverse effects. Fisher et al. (1996) pointed out that making perceptual judgments about voice quality both by listeners and by speakers with ADSD may not be a valid indication of what is actually happening with the vocal folds during phonation, whereas EGG can result in more valid inferences about vocal fold function.

EGG and Parkinson's Disease   EGG has also been used to compare different types of treatment for patients with Parkinson's disease (PD), who often complain of problems with intensity. Ramig and Dromey (1996) compared two treatments designed to increase vocal loudness. One treatment, the respiratory treatment (RT), was designed to increase the activity of the respiratory musculature to generate increased volumes and subglottal air pressure for speech. The other treatment, known as the Lee Silverman vocal treatment (LSVT), targeted increased vocal intensity through improved vocal fold adduction, as well as increased respiratory effort. The EGG measure they used to compare increases in vocal intensity between the two treatments is related to how tightly the vocal folds adduct. In the case of the PD patients, the authors were looking for increased adduction, which would be instrumental in increasing loudness. The LSVT group increased on this EGG measure, whereas the RT group actually decreased. This objective finding allowed the authors to suggest that treatment approaches that focus solely on respiration to increase loudness may even be counterproductive in patients with PD.

Electroglottography has been used to examine the effectiveness of various treatments for increasing intensity in patients with Parkinson's disease.

The effectiveness of fetal cell transplantation (FCT) of dopamine in patients with PD has also been examined by means of EGG measures. Baker et al. (1997) obtained acoustic and EGG recordings for three consecutive days before surgery and some months postsurgery. The patients' limb movements did show notable improvements after surgery. However, the EGG measures did not differ much between the time before and after surgery. This was consistent with perceptual measures that indicated that listener ratings of speech presurgery were not remarkably different from ratings after FCT surgery.

Clinical Study

Background

Frank Lomax, a 36-year-old man from Barbados, suffered a traumatic brain injury secondary to a fall. Upon admission to the emergency room, he was unconscious and having difficulty breathing. He was intubated for eight weeks, at which point he regained consciousness and was able to breathe independently. He was referred to an outpatient neurorehabilitation program for a comprehensive diagnostic workup including speech, occupational therapy, physical therapy, and neuropsychology.

Clinical Observations

During the initial speech evaluation, you were alarmed by the voice quality of this patient. His voice was not only extremely weak and breathy, but severe inspiratory and expiratory stridor were evident. He complained of chronic fatigue and had difficulty enduring the daily treatment program. Talking was clearly effortful and was limited to short phrases when necessary.

Acoustic Measures

Using a Visi-Pitch, you obtained the following acoustic measures for jitter, shimmer, and harmonics-to-noise ratio. It was not possible to obtain accurate F_0 information, due to the excessive breathiness. Jitter measures were abnormally high, with a level of 7.8 percent. Shimmer was also abnormal, at 4.6 dB. Harmonics-to-noise ratio was −3.5 Hz. These measures confirmed and quantified your clinical impressions.

Based on these abnormal measures and the perceptual impression of breathing difficulty, Mr. Lomax was referred immediately to the emergency room of a nearby hospital. The emergency room physician determined that his blood oxygen levels were dangerously low. Subsequent examination by an ENT revealed severe laryngeal scarring and stenosis secondary to the extended period of intubation. Emergency surgery was performed to remove scar tissue and establish an airway, as well as to improve vocal function.

Clinical Questions

1. Upon readmission to your program for voice therapy, what might be your first step in the clinical management process?
2. Suggest two changes that you would expect in the acoustic measures after the surgery, and provide a rationale for each.
3. How might the above two changes be reflected perceptually in the patient's voice?

summary

- Jitter and shimmer measures can be valuable tools in screening programs, in referrals to ENTs, in supplementing diagnostic evaluations, and in monitoring voice changes over time.
- Jitter and shimmer measures may provide a means by which early laryngeal signs of certain neurologic diseases may be detected.
- Jitter and shimmer values have been used to assess the results of surgical procedures in patients with Parkinson's disease, medical procedures in patients with advanced laryngeal cancer, and behavioral techniques in patients with functional voice disorders.
- Electroglottographic measures are helpful in evaluating hyper- and hypoadduction of the vocal folds and have been used to assess laryngeal changes in adductor spasmodic dysphonia and Parkinson's disease.

review exercises

1. Explain how jitter and shimmer measures can be used to supplement perceptual evaluations of vocal function in patients with neurologic diseases.
2. Why would you expect older individuals to have higher levels of jitter and shimmer than young individuals?
3. Why should endotracheal intubation result in high jitter and shimmer values?
4. Explain the relevance of increased shimmer levels in some young children who stutter.
5. Discuss the electroglottographic measures of contact quotient and closed-to-open ratio in relation to vocal disorders involving hyper- or hypoadduction.
6. Choose a vocal disorder and compare the types of information you could obtain about vocal function with jitter, shimmer, harmonics-to-noise ratio, and electroglottography.

The Articulatory System

chapter objectives | *After reading this chapter, you will*

1. Be familiar with the structure and function of the articulators of the vocal tract.
2. Know the traditional classification system of consonants and vowels.
3. Appreciate that the vocal tract is a resonator and know its resonating characteristics.
4. Be able to describe the source-filter theory of vowel production.
5. Understand the acoustic and spectrographic analysis of vowels and consonants.
6. Be able to explain the role of suprasegmentals and coarticulation in connected speech.

We have discussed the power source for speech, which is the air provided by respiration, and the way in which the exhaled air is changed into sound by the process of phonation. However, the sound generated by vocal fold vibration is not the sound that is heard by a listener. More processes need to occur before a sound will be recognizable as a speech sound belonging to a particular language. One of these processes is articulation. To shape specific sounds, organs such as the lips, tongue, and velum move around to come close to or make contact with themselves and other immovable articulators, such as the teeth, alveolar ridge, and palate. Moving the articulators to various locations and positions within the oral cavity modifies the sound wave moving through the vocal tract, giving the sound specific characteristics that are recognized as distinctive speech sounds. Moving the articulators also changes the resonances of the vocal tract. To understand the processes of both articulation and resonation and the ways in which these processes can be disrupted by various types of problems, it is important to have a thorough understanding of the structure and function of the articulators and the vocal tract.

■ *Articulators of the Vocal Tract*

The vocal tract is a tube around 17 cm long in adult males and somewhat shorter in adult females and children. The vocal tract consists of the cavities above the larynx, that is, the pharynx, oral cavity, and nasal cavities (Figure 8.1). The shape of the vocal tract is distinctive in several respects, which are all critical in articulation. First, it is shaped like a bent tube, with the oral and nasal cavities having a relatively horizontal position and the pharynx being relatively vertical. Second, the shape of the vocal tract is highly irregular and complex. Third, the vocal tract is variable in its shape. Every time you move your tongue or lips or mandible, you are changing the shape of the vocal tract.

> The vocal tract is a tube made up of the pharynx, oral cavity, and nasal cavities.

The vocal tract can be thought of as an interrelated system of movable and immovable structures that form a series of valves. For example, the lips form a valve that can open and close. The tongue can form numerous valves by contacting different articulators, such as the alveolar ridge or the velum. The velum forms a valve by touching the posterior pharyngeal wall. These valves channel or constrict the airflow in certain ways to create different types of sounds. To understand how these valves function in speech production, the structure of the articulators that make up the valves must be appreciated.

Oral Cavity

The oral cavity (Figure 8.2) is a space, bounded by various structures. The front boundary of the oral cavity is movable, being comprised of the lips. The sides of the oral cavity are formed by the cheeks, the palate acts as the roof, and the tongue makes up the movable floor of the oral cavity. The back of the oral cavity opens into the pharynx. The oral cavity is critical for many aspects of speech production. First, the opening of the oral cavity in front is the point of exit for most sounds. Second, the oral cavity contains important articulators, including the lips, teeth, alveolar ridge, hard palate, and soft palate (velum), as well as the tongue. Third, the shape of the oral cavity is altered during speech, which is an integral aspect of resonance.

> The boundaries of the oral cavity include the lips, cheeks, palate, and tongue.

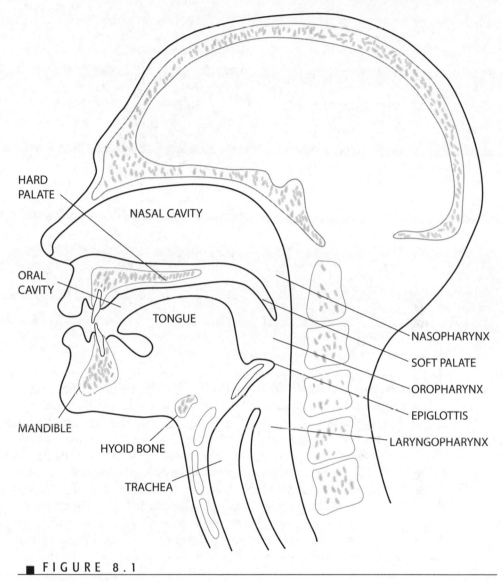

■ FIGURE 8.1

Vocal tract.

Lips

The two lips (adjective: labial; two lips: bilabial) are formed of muscle, mucous membrane, glandular tissues, and fat, all covered by an epithelium. The underlying tissue of the lips is highly vascular, which gives the lips their characteristic red color. The inner surface of the upper lip connects to the midline of the alveolar region by a small flap of tissue called the **superior labial**

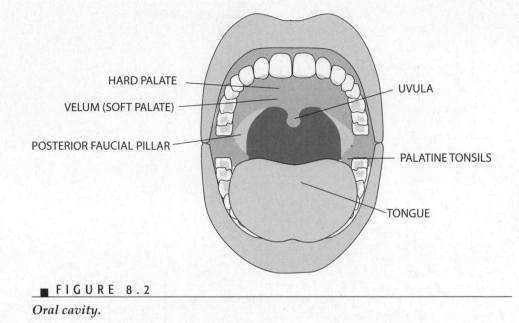

■ F I G U R E 8 . 2

Oral cavity.

frenulum. The lower lip is connected to the midline of the mandible by the **inferior labial frenulum**. The primary muscle making up the lips is the **orbicularis oris**. This is a circular, or sphincteric, muscle surrounding both the upper and lower lips. The orbicularis oris is not an isolated muscle, but fibers from numerous other facial muscles insert onto it. These muscles move the skin wherever they insert. The elevators insert around the upper lip and raise it, while the depressors insert around the lower lip and lower it. Elevators include the levator labii superioris, levator anguli oris, zygomaticus major and minor, and the risorius. Depressors include the depressor anguli oris, depressor labii inferioris, and the mentalis. See Figure 8.3.

> The lips are connected to the upper and lower jaws by the superior and inferior labial frenulum, respectively.

> The orbicularis oris is the primary muscle of the lips, into which fibers from many other facial muscles insert.

The muscles of the lips give them an enormous amount of mobility, allowing them to not only open and close very rapidly, but also to position themselves in many different ways. The lips can pucker more or less tightly, spread out to a greater or lesser extent, and assume many other positions. This flexibility and speed of motion are very important in the articulation of such sounds as /p/, /b/, /m/, and /w/. The lips are also crucial in mastication, acting to keep food and liquid within the mouth. Individuals with low muscle tone or with lip paralysis have difficulty in controlling the flow of saliva out of the mouth, as well as difficulty forming labial sounds.

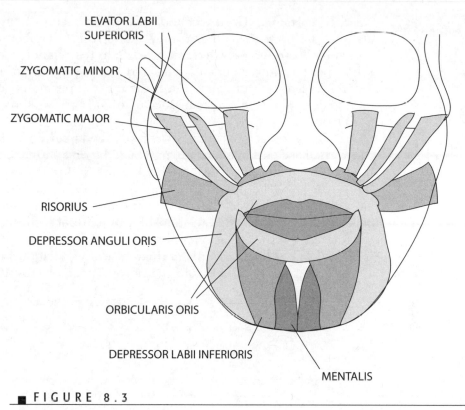

LEVATOR LABII SUPERIORIS

ZYGOMATIC MINOR

ZYGOMATIC MAJOR

RISORIUS

DEPRESSOR ANGULI ORIS

ORBICULARIS ORIS

DEPRESSOR LABII INFERIORIS

MENTALIS

■ FIGURE 8.3

Muscles of the lips and face.

Teeth

Behind the lips are the teeth, arrayed in upper and lower sets (adjective: dental). Children have 20 teeth, 10 in the upper jaw (maxilla) and 10 in the lower jaw (mandible). Adults have 32 teeth, with 16 in both upper and lower sets. Humans have four types of teeth: incisors, canines, premolars, and molars.

> The teeth serve as an immovable articulator that helps to channel the flow of air through the oral cavity.

Teeth are embedded in spaces, called alveoli, within the upper and lower jaws. Teeth are essential for biting, cutting, and chewing food, but they also play a most important role in speech production. They serve as an immovable articulator against which the tongue can form connections, and they also help to channel the flow of air and sound waves in appropriate ways. The teeth are particularly important in directing the airflow for the /s/ sound and acting as an obstacle to increase the turbulence necessary for its correct production. The slushy quality of the /s/ produced by 6- and 7-year-old children with missing front teeth attests to the importance of the teeth in sound production.

Dental occlusion refers to the relationship between the upper and lower dental arches and the positioning of the teeth; occlusal relationships include neutrocclusion, distocclusion, and mesiocclusion.

Dental Occlusion   The upper and lower teeth need to be in appropriate relationship to each other. If they are not, this can affect both eating and speech production. **Occlusion** refers to the relationship between the upper and lower dental arches and the positioning of individual teeth. Problems in upper and lower dental arch position and tooth relationships are referred to as **malocclusions**. There are three classes of occlusions.

Class I occlusion (see Figure 8.4) is also called **neutrocclusion**. This is the normal occlusal relationship, in which the first permanent molar of the upper jaw lies one half-tooth behind the first permanent molar of the lower jaw. The upper arch overlaps the lower one in front. The upper incisors hide the lower incisors so that only a little of the lower teeth show (Seikel et al., 1997). In this relationship, individual teeth may be misaligned or rotated, but the occlusion is normal.

Class II occlusion is known as **distocclusion**. In this relationship the first molar of the lower jaw is posterior to the normal position, resulting in the

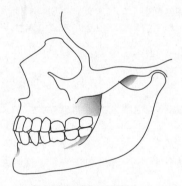

CLASS I OCCLUSION

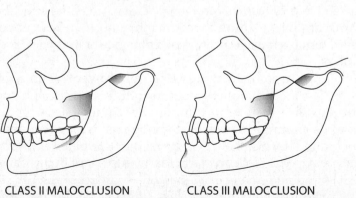

CLASS II MALOCCLUSION   CLASS III MALOCCLUSION

■ F I G U R E 8 . 4

Dental occlusion.

■ TABLE 8.1

Occlusion and Malocclusions

CLASS	OCCLUSION	MOLAR RELATIONSHIP
I	Neutrocclusion	First molar of upper jaw is one half-tooth posterior to first molar of lower jaw.
II	Distocclusion	First molar of lower jaw is posterior to normal position; mandible is retracted.
III	Mesiocclusion	First molar of lower jaw is anterior to normal position; mandible is protruded.

mandible being pulled back or retracted, a condition called *overjet*. This kind of malocclusion often results from micrognathia, a structural problem in which the mandible is small in relation to the maxilla.

Class III occlusion is referred to as **mesiocclusion**. Here the first molar of the lower jaw is anterior to the normal position, with the mandible protruding too far forward, a condition called *prognathic jaw*. Similar to class II problems, this type of malocclusion is often found in craniofacial disorders.

Table 8.1 provides an outline of the occlusion classes.

Hard Palate

The hard palate (Figure 8.5) is a complex bony structure lined with epithelium; it makes up the roof of the oral cavity and the floor of the nasal cavity (adjective: palatal). It serves as a barrier between these two cavities, preventing food, air, and sound waves from escaping the oral cavity.

The hard palate is made up of the palatine processes of the maxilla and the palatine bones and forms a barrier between the oral and nasal cavities.

The anterior three-quarters of the hard palate are formed by the **palatine processes** of the maxilla. The maxilla is a large, complex bone, with projections called processes that articulate with other bones of the skull. The palatine processes join together at the midline and articulate at the **intermaxillary suture**. (A *suture* is an immovable joint.) The posterior one-quarter of the hard palate is formed by the **palatine bones** of the skull. These bones are L-shaped, and the horizontal surface of the L fuses at the midline, forming the posteriormost portion of the hard palate. The meeting of the palatine bones and palatine processes forms a suture called the **transverse palatine suture**. The palate is arched both back to front and side to side. This arch, or *vault*, differs considerably between individuals.

The raised ridge that you can feel running from side to side toward the anterior of the hard palate, about 1/2 inch or so behind the upper teeth, is called the **alveolar ridge** (adjective: alveolar). This ridge is formed by the alveolar process of the maxilla, a projection of bone containing spaces that hold the roots and nerves of the teeth. The alveolar ridge is the point of contact or

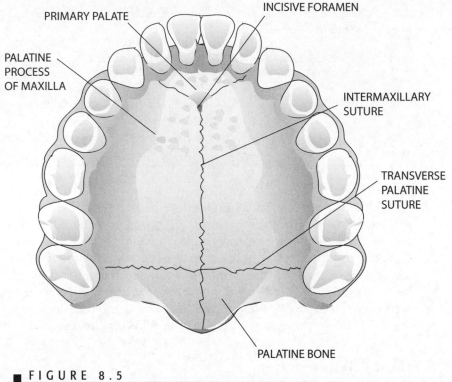

PRIMARY PALATE

INCISIVE FORAMEN

PALATINE
PROCESS
OF MAXILLA

INTERMAXILLARY
SUTURE

TRANSVERSE
PALATINE
SUTURE

PALATINE BONE

■ F I G U R E   8 . 5

Hard palate.

approximation of the tongue for many of the speech sounds of English, including /t/, /d/, /s/, /z/, /l/, and /n/. The hard palate posterior to the alveolar ridge also serves as an immovable point of contact for the tongue in the articulation of many sounds, such as /ʃ/, /ʒ/, and /r/. Because the hard palate is instrumental in the production of many sounds, structural problems such as cleft palate can result in severe speech production difficulties.

Soft Palate

Posterior to the hard palate is the soft palate, so called because it is made of muscle and other soft tissues and contains no bone. It is also known as the **velum**. The velum (adjective: velar) consists of a number of muscles, a large flat tendon, the **aponeurosis**, which attaches the velum to the posterior portion of the hard palate, as well as nerves, blood supply, and glands, all covered by a mucous membrane. Being made primarily of muscle, the velum is able to move, and this movement is of prime importance in biological functions such as swallowing and speech production.

The soft palate, or velum, attaches to the hard palate by means of a tendon called the palatal aponeurosis.

When open, the velo-pharyngeal passage-way allows air to enter and exit through the nasal cavities; when closed, air is forced through the oral cavity.

The velum at rest hangs down into the pharynx, allowing a passageway between the nasal cavities above and the oral cavity below. This passageway between the velum and the posterior pharyngeal wall is the **velopharyngeal passage** or port (Figure 8.6). When the velopharyngeal passage is open, the oral and nasal cavities are said to be coupled. When they are coupled, air is free to enter and exit the respiratory system through the nasal cavities. Sound waves are also free to travel into the nasal cavities. So is food, which can be a problem in cases of cleft palate or paralyzed velum. However, the velum is able to change its position—to raise itself up and back and actually contact the posterior pharyngeal wall. In this raised position it forms a barrier between the oral and nasal cavities, and air, sound waves, and food are prevented from entering the nasal

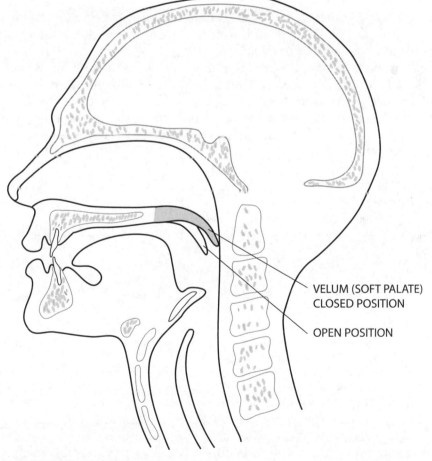

VELUM (SOFT PALATE)
CLOSED POSITION

OPEN POSITION

■ FIGURE 8.6

Velopharyngeal passageway.

cavities. For speech production, exhaled air is thus forced to exit to the atmosphere through the oral cavity.

Most sounds in English are *oral*, that is, they are produced with oral airflow. Only three sounds in English are formed with airflow exiting through the nasal cavities. These *nasal* sounds are /m/, /n/, and /ŋ/. Problems in velopharyngeal function result in air escaping through the nasal cavities rather than through the oral cavity, and this results in distorted oral sounds, or **hypernasality** with excessive nasal resonance.

Problems in velopharyngeal function can result in hyper- or hyponasality.

Problems can also occur when air is prevented from entering the nasal cavities for the production of nasal sounds, resulting in **hyponasality**, or insufficient nasal resonance.

The velum also forms a point of contact for the tongue in the production of the /g/, /k/, and /ŋ/ sounds.

Muscles of the Velum   Five muscles make up the velum; some elevate the velum and others depress it. Table 8.2 lists the muscles of the velum and their functions, and Figure 8.7 shows these muscles.

The **levator veli palatini** muscle makes up the bulk of the velum, and its slinglike arrangement of fibers is instrumental in elevating the velum to close the velopharyngeal port.

The **musculus uvuli** "bunches up" the velum (Seikel et al., 1997) and also raises it. The **tensor veli palatini** used to be considered a tensor of the velum

■ TABLE 8.2

Muscles of the Velum

MUSCLE	ATTACHMENTS	FUNCTION	NOTES
LVP	Temporal bone and medial wall of auditory tube cartilage to palatal aponeurosis	Raises velum	Fibers from left and right sides join; forms a sling for the velum
MU	Posterior part of palatine bones and palatal aponeurosis to mucous membrane cover of velum	Shortens and raises velum	Fibers run the length of the velum on the nasal surface
TVP	Sphenoid bone of skull and lateral wall of auditory tube to tendon that expands to form the palatal aponeurosis	Opens auditory tube	Used to be considered a tensor
PG	Front and sides of palatal aponeurosis to lateral margins of posterior tongue	Depresses velum or elevates tongue	Forms anterior faucial pillars
PP	Various origins, including anterior hard palate and midline of velum to posterior thyroid cartilage	Narrows pharyngeal cavity	Forms posterior faucial pillars

LVP, levator veli palatini; MU, musculus uvuli; TVP, tensor veli palatini; PG, palatoglossus; PP, palatopharyngeus

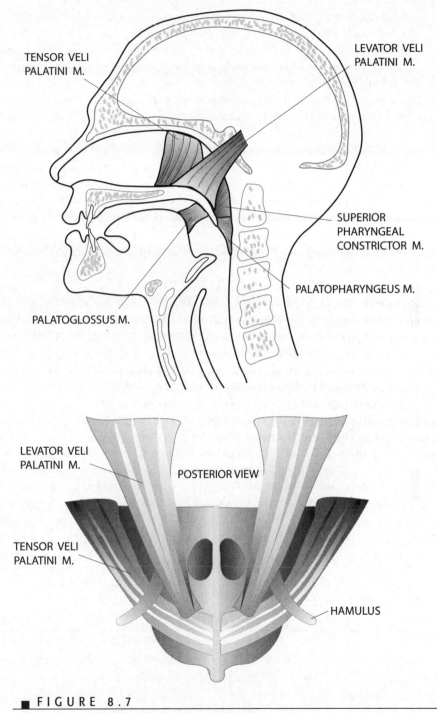

TENSOR VELI
PALATINI M.

LEVATOR VELI
PALATINI M.

SUPERIOR
PHARYNGEAL
CONSTRICTOR M.

PALATOPHARYNGEUS M.

PALATOGLOSSUS M.

LEVATOR VELI
PALATINI M.

POSTERIOR VIEW

TENSOR VELI
PALATINI M.

HAMULUS

■ F I G U R E   8 . 7

Muscles of the velum.

(hence its name), but recent research has shown that this muscle is more involved with the function of the auditory tube. The fibers of the tensor veli palatini course downward and terminate in a tendon. This tendon then changes direction from downward to medial, and the left and right sides of the tendon merge and expand to become the palatal aponeurosis. Contraction of the tensor veli palatini opens the auditory tube, which is normally closed. This opening of the tube occurs when we swallow and allows air pressures within and outside the middle ear to equalize.

The **palatoglossus** muscle depresses the velum. It forms one of the arched pillars that is visible when you open your mouth wide and look toward your throat. There are two of these pillars on either side of your throat, called the *anterior and posterior faucial pillars,* and they mark the posterior boundary of the oral cavity. The **palatopharyngeus** is a muscle of both the velum and the pharynx. It forms the posterior faucial pillars. The palatopharyngeus helps to narrow the pharyngeal cavity and thus helps to guide food into the lower pharynx during swallowing.

Velopharyngeal Closure   To close off the velopharyngeal port, the velum raises itself upward and backward and contacts the posterior pharyngeal wall.

> Velopharyngeal closure involves the velum elevating to contact the posterior pharyngeal wall, as well as inward movement of the lateral pharyngeal walls.

However, this movement of the velum is not a "trapdoor" motion; that is, the velum does not just swing up and down. Rather, the lateral walls of the pharynx are also involved in velopharyngeal motion. Even when the velum is fully in contact with the posterior pharyngeal wall, if there is no movement of the lateral pharyngeal walls, air can escape around the sides of the velum and into the nasal cavities (Golding-Kushner, 1997). The velopharyngeal valve consists of the velum itself, the posterior wall of the pharynx, and the lateral walls of the pharynx.

Four types of velopharyngeal closure have been observed, and they have been categorized on the basis of different contributions of velar and pharyngeal wall motion. Individuals tend to use one particular type of pattern more than the others. Table 8.3 describes these patterns of closure.

■ TABLE 8.3

Types of Velopharyngeal Closure and Relative Contribution of Velar and Lateral Pharyngeal Wall (LPW) Movement

TYPE	CLOSURE PATTERN
Coronal	Mostly velar movement with small amount of LPW movement
Sagittal	Mostly LPW movement with small amount of velar movement
Circular	Approximately equal contribution of velar and LPW movement
Circular with Passavant's ridge	Movement of velum and LPW plus forward movement of Passavant's pad on the posterior pharyngeal wall

Tongue

The tongue is a large, muscular structure occupying a good portion of the oral cavity (Figure 8.8). Because of the number of muscles making up the tongue and the way in which these muscles are intertwined with each other, the tongue has an enormous degree of flexibility and speed in its movements. The tongue is essential in many functions, including chewing, swallowing, and speaking. The tongue is, without doubt, the most important and the most active of the articulators. It modifies the shape and thus the resonance characteristics of the oral cavity. It also acts as a valve by contacting or closely approximating other articulators and modifying the airstream flowing through the oral cavity.

Portions of the tongue include the tip, blade, front, back, and root, which attaches to the hyoid bone.

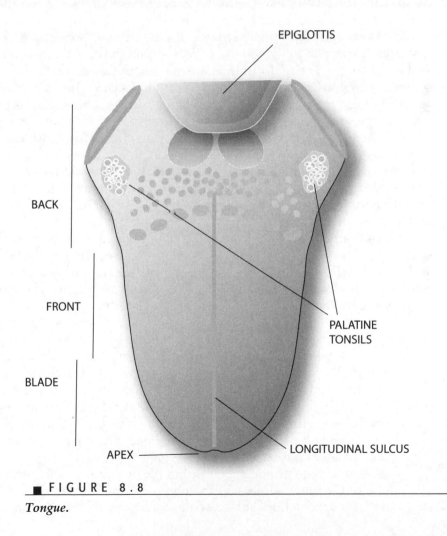

■ FIGURE 8.8

Tongue.

The tongue is an example of a **muscular hydrostat** (Kent, 1997a). This term is applied to muscular organs that do not have a skeleton of cartilage or bone, but provide their own support through muscular contraction. By selectively contracting certain muscles, the muscular hydrostat can make a rigid support for movements of other parts of the tongue (Kent, 1997a). Thus, the tongue can be thought of as consisting of regions that can function semi-independently of each other. The anteriormost portion of the tongue is the *tip*, or *apex*. Just posterior to the tip is the *blade*. The blade is the part of the tongue that lies below the alveolar ridge when it is at rest. The part of the tongue lying just below the hard palate is called the *front*, and the part situated beneath the soft palate is called the *back*. The broad superior surface of the tongue is referred to as the *dorsum*, and the *body* refers to the major mass of the tongue. The root of the tongue attaches to the hyoid bone and extends along the pharynx.

> Two-thirds of the tongue lies within the oral cavity; one-third is located within the pharynx.

The portion of the tongue lying in the pharynx is sometimes called the *base*, and the portion of the tongue surface within the oral cavity is referred to as the *oral tongue*. The oral surface makes up about two-thirds of the total surface of the tongue. The other third of the tongue surface lies within the pharynx and is also referred to as the pharyngeal surface. These references to oral and pharyngeal surfaces are useful when discussing the tongue's role in swallowing; the other terminology (tip, blade, dorsum) is typically used in discussing the tongue's function in speech production processes.

The tongue is divided into right and left sides by a **median fibrous septum**, which provides the origination for some of the muscles. The **lingual frenulum** (or frenum) is a band of connective tissue joining the inferior tongue and the mandible.

The anatomy of the tongue develops over time, in conjunction with other structures of the vocal tract. The newborn's tongue nearly fills the oral cavity and is oriented primarily in the horizontal plane. The posterior third of the tongue gradually descends into the pharyngeal cavity during the first few years of life and attains its adult size at around age 16.

Muscles of the Tongue   The tongue is suspended by muscles from the roof of the mouth and the base of the skull, attaching also to the inner surface of the mandible, the hyoid bone, and the pharynx. The muscles of the tongue are classified according to whether they are intrinsic (both attachments within the tongue itself) or extrinsic (one attachment in the tongue and one in a structure external to the tongue). The intrinsic muscles (Figure 8.9) are involved in adjusting the fine movements of shape and position, whereas the extrinsic muscles (Figure 8.10) act to move the tongue around to different positions within the oral cavity. The intrinsic muscles of the tongue interact in a complex fashion to produce the rapid, delicate articulations for speech and nonspeech activity (Seikel et al.,

> Intrinsic muscles of the tongue adjust fine movements of shape and position, while extrinsic muscles move the tongue to different positions in the oral cavity.

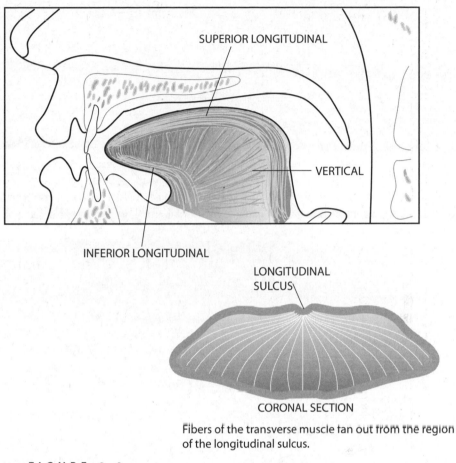

SUPERIOR LONGITUDINAL

VERTICAL

INFERIOR LONGITUDINAL

LONGITUDINAL SULCUS

CORONAL SECTION

Fibers of the transverse muscle fan out from the region of the longitudinal sulcus.

■ FIGURE 8.9

Intrinsic muscles of the tongue.

1997). These muscles are named for the direction that they run within the tongue. The extrinsic muscles move the tongue as a unit and get the tongue into position for articulation. The extrinsic muscles are named for their attachments. Table 8.4 lists the extrinsic and intrinsic muscles.

Tongue Movements for Speech   The tongue is the most important organ of articulation. Because of its muscular structure, you can move your tongue around in an enormous range of ways and at incredibly fast rates. This ability to move in many different ways allows for the wide range of tongue positions and configurations during speech. For instance, according to Hardcastle (1976), the tongue body can move in a horizontal forward-backward plane and in a vertical upward-downward movement. The tip and blade can also move in a horizontal

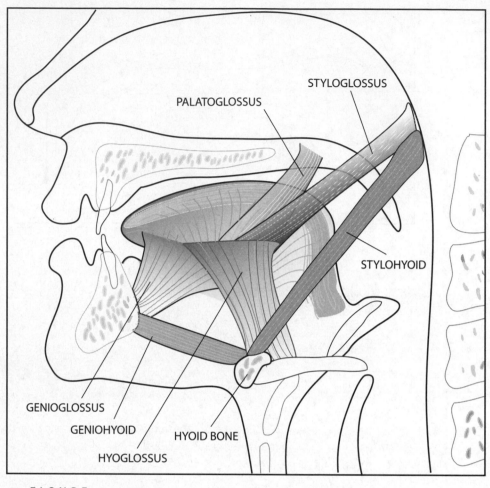

■ FIGURE 8.10

Extrinsic muscles of the tongue.

forward-backward manner, as well as vertically upward and downward. The tongue body can position itself in a convex-concave shape in relation to the palate and can also extend that shape throughout the whole length of the tongue, resulting in a grooving of the central part of the tongue. Finally, the surface area of the tongue dorsum can be spread or tapered.

Speech sounds utilize a combination of these different types of movements. The vowels are motorically the least complex sounds, using primarily horizontal and vertical movements of the tongue body. Alveolar stops /t/ and /d/ involve much more complex movements of the tongue body and tip. Fricatives such as /s/ require even more com-

Because of its complex musculature the tongue is able to achieve a wide range of positions and configurations at extremely rapid rates.

■ TABLE 8.4

Intrinsic and Extrinsic Muscles of the Tongue

MUSCLE	ATTACHMENTS	FUNCTION
Intrinsic		
Superior longitudinal	Hyoid bone and median septum to lateral margins and apex	Elevates tip
Inferior longitudinal	Root of tongue and hyoid bone to apex	Pulls tip down; retracts tongue
Transverse	Median septum to lateral margins in the submucous tissue	Pulls edges toward midline to narrow tongue
Vertical	Mucous membrane of tongue dorsum to lateral and inferior surfaces of tongue	Pulls tongue down
Extrinsic		
Genioglossus	Inner surface of mandible to tip and dorsum of tongue and to hyoid bone	Contraction of anterior fibers retracts tongue; contraction of posterior fibers draws tongue forward
Hyoglossus	Hyoid bone to lateral margins of tongue	Pulls sides of tongue down
Palatoglossus	Front and sides of palatal aponeurosis to lateral margins of posterior tongue	Elevates back of tongue
Styloglossus	Styloid process of temporal bone to lateral margins of tongue	Elevates and retracts tongue

Speech sounds involve different levels of muscular complexity, with the vowels being the least complex and sounds such as /s/ and /r/ being considerably more complex.

plex interactions between the tongue muscles and movements. Understanding the motoric complexity of the /s/ and the many different muscles and movements that are involved in producing the sound helps us to appreciate why so many young children have difficulty with this sound. Similarly, the /r/ sound, because of the muscular dexterity required, is difficult for young children. In fact, it is not uncommon for children to develop the muscular ability to say these sounds properly only at age 7 or 8.

Pharynx

Locations within the pharynx include the nasopharynx, oropharynx, and laryngopharynx.

The pharynx plays a crucial role in many functions, including swallowing, respiration, and speech. In terms of speech, it is particularly important in resonance. The pharynx is a part of the vocal tract that is much more complex than most people think when they look in the mirror and say /a/ to see their throat. The pharynx is a long hollow tube made of muscle, connective tissue, and mucous lining, running behind the nasal cavities, oral cavity, and larynx. It is about 12 cm long and about 4 cm wide at the top end. It narrows, until at its bottom end it is only about 2.5 cm in width (Zemlin, 1998). The portion of the pharynx located behind the nasal

The major muscles of
the pharynx are the
inferior, middle, and
superior pharyngeal
constrictors, which
narrow the pharynx
during swallowing.

cavities is the **nasopharynx**, the section behind the oral cavity is
the **oropharynx**, and the part behind the larynx is known as the
laryngopharynx (see Figure 8.1). The laryngopharynx leads into the
esophagus, posterior to the trachea. This relationship between the laryngopharynx, esophagus, and trachea is extremely important in the development of esophageal speech in the process of voice restoration after
laryngectomy.

Muscles of the Pharynx   The major muscles of the pharynx (Figure 8.11) are
the **pharyngeal constrictors**. These are fan-shaped muscles that overlap one
another rather like shingles (Kent, 1997a). The inferior constrictor is the largest
and strongest of the pharyngeal constrictors. It originates from the sides of the

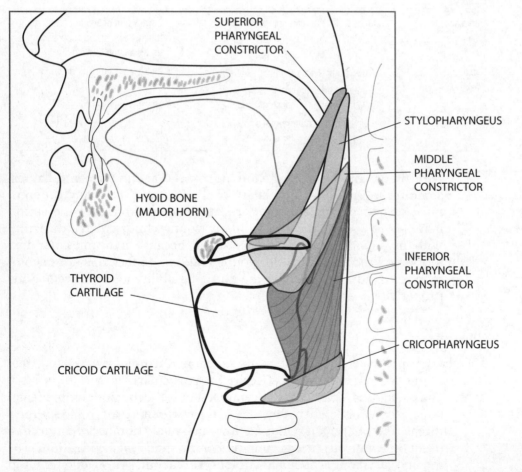

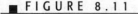 **FIGURE 8.11**

Muscles of the pharynx.

thyroid cartilage and then wraps around the lower to midregions of the pharynx (Kent, 1997a). At the lower margin of the inferior constrictor is another muscle, the **cricopharyngeus**. This muscle arises from the cricoid cartilage and forms a ring around the top opening of the esophagus. The cricopharyngeus muscle is vibrated in esophageal speech, generating the low-pitched sound of esophageal voice.

The middle constrictor extends from the hyoid bone and forms the middle portion of the pharynx. Above the middle constrictor is the superior constrictor. This muscle originates from many locations in and around the soft palate and forms the topmost section of the pharynx. The muscles of the pharynx are closely allied with the tongue, the muscles of the face, and the laryngeal muscles (Seikel et al., 1997). Thus, the pharynx is composed of a complex of muscles that act to constrict the pharynx during swallowing. Other muscles of the pharynx (the stylopharyngeus and salpingopharyngeus) help to elevate and open the pharynx. An important structure located in the lateral walls of the nasopharynx is the auditory tube, which links the pharynx to the middle ear.

Nasal Cavities

The structure of the nasal cavities (Figure 8.12) is surprisingly complex, being formed by the fusion of many of the bones of the skull. The nose is divided into two cavities by the **nasal septum**. The nasal cavities are lined with mucous membrane that has cilia embedded in it. This helps to warm, moisturize, and filter the inhaled air. The nasal cavity is important in the resonating of the nasal sounds in English (/m/, /n/, and /Î/).

Valves of the Vocal Tract

The vocal tract can be conceptualized as a hollow tube that contains a series of valves that regulate the flow of air by opening and closing in various ways (see Figure 8.13). The valves are made up of the articulators, which come together in varying degrees and separate in various manners, thus constricting or obstructing the airstream in specific ways.

There are four such valves in the vocal tract. The first is the **labial valve**, which is formed by the lips. The lips can contact each other completely, come close to each other but not touch, or contact the teeth.

The second is the **lingual valve**, consisting of the tongue. The tongue is an extremely agile and versatile organ, moving around rapidly within and out of the oral cavity, contacting or approximating many different structures to form a variety of different valving positions. For example, the tongue can make full contact with or come very close to the teeth, the alveolar ridge, the hard palate, and the soft palate. The tongue can also protrude outside the oral cavity between the upper and

Valves of the vocal tract include the labial, lingual, velopharyngeal, and laryngeal.

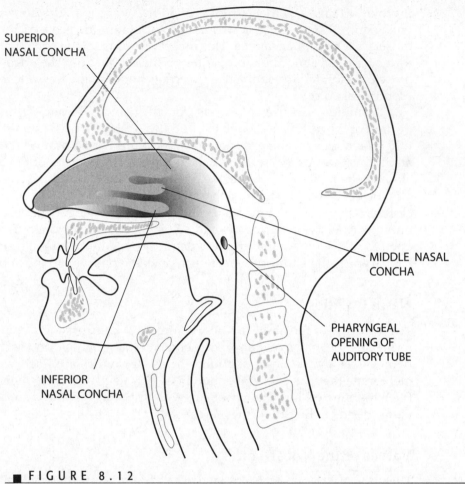

SUPERIOR
NASAL CONCHA

MIDDLE NASAL
CONCHA

PHARYNGEAL
OPENING OF
AUDITORY TUBE

INFERIOR
NASAL CONCHA

■ FIGURE 8.12

Nasal cavities.

lower teeth, forming yet another kind of outlet for airborne sound waves. The
tongue can also change its shape, which also influences the airstream.

The third, the **velopharyngeal valve**, is made up of the velum and the posterior and lateral pharyngeal walls. This valve is of prime importance in directing the flow of air through the appropriate cavity (oral or nasal) for speech
production.

The fourth is the **laryngeal valve**, formed by the vocal folds. This valve
plays a crucial role in the voicing of sounds. Voiced sounds are produced with
vocal fold vibration. For voiceless sounds the valve must be open to allow air
to flow uninterruptedly into the vocal tract.

The sounds of a language are formed by valving the airstream in specific
ways to generate various types of complex periodic and aperiodic sounds. The

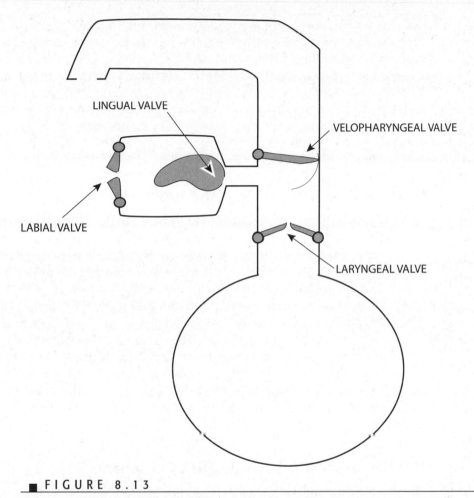

■ FIGURE 8.13

Schematic diagram of valves of the vocal tract involved in regulation of airflow.

way in which the valving occurs and the location within the vocal tract where it occurs form the basis of a classification system for consonants and vowels.

Traditional Classification System of Consonants and Vowels

The consonants of a language are typically classified according to three major dimensions, the **manner of articulation**, **place of articulation**, and **voicing**. Manner of articulation refers to the specific way in which the articulators relate to each other to regulate the flow of air through the oral and nasal cavities.

Place of articulation refers to the location within the vocal tract where the articulators involved in forming the sound contact or approximate each other. Voicing refers to the vibration, or lack of vibration, accompanying the sound. These elements form the traditional classification system for consonants.

The vowels, in this system, are not categorized according to manner, place, and voicing, but primarily according to the position of the tongue body in the oral cavity. For vowels, the tongue body may be positioned higher or lower in the oral cavity, as well as more anteriorly or posteriorly within the oral cavity.

Place of Articulation of English Consonants

There are seven places of articulation in English. In the *bilabial* place the lips either close completely or come close to each other in order to shape the sound wave. In the *labiodental* place the contact occurs between the lips and teeth. In English, typically the meeting is between the upper front teeth and the lower lip. In the *interdental* or *linguadental* place the tongue is positioned between the upper and lower teeth. The *lingualveolar* place (often just called alveolar) is formed by the tongue tip touching or coming close to the alveolar ridge. The *linguapalatal* or palatal place results from the tongue touching or coming close to the hard palate. In the *linguavelar* (velar) place the back of the tongue touches or comes close to the velum. Finally, the *glottal* place is located between the vocal folds when they narrow slightly (but not close enough to vibrate) in the production of a sound.

There are seven primary places of articulation in English: bilabial, labiodental, linguadental, alveolar, palatal, velar, and glottal.

Manner of Articulation of English Consonants

There are six manners of articulation in English, including stops, fricatives, affricates, nasals, glides, and liquids.

Stops   Stops, or plosives, as they are also known, are made when two articulators contact each other and momentarily block the flow of air through the oral cavity. Just behind the blockage oral air pressure (P_{oral}) builds up and is then released explosively when the blockage is released (hence the term plosive). The burst of air that is released is perceived as the stop sound. To generate the high P_{oral}, the velopharyngeal valve must be closed so that air is prevented from exiting through the nasal cavities. For example, the /p/ sound is made by touching the two lips to each other, causing P_{oral} to be built up behind the lips. When you open the lips, the air is forced out in a quick rush, and only then is the sound perceived. See Figure 8.14.

The six manners of articulation in English include stops, fricatives, affricates, nasals, glides, and liquids.

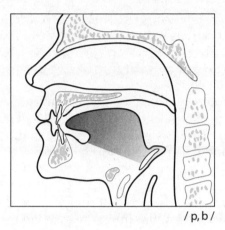

/ p, b /

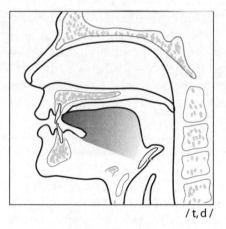

/ t, d /

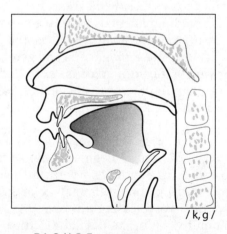

/ k, g /

■ FIGURE 8.14

Tongue position for stops.

There are six stops in English, three voiced and three voiceless, made at three different locations within the vocal tract. Places of articulation are bilabial (/p/, /b/), alveolar (/t/, /d/), in which the tongue tip contacts the alveolar ridge, and velar (/k/, /g/), in which the back of the tongue touches the velum.

The muscles involved in producing stops include the levator veli palatini and the pharyngeal constrictors to raise the velum, the orbicularis oris and other facial muscles for /p/ and /b/, the superior longitudinal muscle for /t/ and /d/, and the styloglossus and palatoglossus for the /k/ and /g/ (Borden et al., 1994).

Fricatives   Fricatives occur when air is forced through a narrow channel somewhere within the oral cavity under high pressure (see Figure 8.15). The narrow channel is formed when two articulators come close to each other, but do not touch. For instance, the /s/ sound is made by bringing the tongue tip and blade close to the alveolar ridge and grooving the center of the tongue by holding the sides slightly upward. Pressurized air is forced through this groove, causing a hissing sound to escape. The velopharyngeal valve is closed to prevent communication between the oral and nasal cavities, allowing high P_{oral} to be built up and released through the channel.

There are nine fricatives in English, five voiceless and four voiced: interdental /θ/ and /ð/, labiodental /f/ and /v/, alveolar /s/ and /z/, palatal /ʃ/ and /ʒ/, and glottal /h/.

The muscles involved in producing fricatives depend on the place of articulation. As with stops, the velum is raised by the levator veli palatini and the pharyngeal constrictors. The labiodental fricatives require contraction of several muscles in the lower part of the face, especially the inferior orbicularis oris. Various tongue muscles are active for linguadentals, with the superior longitudinal muscle playing a primary role. For alveolar fricatives, the muscles of the jaw and tongue are used, particularly the genioglossus and geniohyoid. For the glottal /h/ sound, the narrowing of the vocal folds is controlled by the laryngeal adductors and abductors, while the vocal tract takes the shape of whatever vowel is to follow (Borden et al., 1994).

Affricates   The two affricates in English are made by combining features of stops and fricatives. The sound begins its life as a stop, but changes in midstream to end up as a fricative. For the affricate /t/, the tongue first positions itself in the manner of the alveolar stop /t/ and P_{oral} builds up. However, instead of releasing this pressure explosively, the tongue changes position to that of the palatal /ʃ/ fricative, so the pressurized air is released through the groove. This transition between manners occurs very rapidly, so the resulting /tʃ/ sound is perceived

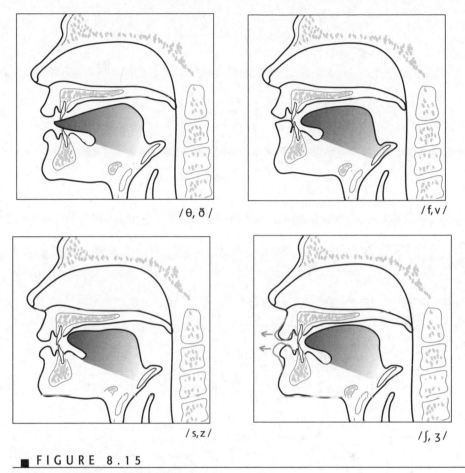

/θ, ð/   /f, v/

/s, z/   /ʃ, ʒ/

Tongue position for fricatives.

not as two separate sounds, but as one unique phoneme. The voiced counterpart of /tʃ/ is /ʤ/, combining the alveolar stop /d/ and the fricative /ʒ/. These sounds are considered to be palatal sounds, because they are released as palatal fricatives, even though they start out as alveolar stops.

For nasal sounds, the velopharyngeal valve is open and the oral cavity is blocked, allowing air to exit through the nasal cavities.

Nasals   Nasals are the only sounds in English that are made by resonating the sound wave in the nasal cavities, rather than the oral cavity (see Figure 8.16). Nasals are similar to stops, in that there is a blockage between two articulators in the vocal tract. The difference is that for nasals the velopharyngeal valve is open. With the oral exit blocked, the outgoing sound wave is forced to exit through the nasal cavities. Oral blockage for the nasals occurs bilabially for /m/, at the alveolar place of articulation for /n/, and at the velar place for /ŋ/. Note that for the

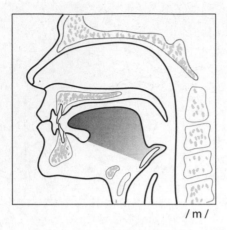

/ m /

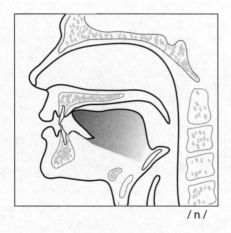

/ n /

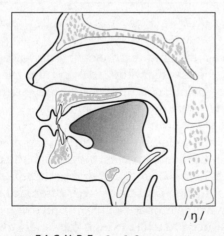

/ ŋ /

■ FIGURE 8.16

Tongue position for nasals.

velar /ŋ/ the velum is still in its relaxed position, with the back of the tongue making contact against it to block the oral cavity.

In terms of muscle activity, the palatoglossus muscle may be used in lowering the soft palate for the nasals, while the levator veli palatini muscle is least active for these nasal sounds (Borden et al., 1994).

Glides   The two English glides, /j/ and /w/, are made on the run, so to speak. The name glide suggests a smooth, flowing movement, and this indeed describes how these sounds are produced, with the tongue shifting smoothly and rapidly from its position for one vowel to a position for another vowel. The glide sound emerges during this shift. Consider the /j/ sound, for example. To produce this sound the tongue starts out high and somewhat forward in the oral cavity, in position for a front vowel, like /i/. The tongue then quickly shifts to the position for a high back vowel, like /u/. We do not actually produce the two vowel sounds on either side of the /j/, but it is during this transition in tongue positions that the /j/ sound emerges. The opposite happens for the /w/ sound, with the tongue rapidly shifting its position from a high back to a high front vowel and the /w/ sound emerging during this quick transition. The lips are often rounded and protruded for the /w/. In terms of place of articulation, /j/ is considered to be palatal, whereas /w/ is considered to be bilabial.

> Glides are formed when the tongue rapidly shifts from the position for a front vowel to the position for a back vowel, or vice versa.

The genioglossus is involved in positioning the tongue for the /j/. For the /w/, the orbicularis oris and other lip muscles are used, as well as the styloglossus to elevate and back the tongue when needed (Borden et al., 1994).

Liquids   It should be noted that some phoneticians do not place liquids in a separate category, but describe them as glides. The term *liquid* is very descriptive, however. Liquids have the property of flowing, so the name of this category of sounds suggests that airflow through the oral cavity is smooth and flowing. For this type of sound, the tongue forms a loose blockage within the oral cavity, allowing air to flow around the blockage and out the mouth. There are two liquids, /l/ and /r/.

> Liquids occur as the tongue forms a loose blockage within the oral cavity and air flows around the sides of the tongue.

For the /l/, the tongue tip contacts the alveolar ridge, but the sides of the tongue are pulled downward, allowing air to flow around the sides of the tongue and out the mouth. The place of articulation for /l/ is the alveolar ridge. For the /r/, the tongue tip is often curled slightly backward (*retroflexed*) and points toward, but does not touch, the hard palate. Tongue position for /r/ can also be "bunched" rather than retroflexed. In either case, air is free to flow around the loose palatal obstruction, exiting through the mouth. The place of articulation for /r/ is palatal.

Since tongue tip position is crucial for the liquids, the superior longitudinal muscle is particularly active. The inferior longitudinal may be more active for /r/ than for /l/, especially if the /r/ is retroflexed. The shaping of the tongue dorsum is probably achieved by the interaction of the vertical and transverse muscles (Borden et al., 1994).

Voicing

In this traditional classification system, consonants are considered to be either voiced or voiceless. Thus, we have a voiced bilabial stop, /b/, and a voiceless bilabial stop, /p/. These two sounds are identical in manner and place of articulation and differ only in their voicing. Pairs of sounds that differ only in voicing are called **cognates**. Other cognates include /t/ and /d/, /s/ and /z/, /f/ and /v/, and others.

> Sounds that have the same manner and place of articulation but differ in their voicing are called cognates.

Thus, any consonant can be uniquely specified by its manner and place of articulation, as well as by its voicing. A voiced alveolar stop, for example, can only refer to the /d/ phoneme, whereas a voiced alveolar fricative must be the /z/. A voiceless palatal fricative is /ʃ/. If you were to classify the /ð/, you would describe it as a voiced interdental fricative, and so on. Figure 8.17 is a chart of English consonants showing manner and place of articulation for each phoneme. For cognates, the voiceless member is placed before the voiced member.

Vowel Classification

In the traditional classification system, vowels are classified primarily according to location of the tongue body within the oral cavity. All vowels are voiced, so there is no need for a separate voicing category. All vowels are produced with a relatively open vocal tract, so there is no need for a separate manner category. Place of articulation does vary for different vowels, in terms of how high or low the tongue body is held within the oral cavity and how advanced or retracted the tongue body is within the oral cavity. *Tongue height* and *tongue advancement* are the two primary dimensions of vowel classification, but other dimensions also play a role in vowel formation, including how tense or relaxed the tongue is and how rounded the lips are; these do not carry as much weight as tongue position.

The vowels are schematized along the two major dimensions in a format called the **vowel quadrilateral** (Figure 8.18), as well as by the tongue positions corresponding to each vowel. This diagram loosely represents the oral cavity.

> The vowel quadrilateral schematizes the anterior-posterior and vertical dimensions of the tongue for different vowels.

The relative vertical position of any phonetic symbol in the quadrilateral represents the position of the highest point of the tongue in the articulation of the vowel that it represents. The relative horizontal position of a phonetic symbol represents the degree of tongue advancement in the oral cavity. In the vertical plane, vowels are classified as *high, mid,* or *low;* in the horizontal plane, vowels are considered to be *front, central,* or *back.* Thus, vowels are classified as high front, or high

	STOPS	FRICATIVES	AFFRICATIVES	NASALS	GLIDES	LIQUIDS
BILABIAL	p / b			m	w	
LABIODENTAL		f / v				
INTERDENTAL		ө / ð				
ALVEOLAR	t / d	s / z		n		l
PALATAL		ʃ / ʒ	tʃ / dʒ		j	r
VELAR	k / g			ŋ		
GLOTTAL		h				

■ FIGURE 8.17

Manner and place of articulation of English consonants.

back, or midfront, or low back, or central, and so on. The highest front vowel is /i/ and the lowest is /æ/. If you produce each front vowel from highest to lowest, you should be able to feel your tongue progressively drop with each sound. The same is true for the back vowels, with /u/ being the highest and /a/ the lowest. The back vowels, in English, tend to be produced with lip rounding, whereas the front vowels are not. If you switch between /i/ and /u/, the highest front vowel and the highest back vowel, you should feel the body of your tongue move from a relatively anterior position for the /i/ to a

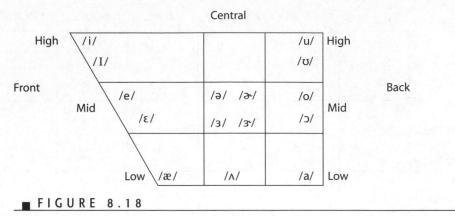

■ **FIGURE 8.18**

Vowel quadrilateral.

more posterior position for the /u/. The central vowels, such as the schwa, are made with the tongue in a neutral position within the vocal tract. This tongue position is extremely important in vocal tract resonance.

■ *Vocal Tract Resonance*

Human anatomy is uniquely suited to producing a wide variety of different sounds. The amazing capacity of our species to produce a range of sounds completely outside the scope of any other species is due to the distinct and unique evolution of the human vocal tract. Our ancestral species, such as *Homo erectus* and other similar species such as Neanderthals, did not possess a vocal tract like ours. The vocal tracts of these species were much shorter, with the larynx positioned much higher in the neck than ours, between the first and third cervical vertebrae. Thus, such species could produce only a limited range of sounds. Only with our own species, *Homo sapiens,* do we find a larynx that is located much lower in the neck (between the fourth and seventh cervical vertebrae). This drop of the larynx resulted in a considerably longer vocal tract. An adult male's vocal tract is approximately 17 cm from the vocal folds to the lips. An adult woman's is about 14 or 15 cm. A very young child's vocal tract is 8 to 9 cm in length and does not have the distinctive right-angled structure seen in adults.

Vocal tract resonance changes depending on the shape of the vocal tract.

Because the vocal tract consists of all the structures of the pharynx, oral, and nasal cavities, it has an extraordinary capacity to change and vary its shape. Every time you move your tongue to a different position, or raise or lower your velum, or open or close your lips and jaw, you change the shape of your vocal tract. This ability to vary the shape of the vocal tract is what allows the wide range of different speech sounds to be generated.

Characteristics of the Vocal Tract Resonator

The vocal tract, basically a tube filled with air, is an acoustic resonator. Therefore, it acts as a filter to selectively transmit frequencies through it, frequencies produced either by the larynx or within the vocal tract itself. The vocal tract falls into a particular category of resonators because of its physical characteristics. Three characteristics are of prime importance.

First, the vocal tract can be thought of as a tube that is closed at one end (at the glottis) and open at the other end (the lips). A tube open at one end and closed at the other is known as a **quarter-wave resonator**.

Second, because the vocal tract is very complex in its shape, it can be thought of as a series of air-filled containers hooked up to each other. Each container acts as a band-pass filter to transmit certain frequencies within its bandwidth and to attenuate frequencies outside its bandwidth. Each container, therefore, has its own resonating frequency (RF), and the overall RF of all these hooked-up containers together is different from each of the single containers. In addition, the irregular shape of the vocal tract makes it a broadly tuned resonator that transmits a wide range of frequencies around each RF.

The vocal tract is a quarter-wave resonator that responds at multiple resonant frequencies known as formants.

Thus, unlike a symmetrical tube, the vocal tract resonates not only at one RF, but at numerous RFs. Also, because the vocal tract is a quarter-wave resonator, the other RFs are *odd-number multiples* of the lowest RF. The lowest RF at which a quarter-wave system resonates has a wavelength that is four times the length of the tube. An adult male's vocal tract is about 17 cm long when it is in its neutral position, that is, when the articulators are in position for the midcentral vowel schwa. In this position, the vocal tract has almost the same cross-sectional width throughout. The wavelength of the lowest RF at which the air within this tube would vibrate maximally would be 4×17 cm, that is, 68 cm. The formula to convert wavelength to frequency is frequency = speed of sound divided by wavelength. The speed of sound is around 34,000 cm/s. Dividing 68 into 34,000 yields 500 Hz. Thus, the lowest RF of the male vocal tract when positioned for the schwa is around 500 Hz. Since the higher RFs are odd-number multiples of the lowest, the next resonance is at 1500 Hz, the one above that is at 2500 Hz, then 3500 Hz, 4500 Hz, and so on. These RFs of the vocal tract are commonly called **formants**.

The third characteristic of the vocal tract is that it is a **variable resonator** whose frequency response changes depending on its shape. Each time you move your articulators into position for a different sound, the formants of the vocal tract change, because the cross-sectional diameter of the different cavities changes. The tube becomes more constricted in some areas and more open in other areas. The different areas of the cavity sizes then resonate at different frequencies. Figure 8.19 shows different vocal tract constrictions and cross-sectional widths when producing the /i/ and /m/ compared with the schwa.

Because the vocal tract can assume different shapes it acts as a variable resonator with changing formant frequencies.

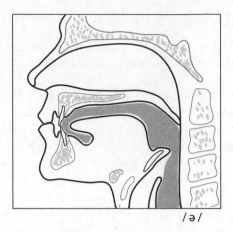

/ə/

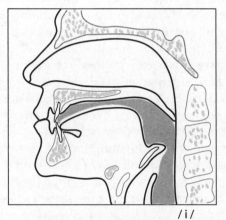

/i/

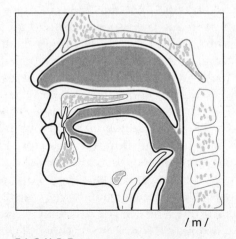

/m/

■ FIGURE 8.19

Vocal tract as a variable acoustic resonator.

The three lowest frequency formants are important in speech production and are numbered F_1, F_2, and F_3.

Changing tongue position from the neutral schwa to the position for a different vowel raises or lowers the formants from 500, 1500, and 2500 Hz to other resonant frequencies. Like any resonator, the vocal tract will resonate more strongly to the harmonic frequencies of the glottal sound that are within its bandwidth. Frequencies outside the band-pass filters of the vocal tract will be attenuated.

The vocal tract has very many RFs. However, because most of the acoustic energy generated by the vocal folds is at frequencies below about 5000 Hz, typically only the first three formants are considered in speech production. The formants are numbered formant 1 (F_1), formant 2 (F_2), and formant 3 (F_3). F_1 is always the lowest in frequency and is usually the most intense.

Vocal Tract Filtering of the Glottal Sound Wave

Recall that the sound produced at the larynx consists of a fundamental frequency that corresponds to the frequency of vocal fold vibration and many harmonics that decrease in intensity as they increase in frequency, at a rate of 12 dB/octave. An adult male's vocal tract in its neutral position for the schwa vowel has formants at 500, 1500, and 2500 Hz. As the sound wave produced at the glottis travels through the vocal tract, the harmonics that are close to any of the RFs and that lie between the upper and lower cutoff frequencies are amplified, and those beyond the cutoff frequencies are attenuated. The vocal tract is a broadly tuned resonator, so the bandwidth of each formant is relatively wide, and many frequencies that are reasonably close to an RF will be resonated. The sound that emerges from this filtering system has the same F_0 and harmonics as the glottal sound. What has changed are the amplitudes of the harmonics: Some harmonics have been amplified and transmitted through the system, while others have been damped. Thus, it is the quality of the sound that has changed from its initial creation at the glottis to its emergence at the lips.

Source-Filter Theory of Vowel Production   The manner in which the vocal tract filters the glottal sound is formalized in the **source-filter theory** of vowel production, proposed by the Swedish scientist Gunnar Fant in the 1960s. The theory takes the three elements involved in vowel production—the glottal sound, the vocal tract resonator, and the sound at the lips—and represents them on three spectra (see Figure 8.20).

The source-filter theory explains how the sound produced at the larynx is modified by changing vocal tract resonances to create different vowels.

The first is the glottal spectrum, showing the sound as it exists at the larynx, before being modified by the filtering properties of the vocal tract. The F_0 has the greatest amplitude, with successively higher harmonics losing amplitude at the rate of 12 dB/octave. Acoustic energy up to around 5000 Hz is present. If it were possible to hear this sound, you would perceive it somewhat like a low-intensity buzz, and not at all like any vowel sound that you are used to hearing. This first spectrum

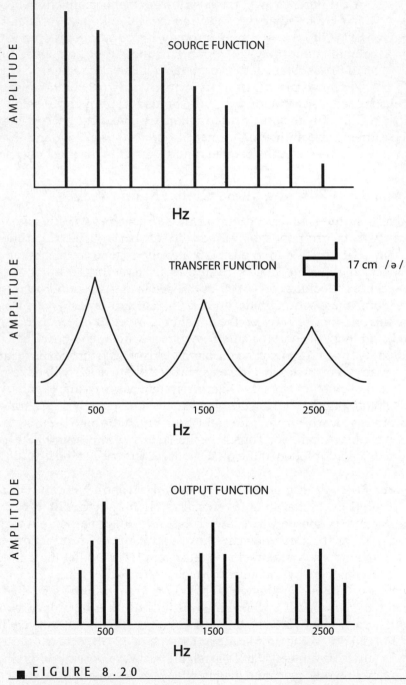

Source-filter theory.

is known as the *source function,* because the glottis is the source of the vowel sound.

The second graph does not represent a sound, but is a resonance curve representing the frequency response of the adult male vocal tract positioned for the schwa vowel, with resonances at 500, 1500, and 2500 Hz. This is known as the *transfer function.*

The third spectrum reflects the sound when it emerges at the lips, the sound output, called the *output function.* In this spectrum the glottal sound has been filtered according to the frequency response of the vocal tract. The same F_0 and harmonics are present in the output as in the glottal source, but the amplitudes of the harmonics have been modified, resulting in a specific sound quality.

These three spectra clearly illustrate how the sound generated by the vocal folds is modified by the resonances of the vocal tract. This theory shows graphically that when an adult male puts his articulators in position for the schwa vowel the sound that emerges from his lips is characterized acoustically by the first three formants of 500, 1500, and 2500 Hz. Perceptually, what is heard is the schwa sound.

The source-filter theory also takes into account the effect that occurs when the sound traveling through the vocal tract is radiated beyond the mouth into the atmosphere. This effect is called the **radiation characteristic** and has to do with the mouth acting like a high-pass filter when it is coupled to the atmosphere. This aspect of the source-filter theory is generally not emphasized to the same degree as the other elements of the theory.

Formant Frequencies Related to Oral and Pharyngeal Volumes   As we have seen, the source-filter theory is based on a male's vocal tract in its position for the schwa vowel, with a relatively constant cross section. In this position the oral and pharyngeal areas, that is, the cavities in front of and behind the constriction in the vocal tract, are equivalent in terms of volume. For the other vowels the vocal tract must change its shape in order to change the formants of the vocal tract. When the vocal tract changes in shape, the relationship between the oral and pharyngeal spaces changes as well. The formant frequencies are related to the volumes of the oral and pharyngeal spaces, because containers of air will resonate at particular frequencies depending on their volume. In general, containers with a larger volume will resonate at lower frequencies, and those with a smaller volume will resonate at higher frequencies. You can hear this by flicking your finger on a bottle or glass. The larger the bottle (the greater volume of air it contains), the lower the pitch of the sound that is heard, and vice versa.

The frequency of F_1 is related to the volume of the pharyngeal cavity as well as to how tightly the vocal tract is constricted. F_2 frequency is related to the length of the oral cavity. These volumes can be changed

Margin notes:

The three elements of the source-filter theory are the source function (the glottal spectrum or laryngeal tone), the transfer function (vocal tract resonant response), and the output function (sound exiting the oral cavity).

F_1 frequency depends on the volume of the pharyngeal cavity: the higher the vowel, the lower the F_1.

F_2 frequency is related to the length of the oral cavity: Back vowels have a lower F_2, and front vowels have a higher F_2.

by moving your tongue to different positions. If you raise your tongue toward your palate, as you would for the high front vowel /i/, you enlarge the pharyngeal cavity behind the tongue constriction and decrease the volume of the oral cavity in front of the tongue constriction. This means that F_1 will be lower, because the greater volume of the pharyngeal cavity resonates more strongly to lower harmonics. F_2 will be higher due to the shorter length of the oral cavity, with resulting amplification of higher harmonics.

Conversely, if you retract your tongue and lower it toward the floor of your mouth as you would for the low back vowel /a/, you lengthen the oral cavity and decrease the volume of the pharyngeal cavity. In addition, because back vowels are often articulated with lip rounding, the oral cavity is further lengthened. Therefore, F_1 will be higher because the smaller volume of the pharyngeal cavity will strongly resonate the higher harmonics in the glottal sound. F_2 will be lower because the lengthened oral cavity will resonate to the lower harmonics in the glottal sound. Figure 8.21 is a schematic of the ratio of oral to pharyngeal volume, as determined by the location of the tongue, and the resulting formant frequencies.

Thus, the F_1 and F_2 of different vowels vary systematically, depending on tongue height and advancement. It is important to keep in mind that formant frequencies change depending on the length of the vocal tract. The source-filter theory is based on an adult male's vocal tract. However, adult females have a shorter vocal tract than adult males, and children's vocal tracts are very much shorter than adults'. The resonances of a tube or pipe resonator such as the vocal tract are related to its length. The longer the resonator is, the lower its RFs, and vice versa. Therefore, a woman's shorter vocal tract will resonate higher frequencies than a man's, and an infant, with a vocal tract approximately half the length of an adult's, will have RFs of around 1000, 3000, and 5000 Hz for the schwa vowel.

Each different vowel is characterized by a different pattern of formants. Thus, the output spectrum of each vowel is different, because different harmonics in the glottal source have been amplified or attenuated, depending on how the vocal tract resonances have changed.

Consequently, each vowel has a different quality, which we perceive as different sounds. Every time you change tongue position for a different vowel, what you are doing acoustically is shaping the filtering characteristics of the vocal tract resonator. Thus, there is a direct connection between articulation of vowels and the acoustic result of changing the resonant filtering properties of the vocal tract to generate different formant patterns.

An important point to keep in mind is that this shaping of the vocal tract in order to generate particular formants is essentially independent of vocal fold vibration. In other words, the source function and the transfer function are

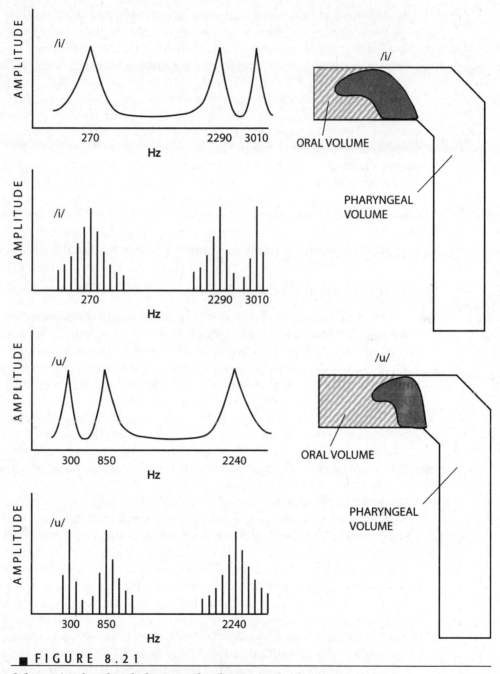

■ FIGURE 8.21

Schematic of oral and pharyngeal volumes.

relatively independent. It is the rate of vocal fold vibration that gives rise to the F_0 of the sound. As we know, the faster you vibrate your vocal folds, the higher the F_0 that results, and vice versa. In addition, the harmonic spacing of the sound wave changes when you change the F_0. But this does not affect your vocal tract. If you are saying the /i/ vowel, no matter what your F_0, your articulators are positioned to generate the formant patterns for /i/. These formants do not change, as long as you keep your tongue in the high front position. If you change your F_0 but keep your tongue positioned for /i/, you have kept the filtering properties of the vocal tract constant, but you have changed the glottal source. On the other hand, you can say /i/ at a particular F_0, perhaps at 150 Hz, and while keeping the F_0 constant, you can change the quality of the sound by moving your tongue to a different position. So you can change tongue position from the /i/ to the /a/ or /u/, while maintaining the same F_0 for all three vowels. In this case, you have kept the source constant, but you have changed the resonance and filtering of the vocal tract.

Vowel Formant Frequencies

Vowels are characterized chiefly by the relationship among the first three formants. This relationship is the major factor in distinguishing between different vowels. In a way, vowels can be thought of as analogous to musical chords. Musical chords typically consist of three or more notes, such as C, E, and G or F, A, and C, and these notes are characteristic of that chord. Each vowel can be thought of as having a corresponding chord that is characteristic of that vowel. This analogy does not hold completely, because the musical chord does not depend on the characteristics of the musician, and vowel formants do. Also, in a musical chord the listener hears all the notes simultaneously, whereas a vowel is perceived as a single note. Nonetheless, this analogy can be a useful way of thinking about the structure of vowels.

Vowels are characterized by different patterns of formants and different qualities.

There are basically three changes in our vocal tract that our articulators can manipulate to change formant frequencies, including the overall length of the vocal tract, the location of a constriction such as a blockage or narrowing along the length of the vocal tract, and the degree of constriction. Constrictions in the vocal tract can result in a lowering of F_1. The tighter the constriction, the more F_1 is lowered. F_2 is lowered by a back tongue constriction, whereas a front tongue constriction will raise the frequency of F_2 and lower the frequency of F_1. Lip protrusion can increase the effective length of the vocal tract by about 1 cm, which will cause a decrease in the frequency of F_1 of about 26 Hz (Zemlin, 1998). In addition, the larynx may be raised or lowered by as much as 2 cm during the production of contextual speech, to increase or decrease the effective length of the vocal tract. This results in a concomitant shift in F_1 by as much as 50 Hz (Zemlin, 1998).

Formant frequencies depend on the length of an individual's vocal tract and typically are lower for adult men and higher for children.

Keep in mind that formant frequencies depend on the length of the individual's vocal tract. Table 8.5 shows clearly that the frequencies of F_1, F_2, and F_3 increase from men's to women's to children's values. What can also be seen from the table is the relationship between vowel height, vowel advancement, and formant frequency. Notice that for the front vowels the highest in the series, /i/, has the lowest F_1. As the tongue decreases in height from /i/ down to /æ/, F_1 increases correspondingly. The same is true for the back vowels. The highest vowel /u/ has the lowest F_1, and the lowest vowel /a/ has the highest F_1. Thus, there is an inverse relationship between F_1 frequency and tongue height: the higher the tongue position, the lower the F_1 frequency, and the lower the tongue position, the higher the F_1 frequency. A high tongue position increases the volume of the pharyngeal cavity, which therefore responds more strongly to lower frequencies in the glottal sound wave. Conversely, a low tongue position enlarges the volume of the oral cavity in front of the tongue constriction, decreasing the volume of the pharyngeal space, which therefore resonates to the higher frequencies in the source. So, high vowels, low F_1; low vowels, high F_1.

■ TABLE 8.5

Formant Values for Adult Men (M), Adult Women (W), and Children (C) for Front, Back, and Central Vowels

	FRONT VOWELS /i/			/I/			/ɛ/			/æ/		
	F_1	F_2	F_3	F_1	F_2	F_3	F_1	F_2	F_3	F_1	F_2	F_3
M	270	2290	3010	390	1990	2550	530	1840	2480	660	1720	2410
W	310	2790	3310	430	2480	3070	610	2330	2990	860	2050	2850
C	370	3200	3730	530	2730	3600	690	2610	3570	1010	2320	3320

	BACK VOWELS /u/			/ʊ/			/ɔ/			/a/		
	F_1	F_2	F_3	F_1	F_2	F_3	F_1	F_2	F_3	F_1	F_2	F_3
M	300	870	2240	440	1020	2240	570	840	2410	730	1090	2440
W	370	950	2670	470	1160	2680	590	920	2710	850	1220	2810
C	430	1170	3260	560	1410	3310	680	1060	3180	1030	1370	3170

	CENTRAL VOWELS /ə/			/ɚ/		
	F_1	F_2	F_3	F_1	F_2	F_3
M	640	1190	2390	490	1350	1690
W	760	1400	2780	500	1640	1960
C	850	1590	3360	560	1820	2160

Source: Peterson & Barney, 1952.

F_2 is related to the length of the oral cavity, that is, the space in front of the tongue constriction for the vowel. The longer the oral cavity is, the lower the frequencies to which it will resonate most effectively. Therefore, F_2 is associated with tongue advancement. Back vowels have a longer distance between the tongue constriction and the lips. Also, back vowels are typically produced with lip rounding, which further elongates the oral cavity. Because of the increased length of the oral cavity in back vowels, they are associated with lower F_2, whereas front vowels, with shorter oral cavities, have higher F_2. Table 8.5 shows that the high front vowel /i/ has the highest F_2, which systematically decreases as tongue height decreases, giving the low front vowel /æ/ the lowest F_2 frequency of the front vowels. However, the lowest F_2 frequency of the front vowels is still higher than the highest F_2 frequency for the back vowels. So, back vowels, low F_2; front vowels, high F_2. In addition to increasing the length of the oral cavity, rounding the lips in back vowels increases the overall length of the vocal tract, resulting in generally lowered formant frequencies for back vowels.

F_1 and F_2 for the central vowels do not follow this systematic pattern relating to tongue height and advancement, but are more evenly spaced, due to the neutral position of the tongue for these vowels.

F_1/F_2 Plots F_1/F_2 *plots* are often used to graph formant information. This kind of plot, or *vowel space*, is a graph with F_1 on the horizontal axis corresponding to tongue height, and F_2 on the vertical axis relating to tongue advancement. You can read the F_1/F_2 chart for a vowel just the same as you would to find the coordinates on any graph, by looking at its position in relation to each axis. The plot in Figure 8.22 shows F_1/F_2 coordinates for the vowels /i/, /a/, /u/, and /æ/ for men, women and children, based on averages determined by Peterson and Barney in 1952. Looking at the /i/ for children, for instance, you can determine its F_1 by going downward and finding its value on the F_1 axis. To obtain its value for F_2, look across to the left at the F_2 axis. A plot like this can be calculated equally as well for individuals as for groups, making it a useful way of comparing individuals' and groups' formant frequency characteristics.

There is considerable variability among speakers in the production of formants. One speaker's F_1/F_2 pattern for a particular vowel may be similar to a different speaker's pattern for a different vowel. The ages and genders of speakers influence their vowel formants. Table 8.5 and Figure 8.22 show that the vowel /a/ can have a F_1 ranging from 730 to 1030 Hz, depending on whether it is produced by an adult male or a young child. Similarly, F_2 ranges for this vowel from about 1090 to 1370 Hz.

F_1/F_2 plots are used to depict an individual's or group's vowel space.

Spectrographic Analysis of Sounds

Spectrography is a method of identifying frequency, amplitude, and duration of sounds. Frequency is displayed on the vertical axis, time is represented on

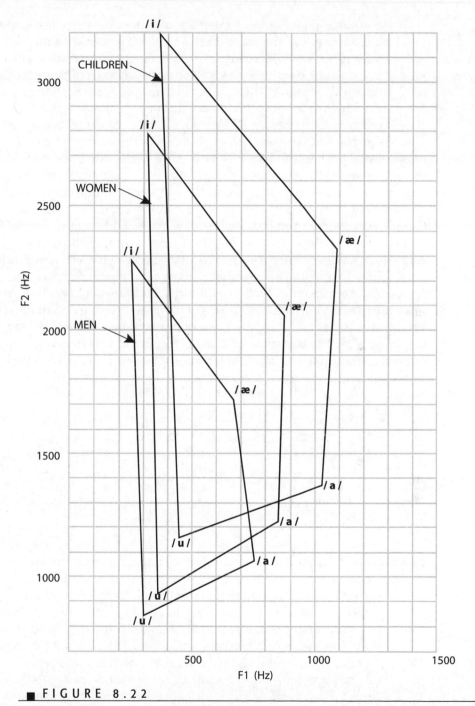

F_1/F_2 *plots for the vowels /i/, /æ/, /u/, and /a/ based on Peterson and Barney (1952) formant data.*

A spectrogram is a visualization of a sound or sounds over time in terms of the amount of acoustic energy at different frequencies.

the horizontal axis, and intensity of acoustic energy is represented by the darkness of the trace on the screen. This kind of display makes it easy to look at the acoustic characteristics of sounds and to see how they change over time. As speech is characterized by rapid changes in the acoustic signal, this kind of visualization is very handy.

The spectrograph has actually been around since the 1940s, but only recently has it become accessible to clinicians as well as researchers, thanks to the explosion of computer technology. Spectrographic analysis used to be a laborious, time-consuming task that was mostly done in university or industrial laboratories. These days, however, spectrographic analysis is used for diagnosis and treatment of many communication disorders in hospitals, university clinics, rehabilitation centers, and the like. Commonly used commercial instruments for spectrography are the Computerized Speech Lab (CSL) and the DSP Sona-Graph, both by Kay Elemetrics. These instruments incorporate microcomputer systems with specialized hardware and software that allows speech to be acquired, analyzed, and displayed on a computer screen as well as auditorily by loudspeakers. The software allows the user to generate waveforms of the speech signal and to measure these waveforms instantaneously by positioning cursors on the screen of the computer monitor. The computer shows the measured values in appropriate units of amplitude and time. Once the waveform has been captured, many different types of analyses can be performed, including spectrography.

Vowels   Spectrographically, vowels are characterized by the first three formants. The formants appear as wide, dark horizontal stripes, reflecting the concentrations of intense acoustic energy at those harmonic frequencies that have been amplified by the vocal tract formants. Because the vocal tract is broadly tuned, many harmonics are amplified near a vocal tract formant, which explains why the bands are so wide. Figure 8.23 shows spectrograms of some vowels.

Diphthongs   A diphthong is a vowel that changes its resonance characteristics during its production. Diphthongs, like vowels, are resonant periodic sounds characterized by their first three formants. Diphthongs are produced by uttering two vowels as one unit. For instance, for the /ai/ diphthong, you put your tongue in the appropriate position for /a/ and quickly shift to the position for /i/. The acoustic result of changing tongue position is that the vocal tract filtering function changes in midstream, resulting in the formants shifting in frequency from the beginning to the end of the sound. These shifts in frequency are called **formant transitions**. Spectrographically, then, diphthongs are characterized by *steady-state formants* at the beginning of the sound, followed by the formant transition, and

Resonant sounds such as vowels, diphthongs, glides, liquids, and nasals are represented spectrographically by their formant patterns.

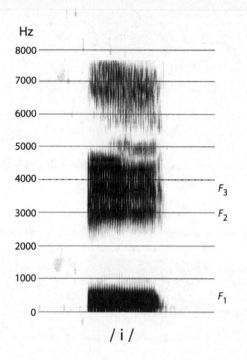

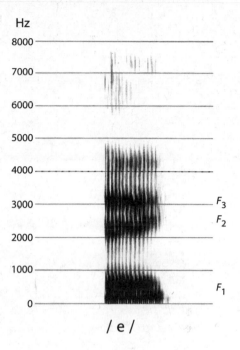

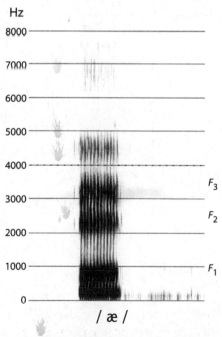

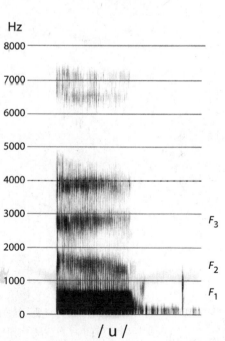

■ FIGURE 8.23

Spectrograms of some vowel sounds.

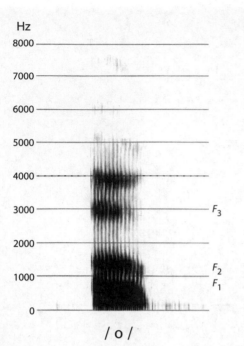

/ o /

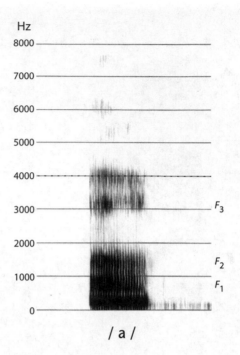

/ a /

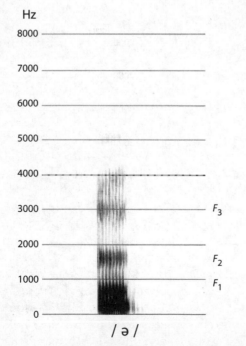

/ ə /

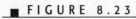 **FIGURE 8.23**

Continued

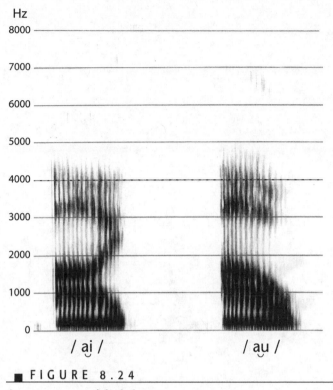

Hz

/ ai̯ /   / au̯ /

■ FIGURE 8.24

Spectrograms of diphthongs.

then another steady-state portion. Figure 8.24 shows a spectrogram of the /ai/ diphthong, which starts out with typical formants for the /a/, with F_1 and F_2 fairly close together and a wide separation between F_2 and F_3. During the transition the frequencies change to those typical for /i/, with a very low F_1 and considerably higher F_2 and F_3. A different pattern of formant transitions is seen for the /au/ diphthong.

Glides   Glides are sometimes classified as semivowels and belong to a class of sounds called **sonorants**. Sonorant sounds are always voiced, and the airflow in this kind of sound is not completely smooth and laminar, but neither is it turbulent. The quick tongue movements that characterize glides result in changing formants. These sounds are therefore characterized by formant transitions that are much more rapid than those of diphthongs. Glides do not show the steady-state portion of the formant that is seen in diphthongs. They are extremely short in duration and often look like little more than a formant transition between two other sounds (see Figure 8.25).

Diphthongs and glides are characterized by formant transitions, which are changes in formant frequency that occur as the vocal tract resonance changes during the sound.

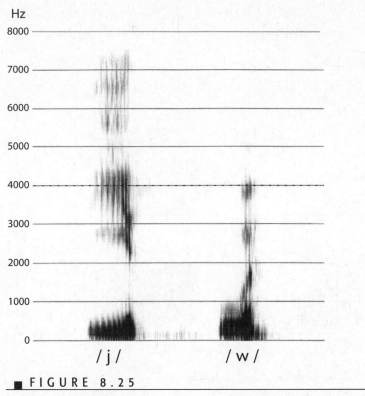

■ FIGURE 8.25

Spectrograms of glides.

The formant transition lasts only for about 75 ms (Pickett, 1999). Typically, the lips are rounded for the /w/, resulting in lower frequencies for all the formants, due to the lengthening of the vocal tract. For both /w/ and /j/, F_1 frequency begins at a very low value, similar to the values for high vowels /i/ and /u/ that form the starting position for the glides. The formants then rise to the F_1 frequency of the following sound. For adult males, F_2 for /w/ starts at around 800 Hz, very close to the average F_2 frequency for /u/; F_2 for /j/ starts at approximately 2200 Hz, also close to the value for /i/. F_3 for /w/ begins at approximately 2200 Hz and that for /j/ at 3000 Hz (Kent, Dembowski, & Lass, 1996). The frequency values for F_2 and F_3 also shift toward the F_2 and F_3 values of the following vowel.

Liquids   The liquids, /r/ and /l/, are also sonorant sounds. They are characterized by more steady-state formants, reflecting the fact that, unlike the glides, these sounds are not made with changing tongue motion. The /r/ sound in English is often retroflexed, with the tongue pointing backward toward the palate. This results in a characteristic lowering of F_3, bringing it close to F_2. F_3 for

The liquid sound /r/ creates a characteristic lowering of F_3.

/r/ is around 1600 Hz, whereas F_3 for vowels ranges between approximately 2200 and 3000 Hz, depending on the specific vowel. The spectrogram in Figure 8.26 shows the steady-state nature of the liquids when they are produced as isolated sounds. The lowering of F_3 for /r/ is clearly seen in the syllables /iri/ and /ili/. Most /r/-colored or **rhotic sounds** show this lowering of F_3. For example, the average F_3 for adult males for the schwa is about 2390 Hz, whereas F_3 for the r-colored version schwar /ɚ/ is about 1690 Hz. F_1 and F_2 for /r/ are similar to those for /l/. The formants for /l/ are approximately 360 Hz for F_1, 1300 Hz for F_2, and 2700 Hz for F_3.

Stops   Like vowels and other sounds, the way in which stops are articulated determines their acoustic characteristics. There are several major differences, though, between stops and vowels. Vowels are always produced by vocal fold vibration, and then the sound wave is filtered through the vocal tract. The vocal tract for vowels and diphthongs is relatively unconstricted, allowing the sound wave to pass through a reasonably wide channel. Glides and liquids are produced with a slightly greater degree of constriction than vowels and also have as their source the periodic glottal vibration.

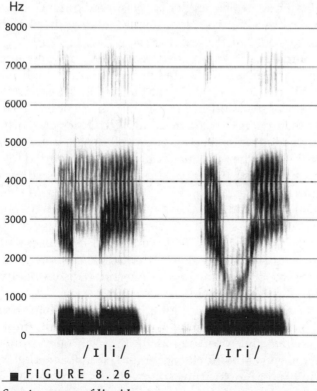

■ FIGURE 8.26

Spectrograms of liquids.

Spectrographic characteristics of stops include the silent gap, release burst, formant transitions, and voice onset time.

Voiced stops include signs of vocal fold vibration such as the voice bar and formants superimposed on the release burst.

The major sound source for stops, on the other hand, is not the nearly periodic vibration of the vocal folds, but the pressurized air forcefully exiting the oral cavity. The manner in which stops are articulated results in four characteristic acoustic features: the **silent gap**, the **release burst**, *formant transitions*, and **voice onset time** (VOT).

The silent gap on a spectrogram reflects the time during which the articulators are forming the blockage and P_{oral} is building up. For a voiceless stop, this interval cannot be seen on the spectrogram. For voiced stops, a band of low-frequency energy, the **voice bar**, is sometimes apparent. The voice bar is an indication that vocal fold vibration is occurring during the articulatory closure and pressure buildup.

The second feature is a burst of aperiodic sound, which follows the silent gap. On the spectrogram in Figure 8.27, you see the burst as a vertical line extending into the high frequencies, representing the broad range of frequencies characteristic of aperiodic sounds. The line is short in duration, because the release of the stop is transient, lasting around 10 to 30 ms. Bursts are usually seen for stops in initial and medial position, but may not occur for stops in final position, which tend to be unreleased in English. Most of the energy in the burst spectrum for /p/ and /b/ is low in frequency, between 500 to 1500 Hz, or else the acoustic energy may be spread out over a wide range of frequencies (see Figure 8.27). The alveolar /t/ and /d/ have a small area in front of the constriction, called the *front cavity*, that acts as a high-pass filter (Pickett, 1999), emphasizing the higher frequency components in the noise source. Alveolar stops therefore have high-intensity and high-frequency energy, around 2500 or 3000 to 4000 Hz (Baken, 1996; Pickett, 1999). The velar /k/ and /g/ have a larger cavity in front of the constriction. This has the effect of concentrating their energy in the midrange of frequencies, around 1500 to 4000 Hz, depending on the tongue position for the following vowel.

Voiceless stops have a greater degree of aspiration than voiced stops; aspiration is noise generated by turbulent airflow.

Keep in mind that these frequencies, like those reported for vowels, are based on male vocal tract acoustics and vary depending on the person's gender and age.

Bilabial stops tend to show a diffuse spectrum, with energy spread out over a wide range of frequencies and more energy in the lower frequencies than in the higher. Alveolars are also diffuse, with energy either increasing toward the higher frequencies or spread out relatively evenly. Velars are compact, with energy concentrated in a relatively narrow frequency region (Ryalls, Baum, & Larouche, 1991).

The bursts of voiceless stops are longer in duration than those of voiced stops, because voiceless stops are also characterized by **aspiration**. Aspiration refers to noise generated by turbulence as air moves through the glottis during the time in which the vocal folds are starting to close for the following voiced sound. The turbulent air moving through the glottis delays vocal fold closure, resulting in a longer burst. Voiced stops do not show this aspiration noise,

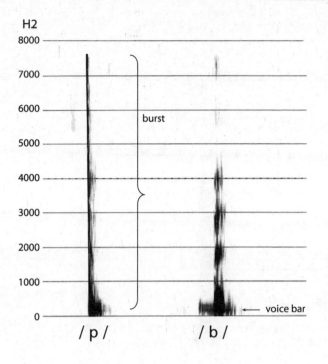

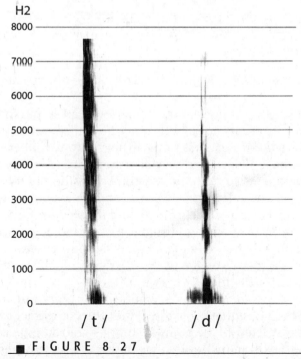

■ FIGURE 8.27

Spectrograms of stops.

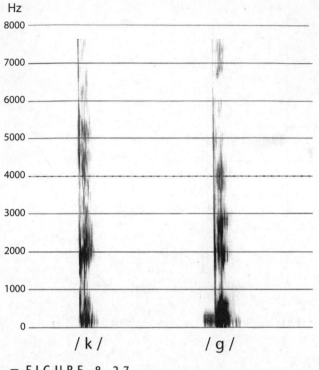

Hz

/ k /   / g /

■ FIGURE 8.27

Continued

because the vocal folds are already closed and vibrating during the initial part of the stop.

The third feature of stops is formant transition. Voiced stops have formants superimposed on the transient noise, reflecting the contribution of voicing to the production of the sound. Voiceless stops do not show any inherent formant structure. However, both voiced and voiceless stops are associated with formants as the articulators move from the constricted position of the stop to the more open position of the following voiced sound. Formant transitions can occur either from a voiced sound occurring before the stop, or from the stop to a following voiced sound, or both, and usually last around 50 ms. The slope of the formant transition—that is, whether it increases, decreases, or does not change in frequency—depends on the place of articulation of the stop and the vocal tract positioning for the following sound.

In general, a very low F_1 frequency signifies that the vocal tract is constricted. The lower the F_1 frequency is, the tighter the vocal tract constriction. Because stops are constricted to the point of complete blockage, the transition for F_1 always starts off extremely low in frequency, close to zero, and therefore always increases in frequency to the appropriate frequency for the following vowel or voiced consonant. No matter what the place of articulation of the stop, F_1 formant transitions are always rising when a stop is followed by a vowel. Similarly, when moving the articulators from a vowel to a stop position, F_1 will decrease in frequency from that of the vowel to almost zero for the stop. Therefore, F_1 transitions always fall in a vowel-to-stop situation.

Frequency of the F_2 transition is related to the length of the oral cavity and therefore reflects the movement of the tongue and lips in a backward–forward direction. This means that F_2 frequency transitions in stops are correlated with place of articulation of the stop. The bilabial stops show F_2 frequency transitions increasing from their starting value of approximately 600 to 800 Hz to the F_2 value for the following vowel. The starting value for the alveolars is about 1800 Hz. A velar stop can be associated with a starting frequency of either about 1300 Hz, if it is followed by a back vowel, or a much higher starting frequency between 2300 and 3000 Hz if it is followed by a front vowel. /k/ is articulated more posteriorly in the oral cavity when followed by a back vowel and more anteri-

Bilabial, alveolar, and velar stops are associated with different F_2 frequency transitions.

orly when followed by a front vowel. Because F_2 is correlated with the length of the oral cavity, the position of the following vowel determines the F_2 frequency for the /k/. When followed by a back vowel, a larger front cavity is created, which therefore resonates lower frequencies; when a front vowel follows the /k/, a smaller front cavity results, which resonates the higher frequencies. These F_2 frequencies are based on the adult male vocal tract and will vary depending on age and gender.

Voice onset time (VOT) refers to the time between the beginning of the stop burst and the onset of vocal fold vibration for the following vowel; VOT can be positive or negative, depending on the timing of the initiation of vocal fold vibration in relation to the burst.

The fourth acoustic aspect of stops is the difference between voiced and voiceless stops, indicated partially by voice onset time (VOT). VOT refers to the time between the release of the articulatory blockage (i.e., the beginning of the burst) to the beginning of vocal fold vibration for the following vowel. This interval of time is measured in milliseconds and is commonly taken as an indication of the coordination between the laryngeal and articulatory systems. VOT is usually measured in initial stops, and its values can fall into one of four categories, depending on the timing between the release of the burst and the onset of vocal fold vibration. The value can be negative, indicating that the vocal folds are vibrating before the articulatory release takes place. This is known as *prevoicing VOT lead* and sometimes occurs for voiced stops. Another category involves simultaneous voicing, in which voice onset and articulatory release occur at the same time, yielding a VOT of zero. The third category includes VOT with a *short lag,* in which the onset of vocal fold vibration follows shortly after the release burst. These latter two categories are common for voiced stops in English. The fourth category includes voiceless stops that typically show a *long lag* time; vocal fold vibration is delayed for a relatively long time after the articulatory release. VOTs for voiced stops range from about −20 ms to about +20 ms. Voiceless stops have longer VOTs that range from about 25 ms to 100 ms. VOT spectrograms are shown in Figure 8.28.

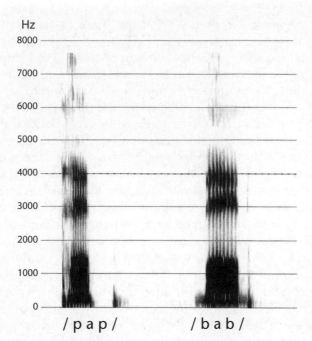

/ p a p /   / b a b /

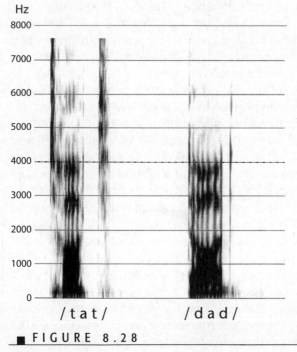

/ t a t /   / d a d /

■ F I G U R E 8 . 2 8

Voice onset time.

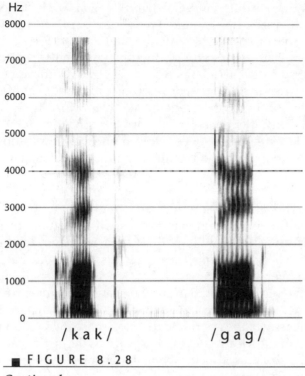

■ FIGURE 8.28

Continued

It has been found that VOT depends on the place of the stop articulation and increases as place of articulation moves backward in the oral cavity. In general, bilabials have the shortest VOTs (including frequent prevoicing), alveolars have intermediate VOTs, and velars have the longest VOTs. VOT is not as important in signaling the voicing distinction in final position as it is in initial position. When the stop occurs in the final position of a word, the duration of the vowel preceding the stop, rather than the consonant itself, is an important acoustic cue for the voiced–voiceless contrast. Vowels are longer before voiced stops and shorter before voiceless stops.

There are other acoustic measures, as well, that help speakers make the distinction between voiced and voiceless stops. For instance, F_0 can help to signal the voicing distinction, because vowels following voiceless stops are associated with a higher F_0 than vowels following voiced stops. Other cues include the presence or absence of voicing during closure; the duration of the silent interval, which is longer for voiceless than for voiced stops; and the strength of the release burst and the presence of aspiration, with voiceless stops showing a stronger burst than voiced stops, as well as aspiration noise.

Other languages have different VOTs from English. For instance, VOT values for /ptk/ in Spanish, Italian, and French are similar to the values for /bdg/ in English. In fact, speakers of Spanish, Italian, and French often sound to English-speaking listeners as though they produce only voiced stops, because none of the stops in these languages is aspirated (Borden et al., 1994). VOT has also been used to document developmental changes in motor control. Young children do not produce voiced and voiceless stops with clearly separated VOT values. Only after the age of 6 years or so (Baken, 1996) do children show a more adult distinction between voiced and voiceless stops. In the elderly population, variability in VOT values is much greater than in younger speakers.

Fricatives   Fricatives are produced when pressurized air becomes turbulent, resulting in random variations in air pressure. The acoustic result of this turbulent flow is noise, called **frication**, that sounds like hissing. On a spectrogram, a fricative looks like a wide band of energy distributed over a broad range of frequencies. The energy in fricatives is much longer in duration than stops, because fricatives are continuous sounds, whereas stops are transient. The specific range of frequencies and the intensity of the aperiodic frication noise depend on the place of articulation of the fricative. In many fricatives the airflow also comes up against an obstacle, such as the teeth, that increases the amplitude of the noise produced at the constriction.

> The turbulent flow of air in a fricative results in noise called frication, depicted spectrographically as a wide band of energy distributed over a broad range of frequencies.

Fricatives are characterized by **white noise**, which is aperiodic sound that has its energy distributed fairly evenly throughout the spectrum. However, this sound is not only produced within the vocal tract, but is also resonated and shaped by the vocal tract as the sound travels through it. Depending on the position of the articulators for production of the fricative, certain frequency ranges in the aperiodic complex sound will be reinforced, and other frequency ranges will be attenuated. This happens because the fricative noise is resonated most strongly in the front cavity, the area in front of the location of the narrow channel that forms the constriction. The size of the front resonating cavity shapes the resulting spectrum, because the smaller the size is, the higher the RF of the cavity. Fricatives that are produced most anteriorly, the /f, v, T, and ð/, do not have much of a front resonating cavity, and so they have a very low-intensity spectrum spread out over a broad range of frequencies. The strongest resonance for /f/ ranges from about 4500 to 7000 Hz and that for /θ/ occurs at around 5000 Hz (Pickett, 1999). For the /f/ and /θ/, the peaks of spectral energy are so high that they essentially do not play much of a part in how these sounds are perceived. See Figure 8.29.

> The spectrum for fricatives depends on place of articulation because fricative noise is resonated most strongly anterior to the articulatory constriction.

For the /s, z, ∫, and ʒ/, it is possible to calculate the RF of the front cavity in the same way as for the resonances of the vocal tract. The front cavity for

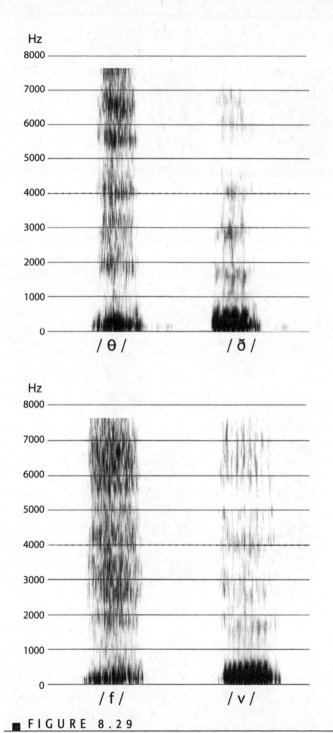

■ FIGURE 8.29

Spectrograms of fricatives.

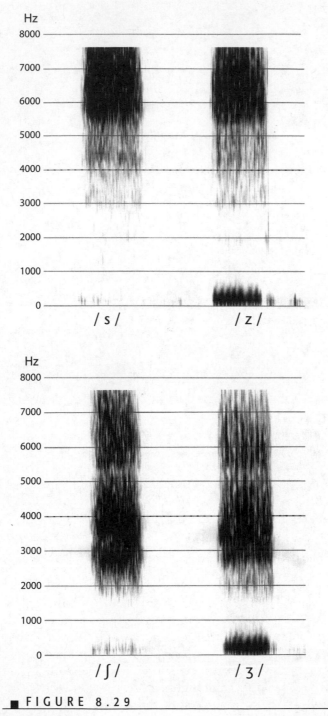

Continued

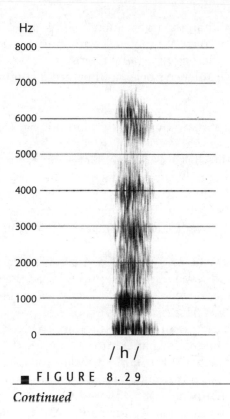

Hz

/ h /

■ FIGURE 8.29

Continued

these sounds is basically a tube open at one end (the lips) and closed at the other (because the constriction behind the front cavity is very small), making it a quarter-wave resonator. The front cavity for the alveolar fricative /s/ has been measured to be around 2.5 cm, so using the formula frequency = velocity divided by wavelength, the lowest RF of the front cavity is 3400 Hz (2.5 cm × 4 = 10 cm; 34,000/10 = 3400 Hz). There are also higher RFs that are odd-number multiples of the lowest, but it is the lowest RF that is most important for the perception of fricative sounds. Thus, the /s/ has its greatest amplitude at these very high frequencies, as can be seen in Figure 8.29.

The palatal fricatives /ʃ/ and /ʒ/ have a longer resonating front cavity than the alveolars, and their major resonant region is therefore lower than that for /s/. In addition, /ʃ/ and /ʒ/ are usually made with lip rounding, which further lengthens the front resonating cavity. You can hear the effects of the lip rounding by saying /ʃ/, first with your lips spread out as if for the /i/ sound, and then with lip rounding. The pitch of the /ʃ/ shifts from higher in the unrounded condition, to lower in the lip-rounded production. Most of the sound energy for /ʃ/ is concentrated around 2000 Hz and above. /s, z, ʃ, ʒ/ are classified as **stridents** and

The alveolar and palatal fricatives have more intense acoustic energy at high frequencies because of the way that they are resonated.

have much more intense energy than the nonstridents, /f, v, θ, ð/. Fricatives can be voiced or voiceless, with voiced cognates showing a voice bar on the spectrogram. Voiced fricatives also have periodic energy from vocal fold vibration superimposed on the turbulence noise, so they are a combination of aperiodic and periodic sound.

Affricates   Affricates are made by quickly combining a stop with a fricative, so the acoustic characteristics of affricates have elements of both stops and fricatives. Affricates have a silent gap associated with the stop part of the sound, but in connected speech this interval is often not really noticeable. Frication noise related to the fricative portion of the affricate follows the silent gap. Fricatives and affricates look very similar on a spectrogram, except that affricates are shorter in duration.

> The coupling of the oral and nasal cavities results in the characteristic nasal spectrogram.

Nasals   The nasals are the three sounds in English that are produced by lowering the velum and resonating the sound wave in the nasal cavities. In acoustic terms, when we lower the velum, we couple the nasal cavities to the rest of the vocal tract, and this produces some interesting acoustic effects. In particular, coupling the oral and nasal cavities introduces **antiresonances** or **antiformants** into the picture. It also introduces an extra formant, the **nasal formant** or **nasal murmur**.

> Acoustic characteristics of nasals include antiresonances and an additional nasal formant.

Antiformants, also known as antiresonances or zeros, are bands of frequencies in which the acoustic energy has been damped. On spectrograms, antiformants look like extremely weak intensity formants. Antiformants occur mainly because the nasal cavities are extremely sound absorbent, due to their soft, moist lining and cilia and their convoluted internal structure. Sound waves traveling through the nasal cavities are therefore damped, at around the frequencies of the antiformants. Antiformants filter frequencies in the exact opposite way to formants. A vocal tract formant amplifies frequencies in its bandwidth and attenuates those outside its cutoff frequencies. An antiformant attenuates frequencies within its bandwidth and amplifies those outside its bandwidth. Nasals are therefore acoustically very complex sounds, because they have both formants and antiformants in their spectrum. The nasal formant is the most intense, while the antiformants are very weak in acoustic energy. The actual frequencies of the antiformants depend on how widely opened the velopharyngeal passage is. The degree of opening changes during a nasal sound, resulting in variable frequency locations of the antiformants. Figure 8.30 shows spectrograms for the nasal sounds.

To produce a nasal sound, the oral cavity is blocked momentarily either at the lips, alveolar ridge, or velum. This oral blockage, in combination with the lowered velum, is what generates the nasal murmur. The nasal murmur consists of extra resonances that are generated because the vocal tract now has two branches leading off the pharynx, instead of just the one branch for oral sounds.

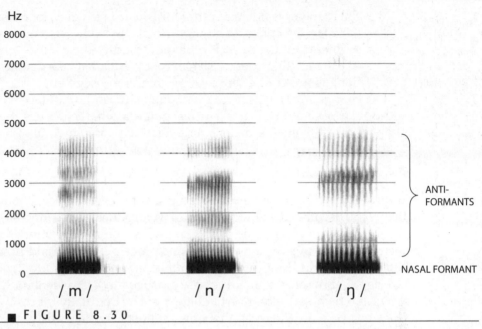

■ FIGURE 8.30

Spectrograms of nasals.

The murmur is strong in low-frequency energy of less than 500 Hz for an adult male. There are energy regions at higher frequencies of the murmur, but these are much weaker than the low-frequency resonance. This high-intensity, low-frequency portion of the murmur is often called the nasal formant. The murmurs for each nasal sound are not exactly alike, but they are very similar. Because the nasal cavities do not change their size or shape for each sound, the resonating characteristics of the nasal cavities remain essentially the same for all the nasal sounds. Nasals have little intensity, because sound energy is absorbed by the mucous lining and cilia in the nasal cavities and also because the sound has a longer way to travel from the larynx to the nasal cavities.

From our discussion it is clear that the acoustic characteristics of speech sounds result from the movement of air through the vocal tract. The way that the air moves, in turn, depends on the actions of the various articulators. The actions of the articulators create variations in the pressures, flows, and resistances within the vocal tract. Speech acoustics, thus, arise from the interaction of articulatory and aerodynamic factors.

The Production of Speech Sounds in Context

So far we have discussed the individual phonemes of speech, the segments of speech that we combine in different sequences to form words and sentences.

Coarticulation occurs when articulators move almost simultaneously in the production of adjacent sounds.

This process is not just a straightforward stringing together of individual speech sounds. As sounds are produced to form words, individual segments influence each other and modify the acoustic characteristics of the resulting sounds. This process is called **coarticulation**. In addition, as we form a sentence by combining segments, we continuously change many aspects of pitch, intensity, and other factors. Changes in these features are known as **suprasegmental** characteristics, because these changes affect many segments over a relatively long interval of time.

Coarticulation

From our discussion of the acoustic nature of vowels and consonants, it would be easy to assume that when we speak we produce each sound singly, moving our articulators precisely in the way described for each sound. This is not, in fact, the case. Speech is a very dynamic process. It is fast and flowing. Rather than each sound being produced in a sequence, sounds are produced in an overlapping manner; that is, they are coarticulated. Coarticulation refers to the ways in which two or more articulators move at virtually the same time to produce two or more different phonemes almost simultaneously.

For example, to say the word *cat,* you do not produce all the articulatory movements with their corresponding acoustic features for the /k/, moving on to the vowel only when the /k/ is completely finished. Likewise, you do not go through the entire process of putting the tongue into its position for the vowel and creating the appropriate resonance characteristics of the vocal tract, and only once this is done, moving on to the /t/.

What actually happens is that the articulatory movements overlap in time. As you are moving the back of your tongue upward to contact the velum for the /k/ sound, the blade of your tongue is simultaneously moving downward for the low front vowel /æ/. Before the vowel is complete, and possibly while the back of your tongue is still contacting the velum for the /k/ sound, you move the tip of your tongue upward to contact the alveolar ridge for the stop /t/. Because the articulatory movements overlap, the resulting acoustic features overlap as well. This is easy to see on a spectrogram, where sounds made in connected speech look somewhat different from the same sounds produced in isolation. See Figure 8.31.

Basically, elements of preceding and following sounds are incorporated in any target sound in the utterance. The effects of coarticulation can be seen in numerous ways. For example, in the word *sue,* the lip rounding that is associated with the back vowel /u/ is already present during production of the /s/. In the word *see,* lip rounding is not seen on the /s/, because the following /i/ vowel is unrounded. Acoustically, the two /s/ sounds have their spectral peaks at slightly different frequency locations because of the influence of the following vowel.

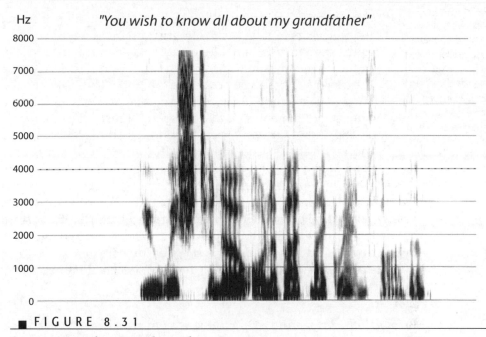

Hz *"You wish to know all about my grandfather"*

■ FIGURE 8.31

Spectrogram of connected speech.

Another example of coarticulation occurs when a preceding vowel is nasalized because of an upcoming nasal consonant. Thus, in the word *thumb,* the /^/ would show spectrographic evidence of nasalization, such as a nasal formant and weak F_1, F_2, and F_3. This nasalization occurs because the velum is already lowering during the vowel production, in anticipation of the following /m/ sound. On the other hand, in the word *thud,* the vowel is not nasalized.

Coarticulation works both ways. That is, an upcoming sound can influence the preceding sound (**backward coarticulation**), as in the preceding examples of the nasalized vowel and the different productions of the /s/ in *sue* and *see*. Preceding sounds can also modify ensuing sounds (**anticipatory coarticulation**). The /a/ in the word *not* would show nasalization effects because of the preceding /n/, whereas such effects would not be seen in the word *dot.* Coarticulation is an important feature of connected speech that makes speech transmission extremely rapid and efficient.

Backward coarticulation refers to an upcoming sound influencing a preceding sound; anticipatory coarticulation occurs when a preceding sound modifies an ensuing sound.

Suprasegmentals

When you speak, you are conveying a lot of information to your listener. Some of the information is carried in the actual words you use, but a lot of the information is carried in the melody, or prosody, of your speech. As you speak, you

Suprasegmental features of speech include intonation, stress, and duration. Intonation refers to the variation in fundamental frequency levels throughout a breath group.

vary your F_0 and intensity levels continuously. For instance, in a sentence such as "I'll be home late tonight," you lower your F_0 at the end of the utterance to signal that this is a declarative sentence, a statement of fact. For a question, speakers typically raise their F_0 at the end, as in the question "You'll be home late tonight?" These F_0 changes are not restricted to a single phoneme or segment, but usually occur over a sequence of phonemes, such as a word, phrase, or sentence.

Speakers also vary their F_0 and intensity levels to express different moods, feelings, and attitudes. If you are feeling exuberant, for instance, you are likely to show much more marked F_0 changes than if you are feeling depressed. In fact, some research suggests that anger is characterized by a faster speech rate, higher average F_0, wider F_0 range, abrupt F_0 changes, and higher intensity and a breathier voice quality. Sadness seems to be associated with a slightly slower speech rate, lower average F_0, narrower F_0 range, downward F_0 inflections, and lower intensity.

The primary suprasegmental features of speech are **intonation**, **stress**, and **duration**.

Intonation   Intonation refers to the way in which speakers vary their F_0 levels to signal linguistic aspects of speech, such as the type of utterance (declarative, question, etc.). This variation in F_0 level is often referred to as the F_0 *contour* or *pitch contour*. English is characterized by a rise–fall F_0 contour for declarative sentences, in which the F_0 starts off at a higher level at the beginning of the utterance and lowers toward the end of the sentence. So, for instance,

> Harry's
>   going
>   home.
> I had eggs
>   for
>   breakfast.

It has been theorized that one of the reasons speakers drop their F_0 at the ends of sentences relates to the physiology of coordinating respiration for speech with phonation. The theory is based on **breath groups**. A breath group refers to a phrase or sentence that is produced on one exhalation. Throughout a typical declarative breath group, subglottal pressure stays fairly steady until the last portion of the utterance, when it drops. As P_s drops, so does F_0. For a question, which is marked by a rising F_0 at the end of the utterance, the speaker must increase the tension on the vocal folds by muscular action to counteract the drop in P_s that occurs naturally at the end of the breath group. The F_0 for declarative utterances seems to start at a wide variety of F_0, but the endpoints typically fall to around the same frequency (Borden et al., 1994). Thus, a pattern of falling F_0 seems to result from the natural functioning of the speech subsystems, but we can override the system for linguistic purposes.

Intonation patterns can be displayed on instruments such as the CSL and the Visi-Pitch. The Visi-Pitch and CSL have programs that track F_0 over time and show graphically the changes in F_0 in an utterance. Figure 8.32 is a schematic representation of the F_0 contours of the utterance "Harry's going home" said as a declarative and as a question.

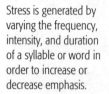

Stress is generated by varying the frequency, intensity, and duration of a syllable or word in order to increase or decrease emphasis.

Stress Stress is another important way of signaling different types of information in an utterance. Stress involves varying the frequency, intensity, and duration of a syllable or word in a way that highlights a particular portion of the utterance. A stressed syllable has a higher F_0, higher intensity, and longer duration than an unstressed syllable, and it is typically the vowel that carries the increased stress. The greater the level of stress is, the higher will be the F_0 and intensity of the vowel, the longer its duration, and vice versa. Stress patterns differ among

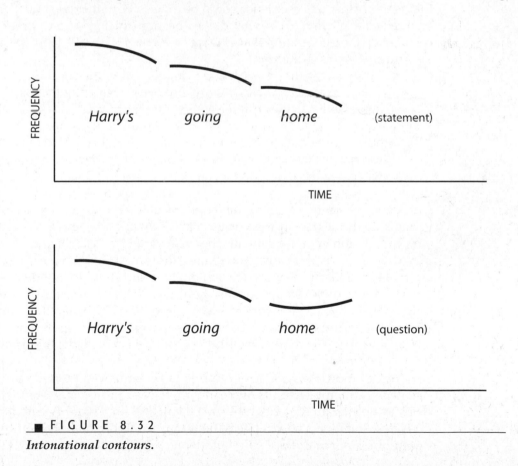

■ FIGURE 8.32

Intonational contours.

languages, and it can be easy to detect a foreign speaker of a language by his or her nonstandard use of stress. For instance, in English, the word *HAMburger* has stress on the first syllable. Someone who stressed the second syllable, *hamBURGer* would be instantly identifiable as a nonnative speaker of English.

Stress also functions on a linguistic level to signal the meaning of a word (called *lexical stress*). For example, the words *PREsent* and *preSENT* have completely different meanings. The first word, with stress on the first syllable, means either a gift or being at a particular place at a particular time. The second word, with stress on the second syllable, means to give. There are many pairs like this in English, or **heteronyms**, in which stress on the first syllable indicates a noun and stress on the second syllable indicates a verb. Some examples include *REcord–reCORD, ADDress–addRESS,* and *IMport–imPORT,* and there are numerous others.

Another function of stress occurs at a discourse (conversational) level when emphasis is placed on the most salient information in an utterance. For example, in the sentence "He sat on a GREEN chair," it is the color of the chair that is important. This sentence could be in answer to the question "Did he sit on a red chair?" On the other hand, the question "Did he sit on a green table?" might elicit the information that "He sat on a green CHAIR." Here it is the type of furniture that is in question.

Vowel reduction occurs when the formant patterns of a vowel become neutralized and shift toward the schwa.

However the stress is used linguistically, the formant patterns of vowels in stressed syllables are clear and distinct, whereas vowels in unstressed syllables often demonstrate more neutral (i.e., more like a schwa) formant frequencies. The term **vowel reduction** is used when the formant patterns of a vowel become neutralized. Vowel reduction is common in the speech of individuals with communication disorders due to deafness, neurological problems, and other causes.

Duration   Duration refers to the length of time of a speech sound. Duration varies with the degree of stress on a syllable or word. However, phonemes also vary in their inherent duration just because of the way in which they are articulated. Stops, for instance, are extremely short in duration, whereas fricatives are longer. Similarly, diphthongs are longer in duration than glides.

The duration of a sound can also be a cue to voicing. In English, vowels are longer when they come before a voiced consonant than when the same vowel precedes a voiceless consonant. Thus, the vowel /I/ is longer in the word *hid* and shorter in the word *hit*. Likewise, the /a/ in *hard* is longer in duration than the /a/ in *heart*.

The duration of a syllable or word in the stream of connected speech is associated with complete units of meaning, such as a phrase or sentence. The last word in a phrase or sentence tends to be longer than it would be in other positions in a sentence, and this helps the listener to figure out the boundaries between phrases. For example, in the utterance "I saw the tree," the word *tree* is fairly long in duration. When the word *tree* occurs in the middle of a sentence, it is shorter in duration, as in the example "I saw a tree being cut down."

These suprasegmental features are vitally important in clarifying the grammatical aspects of speech, in providing an emotional framework for the idea being expressed, and in enhancing the intelligibility of speech. Speech that lacks suprasegmental variation is perceived as flat and uninteresting, and speech in which the suprasegmental aspects are distorted in some way can be very difficult to understand.

s u m m a r y

- The articulatory system includes the vocal tract and the structures within it.
- The articulators act as a series of valves that regulates the flow of air through the vocal tract to produce different speech sounds.
- In the traditional classification system, consonants are categorized according to place of articulation, manner of articulation, and voicing; vowels are classified in terms of tongue height and tongue advancement.

- The vocal tract is a variable quarter-wave resonator with multiple resonant frequencies.
- The source-filter theory explains vowel production in terms of the laryngeal source function, the vocal tract transfer function, and the output function.
- Acoustic characteristics of vowels and consonants depend on their articulation and can be seen on spectrograms.
- Connected speech is characterized by coarticulation and suprasegmentals.

r e v i e w   e x e r c i s e s

1. Compare and contrast the tongue and velum in terms of their structure and function.
2. Discuss the six ways in which consonants are formed in English.
3. Explain why the lowest resonant frequency of an adult male's vocal tract is approximately 500 Hz for the schwa vowel and why a young child's is approximately 1000 Hz.
4. Identify the three spectra in the source-filter theory and explain how each relates to the theory.

5. Explain the relationship of F_1 and F_2 to the oral and pharyngeal spaces of the vocal tract.
6. Describe the articulatory and acoustic similarities and differences between diphthongs, glides, stops, fricatives, and nasals.
7. Explain what is meant by the terms *suprasegmental* and *coarticulation*.

chapter

9

Clinical Application
Breakdowns in Production of Vowels and Consonants

chapter objectives

After reading this chapter, you will

1. Be aware of the relationship of the source-filter theory to problems in speech production.

2. Understand how measures of vowel duration and vowel formants are used to describe dysarthric speech.

3. Appreciate the role of spectral analysis of consonants in dysarthria.

4. Be able to describe segmental and suprasegmental speech production problems in speakers with hearing impairment.

5. Understand the importance of spectrography, palatometry, and glossometry as visual biofeedback for speakers with hearing impairment.

6. Be familiar with spectral analysis of speakers with phonological disorders.

7. Know how acoustic analysis is used to describe speech in tracheotomy and cleft palate.

Correct articulation is a fundamental basis of intelligible speech. Intelligibility is a multidimensional concept, involving the degree of precision of articulation, the person's rate of speech, and factors such as the length of the utterance, the familiarity and predictability of the words used, and the listener's experi-

232

Scaling procedures and identification tasks are perceptual methods of measuring a person's speech intelligibility.

ence with the speaker's speech patterns. Poor or reduced intelligibility due to any of these aspects results in poor communication. Reduced intelligibility can be socially, professionally, and educationally devastating, so improving intelligibility is often one of the most important goals of clinical management.

Intelligibility has been measured perceptually by two kinds of techniques: **scaling procedures**, by which listeners rate the individual's overall speech intelligibility, and **identification tasks**, in which listeners transcribe what the speaker says. These scores are used clinically to evaluate how effectively a patient communicates and to document any changes in the speaker's intelligibility over time. However, they provide little information about the acoustic or phonetic factors responsible for variations in intelligibility scores (Ansel & Kent, 1992). For example, two individuals with exactly the same score or rating on an intelligibility test can have very different articulation errors that contribute to that score. These kinds of ratings usually yield only an overall estimate of a speaker's intelligibility, and it is not possible to determine from this score what the speaker is actually doing in terms of articulation. This makes it difficult to use the score as a starting point for therapy.

By determining exactly how the speaker is articulating, treatment can be geared to the individual's speech production patterns to ensure that therapy is as effective and efficient as possible. Knowledge of the movements of the articulators in producing different sounds and the acoustic consequences of these movements is therefore highly useful clinical information. Acoustic information reflecting articulation function can be used diagnostically to infer how the patient is articulating. It can be used for treatment to help the patient visualize correct and incorrect manners of sound production. And it can be used as a means of monitoring changes in the person's function and progress (or lack of progress) during the course of treatment. This is not only essential information for the clinician and patient, but, in these days of cost consciousness, this kind of documentation of progress is an important way of assuring treatment effectiveness for third-party payers.

Source-Filter Theory and Problems in Speech Production

The source-filter theory provides a way of conceptualizing problems of speech production. Problems can occur either at the source or at the filtering stage of sound production, or at both. Problems at either of these stages would affect the output. Source problems include anything that interferes with vocal fold vibration, resulting in vocal problems such as hoarseness and breathiness. For example, the rigidity of the laryngeal muscles that often occurs in Parkinson's disease is a source problem, affecting vocal fold vibration. The source of the sound may also be within the oral cavity, as occurs for stops, fricatives, and affricates, so source problems in this case would affect articulation and intelligibility. Problems with the filtering and modification of the sound wave created either at the glottis or within the oral cavity result in articulation and intelligibility problems. The output function can be measured in terms of durations of vowels and consonants, vowel formant information, and spectral measures of phonemes.

Dysarthria

Dysarthria is the name for a group of neurological disorders in which the speech musculature is weak, paralyzed, or uncoordinated. Dysarthria often results from stroke, head injury, or progressive neurological diseases such as Parkinson's disease (PD) and amyotrophic lateral sclerosis (ALS). Much research has been done on the acoustic characteristics of the dysarthrias related to these diseases, and this information is very helpful in understanding the underlying articulatory function. Measures such as duration of vowels and consonants, formant frequency information, and spectral analysis of phonemes help to supplement and complement perceptual judgments about the intelligibility of an individual's speech. In addition, such measures can show how a person may be compensating for the impairment. This is clinically vital information, because two people who sound similarly and who score similarly on an intelligibility test can have very different articulatory movements and compensatory strategies, which result in similar perceptual ratings. Clearly, the treatment plan for each individual should target the specific underlying problem.

> Acoustic measures such as vowel duration, formant frequency information, and spectral analysis complement and supplement perceptual evaluations of speech production.

Vowel Duration Measurements   Durations of vowels and consonants have been compared in normal speakers and dysarthric patients as a way of determining if dysarthric speakers have problems with the timing of their articulatory movements. Duration of both vowels and consonants has been found to be longer and more variable in speakers with different types of dysarthrias. For instance, Caruso and Klasner Burton (1987) looked at duration of vowels in speakers with ALS who were perceptually rated 80 to 85 percent intelligible during conversation. The ALS speakers' vowel durations were significantly longer than normal, indicating that these individuals may have weak, slowly moving tongue gestures. These changes in the speed of tongue movement may be an early indication of ALS, before speech is perceived to be distorted. Therefore, these acoustic measurements that reveal timing abnormalities in articulatory function may help in the early detection of this disease.

Similar findings have been reported for speakers with other types of neurological problems (Seddoh et al., 1996). Longer durations of vowels and consonants can also show up as an overall slowing of the rate of speech. Normal speakers typically have a rate around 5 syllables per second. LeDorze et al. (1994) found that their nondisordered speakers had an average rate of 4.7 syllables per second, while the rate for the dysarthric speakers was considerably slower, at an average of 3.1 syllables per second. Figure 9.1 shows spectrograms of a dysarthric speaker saying "You wish to know all about my grandfather." Notice that the durations of all the sounds are considerably longer in the dysarthric speaker's production than in the normal production of the same sentence shown in Figure 8.31.

A dysarthric speaker may have a reduced vowel space, indicating that his or her tongue is not reaching appropriate positions for nonneutral vowels.

Vowel Formant Measurements   Other acoustic analyses measure various aspects of formant frequencies and formant transitions. For instance, F_1/F_2 vowel charts can be created for various vowels (see Figure 8.22). A vowel space results from the plot, and inferences are made about the speaker's tongue movements from the size of the space.

Some dysarthric speakers have been shown to have a reduced vowel space, in which formant values for nonneutral vowels, such as /i/, /a/, and /u/, shift to a more neutralized pattern. This compression of the vowel space indicates that speakers with dysarthria have reduced ranges of F_1 and F_2 frequencies. At the articulatory level, the reduced vowel space indicates that speakers are not reaching appropriate tongue

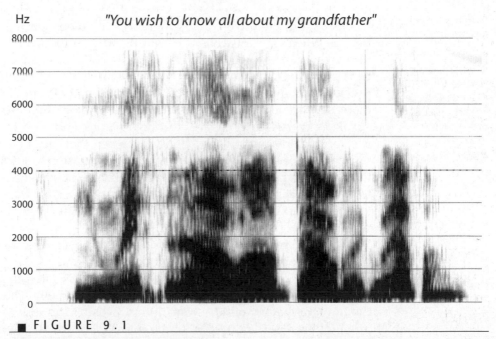

■ FIGURE 9.1

Spectrogram of dysarthric speech.

positions for the nonneutral vowels, but are keeping their tongues closer than normal to the neutral schwa position. An F_1 that is higher or lower in frequency than normal means that the tongue is not achieving the appropriate height for that particular vowel; a higher or lower than normal F_2 frequency indicates that the tongue is too far forward (in the case of a back vowel) or too far back (in the case of a front vowel).

This kind of vowel distortion can have a dramatic impact on speech intelligibility. Using this kind of formant analysis, Ziegler and von Cramon (1983) demonstrated changes in articulatory function over time for speakers with closed head injury and resulting dysarthria. Many of the patients started out being completely mute. In the period immediately following mutism (first eight weeks), some patients showed a marked shift of formants toward the center of the formant chart, particularly for F_2. From eight weeks to six months postinjury, patients showed a gradual widening of vowel spaces, and after six months, there was an appreciable increase in vowel space. Acoustic evidence thus demonstrated the gradual recovery of articulatory function. Specifically, it could be inferred that the patients' tongues became more mobile over time and were better able to reach appropriate positions for different vowels. This information not only provides objective evidence of progress in speech production, but also the specific degree of progress can be documented.

In a similar study, Turner, Tjaden, and Weisner (1995) constructed vowel spaces for speakers with and without amyotrophic lateral sclerosis (ALS). Not only did the dysarthric speakers have a reduced vowel space compared to the normal speakers, but there were also differences in vowel space between the groups when the researchers manipulated rate of speech. When the normal speakers slowed their rate of speech overall, their vowel spaces increased, showing that their tongue movements became even more precise in reaching vowel targets. Perceptually, their intelligibility also increased accordingly. This relationship did not hold for the ALS speakers, whose vowel spaces did not enlarge, and who therefore did not consistently improve intelligibility when they used a slower than normal rate of speech. This is important information to know, because teaching dysarthric speakers to slow their rate of speech is a popular technique for increasing intelligibility. Information about vowel space can be helpful in deciding whether a clinical strategy such as slowing rate is effective for a particular individual.

Another way that formant information has been used to infer articulatory function in people with neurological disorders is by measuring F_2 transitions in various ways. F_2, as we know, is related to place of articulation, because it is linked to tongue advancement. The portion of the formant that contains a transition is measured in terms of its slope (see Figure 9.2). That is, the duration of the transition is measured in milliseconds (ms), and the extent of the transition is measured in hertz (Hz), resulting

Information about vowel space can help a clinician to decide whether a particular strategy, such as slowing speech rate, is effective for a client.

The slope index, measured in Hz per ms, is based on the relationship between F_2 transitions and place of articulation.

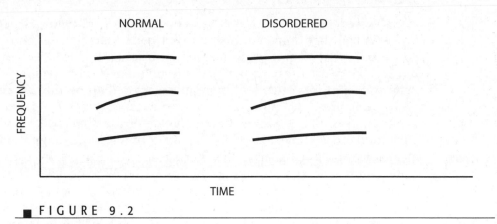

NORMAL   DISORDERED

FREQUENCY

TIME

■ FIGURE 9.2

Formant trajectories.

in a **slope index** measured in hertz per millisecond (Hz/ms). A flatter slope reflects an articulatory movement that is made over a greater period of time. This indicates that tongue movement is slower with less range of movement.

The slope index provides diagnostic information regarding whether tongue movement is close to or far from normal and also provides ongoing information regarding the course of the disease and its effect on speech. Similar to measures of vowel space, information about a patient's formant transitions may also help to detect early signs of the disease, before a decrease in intelligibility can be heard perceptually. Kent et al. (1991) reported that women without any neurological problems have a slope of 3.76 to 5.4 Hz/ms. This is a very steep slope, showing that F_2 frequency changes rapidly within a short period of time as the tongue makes quick adjustments for the particular sound. In fact, a slope of 3.0 Hz/ms seems to be a dividing point between normal speakers and those with ALS, and a slope index of 2.5 Hz/ms appears to distinguish dysarthric patients with good intelligibility from those with poor intelligibility (Kent et al., 1989).

To illustrate how a slope index provides information about underlying articulatory factors, Kent et al. (1991) reported on a woman with ALS who showed a much less steep slope than normal, which became even more shallow as her disease progressed. At the beginning of a two-year interval during which the woman's speech was analyzed, her average slope was 3.17 Hz/ms. By the end of two years, the slope declined by about 40 percent, to 1.32 Hz/ms. The reduced slope reflected the patient's weaker and slower tongue movements and her reduced range of articulatory motion. During the same period, her speech deteriorated perceptually in intelligibility, dropping on an intelligibility word test by about 50 percent.

Weismer, Martin, Kent, and Kent (1992) looked at F_1/F_2 data in normal speakers and in two groups of ALS subjects: those whose speech intelligibility scores exceeded 70 percent and those whose scores were below 70 percent. The ALS speakers had longer transition durations than normal and shallower slopes. In both ALS groups, formant trajectories tended to cluster around 500 and 1500 Hz for many of the words, reflecting vowel centralization. However, some ALS speakers often had more movements than normal for certain formant trajectories. This was particularly true for F_1, which is related to degree of mouth opening, as well as to the volume of the pharyngeal cavity. These aberrations in F_1 trajectories, according to the authors, suggested that the speaker was producing larger than normal jaw movements. In ALS the tongue is often more involved than the jaw or lips, so the ALS speakers may have been compensating for the decreased tongue movement by using more jaw movement to produce the sound.

Analysis of formant trajectories has also been used clinically to document treatment effectiveness. For example, Dromey, Ramig, and Johnson (1995) treated vocal loudness in a man with Parkinson's disease and examined his articulatory movements as his intensity increased throughout treatment. For all the vowels studied, the degree of the frequency change of the F_2 transitions increased, particularly for words containing high front vowels. The authors used this acoustic information to highlight the fact that their vocal intensity treatment was effective in increasing articulatory movement, even though articulation was not a focus of the treatment.

Consonant Measures   Distortion of consonants is another major feature of dysarthric speech and also contributes to poor intelligibility. Many people with dysarthria have particular difficulty in producing fricatives and affricates, which require a high degree of tongue movement precision. Such individuals often also find it difficult to distinguish between place of articulation for fricatives, such as between the palatal /ʃ/ and the alveolar /s/, probably because

Acoustic measures of consonants focus on aspects such as the spectrum of a stop and the duration of frication noise in a fricative.

the lack of precise tongue control makes it hard to maintain the narrow and more anterior tongue position for the /s/. Researchers have reported that the spectrum of the /s/ produced by dysarthric speakers may show lower frequency peaks than normal, indicating a more posterior constriction, a wider or longer constriction, reduced flow through the constriction, or some combination of these factors (Tjaden & Turner, 1997). On the other hand, some dysarthric individuals may not be able to keep the tongue positioned more posteriorly for the /ʃ/, resulting in a spectrum with higher frequency peaks similar to those for /s/.

The duration of the noise interval in fricatives has also been studied for clues to the specific kinds of speech production deficits shown by patients with various types of neurological problems. Harmes et al. (1984) found that the frication noise duration of /s/ and /z/ did not differ between individuals with Broca's aphasia and neurologically intact individuals, showing that the patients with aphasia did not lose control of the timing aspects of fricative pro-

Based on acoustic measures, researchers have found inadequate closure for stops in individuals with Broca's aphasia, multiple sclerosis, and Parkinson's disease.

duction. However, spectral analysis of the friction noise showed that some of the aphasic speakers produced their /s/ sounds with a lower frequency spectrum than the normal speakers. Also, the noise energy was more spread out over a wider range of frequencies than is usual for /s/. Physiologically, the aphasic individuals were producing their /s/ sounds with a more posterior tongue position that was also less tightly grooved.

Spectral analysis of stop consonants has shown similar articulatory problems in the speech of dysarthric individuals. For example, Shinn and Blumstein (1983) found changed spectral characteristics in the alveolar stop /t/ in the individuals with Broca's aphasia whom they tested. If the closure for a stop is not complete due to a lack of articulatory control, there will be a continuous release of pressure, similar to a fricative. Spectrographically, the silent gap that is characteristic of stops is obliterated. Shinn and Blumstein observed a gradual buildup of noise, with no burst corresponding to the release of the blockage. This suggests that the patient with Broca's aphasia never completely closed off his vocal tract for the stop.

Some individuals with multiple sclerosis (MS) show similar inadequate closure for stops, reflected in continuous frication. Speakers with MS in a study by Hartelius, Nord, and Buder (1995) also showed continuous voicing throughout the voiceless stops /p/ and /k/. Also, the stops were nasalized, with a nasal formant occurring during the occlusion of the voiced stop /d/.

The importance of finding out the precise articulatory movements that contribute to reduced intelligibility becomes very clear from a study of speech rate in Parkinson's disease. In most types of dysarthria, speech rate is slowed, but in Parkinson's the speech rate is often perceived as faster than normal. This is known as **accelerated speech**. The increased rate of speech is particularly damaging to intelligibility, and reducing speech rate is often used as a clinical tool.

Ziegler, Hoole, Hartmann, and von Cramon (1988) examined speech rate in patients with PD and found that most of the patients with accelerated speech actually had average rates within or close to the normal range. However, other aspects of their articulation were affected. For instance, they had difficulty in completely stopping sound production during stop closures, demonstrated by the presence of frication noise during the articulatory closures for voiceless stops. They also took a shorter than normal time to switch from an opening movement for a vowel to a closing movement for a consonant, suggesting that the articulators began to close for the consonant before the vowel had been satisfactorily achieved. However, the vowels themselves were normal in duration. Thus, these patients actually showed normal movement times, but the articulators were not reaching their targets within those intervals, a condition called **articulatory undershoot**.

The authors argued that the perceptual impression of faster than normal speech rate must have been based on acoustic cues aside from the actual rate of speech itself, such as the articulatory undershoot. They noted that when normal speakers increase their speech rate, the articulators do not reach their target positions with as much accuracy as they do at slower rates. Therefore, it is likely that articulatory undershoot by a dysarthric speaker with a normal or near normal rate of speech may lead to the impression of an accelerated speech rate. With this kind of information, a clinician can plan treatment to teach the patient with Parkinson's disease to be more precise in reaching articulatory targets. This kind of treatment may be more efficient than teaching the patient to slow down speech that is actually within normal limits for rate. Thus, inferring the articulatory basis for the unintelligible speech helps to understand precisely which aspects of articulation should be targeted in therapy.

Hearing Impairment

Another area that has benefited greatly from a knowledge of the relationships between articulation, aerodynamics, and acoustic output is deafness. Deaf or hearing-impaired individuals typically have a great deal of difficulty with articulation, because normal articulation depends to a large extent on hearing the sounds of the language. Clinical experience and research have shown that hearing-impaired and deaf speakers often have problems with various aspects of speech production, resulting in loss of intelligibility. The range of intelligibility impairment varies from mild to extremely severe. The kind of distortion in speech that is perceived is often labeled *deaf speech,* and it can be very easy to recognize a deaf or hearing-impaired speaker by the sound of his or her speech. Speakers may have difficulty producing vowels and consonants and may also be unable to control the suprasegmental aspects of speech. Some speakers may not be able to coarticulate the speech sounds appropriately and may produce speech as a series of separate phonemes (Tye-Murray, 1987). For example, hearing-impaired children often start to move their articulators in anticipation of an upcoming vowel later than normally hearing children (Waldstein & Baum, 1991). These problems in articulatory coordination may account for many of the intelligibility deficits of some deaf talkers.

Vowel spaces for hearing-impaired and deaf speakers are often reduced, indicating limitations in anterior-posterior and vertical degrees of tongue movements.

Segmental Problems   The most frequent errors in deaf speech are vowel problems, particularly neutralization of vowels. F_1/F_2 charts show marked limitations in both horizontal and vertical degree of tongue movements for vowels in deaf speakers, even those who are intelligible or semi-intelligible. Consonant errors are also common, such as omissions and substitutions involving voicing and manner of articulation. Place of articulation errors also often occur and may be particularly difficult for many individuals with hearing impairment, because of their imprecise tongue position and reduced articulatory movement.

Acoustic analysis shows that speakers with profound hearing impairment produce alveolar and velar stops farther back in the oral cavity than hearing speakers.

Acoustic analysis of phonemes has been helpful in determining how hearing-impaired speakers distort place of articulation. We saw in Chapter 8 that stops produced by normal speakers show different spectra depending on place of articulation. Analysis of the spectra of profoundly hearing-impaired speakers' stop consonants indicates that they produce alveolar and velar stops with the constriction farther back in the vocal tract than normal. This information is clinically applicable, because it suggests a physiologically based starting place for achieving more precise acoustic targets. If a child is distorting consonants by producing them too far back in the vocal tract, treatment can focus on helping the child to bring the articulators to a more forward position for the sound. Also, the effectiveness of this strategy can be checked perceptually and with similar acoustic analysis during the course of treatment.

Suprasegmental Problems Suprasegmental problems are another feature of deaf speech, including inappropriate, excessive, or insufficient variations in F_0 and intensity. For instance, Monsen (1979) tested 3- to 6-year-old severely and profoundly hearing-impaired children imitating words. He examined the duration of the word and the F_0 contour of the word. The children's task was to imitate a word with a smoothly falling, declarative contour. A falling contour should be easy to produce, since F_0 typically decreases as subglottal air pressure falls at the end of the word. However, most of the deaf children did not produce the smoothly falling F_0 contour. Some of the children produced a *flat contour*, and others showed a *changing contour*. In the changing contour pattern the direction of the frequency change appears to be uncontrolled. F_0 may first rise, then fall, then be level, then rise, all over the course of a single syllable. Another suprasegmental problem is that deaf talkers often do not produce enough variation in F_0 to differentiate between declarative versus interrogative utterances. These atypical contour patterns can seriously degrade a speaker's intelligibility.

Deaf speakers tend to have problems with the suprasegmental aspects of speech, including inappropriate, excessive, or inadequate variations in fundamental frequency and intensity.

Many programs for deaf and hearing-impaired speakers focus on improving speech intelligibility as a major part of the program. An important question in many training programs is how much emphasis should be placed on different aspects of speech production to achieve optimal intelligibility. For instance, some programs may focus more on segmental aspects of speech, while others may devote more time and effort to suprasegmental aspects. Acoustic analysis has been used to try to determine whether segmental or suprasegmental aspects of speech production contribute most to improved intelligibility. In an interesting experiment, Maassen and Povel (1985) took speech samples of deaf children and resynthesized them acoustically with correctly produced vowels and consonants. They played the original speech and the resynthesized speech samples to listeners who evaluated the intelligibility of the utterances. Correcting the segments (phonemes) caused a dramatic 50 percent increase in intelligibility, with a major part of the increase resulting from correcting the vowels. The investigators used the same protocol to change the suprasegmental aspects of the speech samples. This also increased intelligibility scores, but only by about 10 percent. The authors advocated focusing on vowel articulation. They proposed that, once the segmental aspects have been improved, work can be done on the suprasegmental aspects to fine-tune the child's intelligibility and naturalness of speech.

Using a different acoustic protocol, Metz, Schiavetti, Samar, and Sitler (1990) also emphasized training children in the segmental aspects of speech production to improve intelligibility. They examined acoustic measures representing both segmental and suprasegmental aspects of speech production. These included VOT, F_2 transitions, difference between F_1 of /i/ and /a/, difference between F_2 of /i/ and /u/, and F_2 change associated with the diphthong /ai/. The suprasegmental aspects included change in F_0 associated with statements and questions, differences in vowel F_0, vowel duration, and vowel intensity between stressed and unstressed syllables, and overall duration of sentences. The deaf speakers' intelligibility was rated by normal hearing listeners. The authors found that the acoustic events related to segmental control were the most important factors in how intelligible the speakers were rated, whereas suprasegmental aspects were secondary.

Instrumentation in Treatment Programs for Deaf Speakers   Speech training programs often emphasize the combination of residual hearing and visual cues to compensate for the individual's hearing loss. Although this kind of training can be helpful in improving speech sounds that are easy to see, such as bilabials, linguadentals, and labiodentals, which are produced in the front of the mouth, less improvement tends to occur for speech sounds that are produced in the middle or back of the mouth, including many vowels. Another disadvantage of relying solely on residual hearing and speechreading cues is that the child does not receive instant feedback about his or her articulatory movements as they occur. This makes it more difficult for the child to associate the articulatory movement with the tactile feedback from the tongue or other articulators, which is an important aspect of learning speech sound production.

Visual feedback from acoustic measures such as spectrograms can be used to train speakers to produce more precise articulatory targets.

Instrumental devices have the advantage of instantaneous visual feedback as the child produces the target sound. For example, Ertmer, Stark, and Karlan (1996) used spectrographic displays to train two 9-year-old children with profound hearing loss to produce vowels. The children were taught to recognize the formants of different vowels and were then shown how to position their tongues to achieve the target. Analysis of the children's formants after treatment demonstrated that they improved their vowel productions.

Similarly, Ertmer and Stark (1995) used spectrograms with a 3-year-old boy who used mainly gestures and signs to communicate. When he did attempt to communicate orally, his utterances usually consisted of isolated vowels or isolated consonant–vowel sequences. The child produced spontaneous utterances in only three contexts: to gain attention, to label objects, and during games and puzzles. However, when he was provided with spectrographic feedback, he vocalized more to see how his sounds changed the visual display. In other words, he learned to become interested in and to explore different sounds, almost like playing a game. In fact, normally hearing babies and young children use this kind of vocal play in learning to associate the way it feels to make a particular sound and the acoustic output of that sound. Because treatment using acoustic visual feedback encourages this kind of self-stimulatory vocal behavior, it allows treatment activities to be spontaneous, play oriented, and child directed. The instrumentation provides the child opportunities to discover the relationship between acoustic output and tactile feedback within the vocal tract and therefore affords much greater opportunity for internalizing the sounds of speech.

Palatometry and Glossometry   While spectrography provides individuals with visual displays of acoustic information, it does not directly correlate with articulatory function. Two recently developed techniques, **palatometry** and **glossometry**, provide direct information about the movements of the articulators. This can be extremely valuable for deaf speakers. A palatometric system consists of electrodes that are mounted on a thin acrylic plate called a **pseudopalate**, which is custom-made to cover the individual's hard palate and upper teeth. A surface electrode is attached to the person's wrist. This electrode generates a small, nonharmful, nondetectable charge. A current flows to the pseudopalate electrodes when the speaker's tongue makes contact with them. The palatometric contacts can be relayed to a video monitor to provide visual feedback of the patterns of contact between the tongue and palate.

Palatometry and glossometry can provide useful clinical information about specific movements and contacts of the tongue and other articulators during speech.

Fletcher, Dagenais, and Crotz-Crosby (1991a) used this method of training with profoundly hearing-impaired, unintelligible girls ages 10 to 16 years. They taught the girls the place and manner of articulation for various stops and fricatives. Through the palatometric display on the video screen, the girls could see exactly where their tongues were making contact on the alveolar ridge and palate and were able to modify their positions as appropriate. This instantaneous visual feedback regarding tongue position was effective in helping the girls become more accurate in reaching articulatory positions, and their intelligibility increased correspondingly.

Palatometry is suitable to train consonants by displaying contact patterns between the tongue and palate. However, for vowels the tongue does not make contact against another articulator. Glossometry is another technique used to visualize tongue positions and shapes anywhere within the oral cavity and can therefore be used for vowel training. As with palatometry, the speaker is fitted with a pseudopalate, which is customized to fit his or her hard palate and upper teeth. Mounted on the pseudopalate are four pairs of light emitting diode (LED) photosensors. Hardware and software outside the speaker's mouth are used to calculate the distance between the sensors and the tongue at 10 ms intervals. These distance values are stored on a hard disk and are also displayed on a video monitor.

Fletcher, Dagenais, and Crotz-Crosby (1991b) used this method to train 4- to 16-year-old profoundly hearing-impaired girls to produce less centralized vowels. The glossometric display provided immediate visual feedback of the vertical location of the girls' tongues in the oral cavity. Using this technology, some of the girls learned to produce more intelligible vowels and expanded their use of the oral space. They showed greater differentiation between vowels, with marked changes in tongue positions and shapes toward normal.

Phonological Disorders

Speech intelligibility is the prime focus in the remediation of phonological disorders. When very young children start learning to produce the phonemes of their language, they very often do not have the sophisticated perception or the fine motor control necessary to produce the sounds in the adult manner. It is very common for young children to use simpler articulatory gestures, known as **phonological processes**, in place of the adult model. The phoneme /k/, for example, requires a high degree of neurological control of the articulators, and many young children find the /t/ sound easier to produce in its place. Substituting a sound with a more anterior place of articulation, such as /t/, for one with a more posterior place of articulation, such as /k/, is called **fronting**; so, for example, the /k/ in *candy* is fronted to /tændi/. Another common phonological process is for the child to omit the final consonant in a word, known as **final consonant deletion**. Thus, *cat* might become /kæ/, or *seat* turns into /si/.

> Children use phonological processes such as fronting and final consonant deletion to simplify the articulatory gestures for more complex sounds.

Children use numerous phonological processes, some more typical of normally developing children and others less so. The use of phonological processes tends to varying degrees to have an effect on children's intelligibility. Most children decrease and eventually eliminate these types of phonological processes as they develop more refined neurological control of perception and production. Some children, however, continue to use phonological processes beyond the usual age of around 3 years and require remediation to develop more intelligible speech. In this case, it is important to find out the extent of the child's knowledge of the sound system of the language.

Acoustic measures are helpful in revealing underlying patterns of difficulty in children with phonological problems, resulting in targeted treatment strategies.

In other words, if a child fronts the /k/ sound to a /t/, is it because he or she does not perceive the /k/ as a unique phoneme distinct from /t/ and therefore does not differentiate between the production of these two sounds? Or does the child actually perceive the contrast between /k/ and /t/, but uses a different way of marking the /k/ sound to differentiate it from the /t/, a way that is not audible to listeners? If this is the case, then the child has what is called *productive knowledge* of the contrast between the sounds. Another example of productive knowledge is a child who seems to omit a final consonant, but who may actually be producing the consonant in a way that is not perceptible to adults. Another child, on the other hand, may indeed completely omit the consonant.

Acoustic measurement has been very helpful in answering these kinds of questions and revealing the underlying patterns of speech difficulty. Acoustic analysis is particularly valuable in differentiating places and manners of production that reveal whether a child has productive knowledge of the target sound. This kind of information is important, because treatment strategies differ for a child who has productive knowledge of a contrast and one who does not. This information can also help to predict how quickly a child will acquire the sound.

For example, Forrest et al. (1990) tested four phonologically disordered children who all fronted /k/, producing /t/ for /k/ in all word positions. Three of the four showed no distinction between the spectra for /k/ and /t/. The remaining child (KR) showed significant distinctions between /t/ and /k/ spectra. Thus, only one of the children made an acoustic distinction between /k/ and /t/. However, this distinction was not the same one made by normally articulating children and did not result in an audible contrast between the sounds. That is, KR's /k/ still sounded perceptually like a /t/, even though it was different acoustically. What was interesting was that treatment for all four of the children focused on sounds other than /k/. However, even though the /k/ sound had not been worked on directly, KR produced it correctly after therapy. This child, who had some knowledge of the velar–alveolar contrast as measured acoustically, acquired /k/ without treatment, whereas the other children did not.

These kinds of inaudible acoustic differences suggest that the child may have a more sophisticated knowledge of the sound system than would be assumed by just doing a phonetic transcription of his or her speech (Tyler, Figurski, & Langsdale, 1993). Furthermore, children with this knowledge seem to respond more quickly to treatment than children who do not show these subtle acoustic differences. Similar research has been done on other phonetic contrasts, such as voiced versus voiceless stops. Using VOT as an indication of voicing, Tyler et al. (1993) showed that of four boys with voicing difficulties three had no significant differences in VOT between voiced and voiceless stops. One boy, however, produced significantly different VOTs for voiced and voiceless sounds, although this distinction could not be detected perceptually. This child required the shortest treatment period to acquire the voicing contrast, whereas the other three boys took much longer.

This kind of information is important, because it can suggest a logical starting point for therapy. Children who show no acoustic differentiation between sounds may benefit from activities designed to enhance their awareness of differences between sounds (e.g., voiced and voiceless and velar versus alveolar). Children who show by acoustically marking a contrast that they do perceive differences could focus more on actual sound production, using phonetic placement cues, minimal pairs activities, and so forth.

In terms of treatment strategies, spectrographic or other visual displays of speech sounds are extraordinarily helpful. They can help the child to perceive visually the differences between sounds that they may have difficulty in perceiving auditorily. The spectrogram can serve as a model against which the child can compare his or her own productions and can be very motivating in terms of checking progress.

Tracheotomy

Medically fragile children are now living longer due to advances in medical technology. Such children often have respiratory problems and must be on ventilators. This requires a tracheotomy, and long-term tracheotomy (longer than six months) is associated with anatomic and physiologic alterations of the speech production mechanism (Kamen & Watson, 1991). For instance, the vocal tract does not undergo normal developmental changes. During the first year of life, the tracheal cannula, that is, the tube that is inserted into the trachea through the stoma created in the child's neck, prevents the larynx from making its developmental descent. The vocal tract, therefore, retains its less mature shape. This in turn limits movement of the tongue, because the tongue body is kept in a retracted position. Two problems arise from the tongue position. One is a reduced number of articulatory movements that the child is able to make, and the second is alteration of the resonance characteristics of the vocal tract.

Long-term tracheotomy during infancy can affect the child's articulation and resonance characteristics.

Some early interventionists believe that long-term tracheotomy does not have a negative impact on subsequent speech production development. However, acoustic analysis based on F_1 and F_2 information has documented the differences in articulatory functioning in children who have had tracheotomies and those who have not. Kamen and Watson (1991) found that children who had had long-term tracheotomies used a reduced vowel space and did not achieve adequate vocal tract opening for /a/. F_1 and F_2 for /i/ were significantly lower for these children, suggesting a less open oral cavity position and less fronting of the tongue. What was striking to the authors was how long these articulatory differences lasted and their impact on overall speech patterns. The problem is that the old patterns of articulatory movement left over from the tracheotomy distort newly acquired speech sounds. The articulatory patterns inferred from acoustic measures indicated that the tracheotomy limited both the quantity and quality of normal speech developmental experiences.

The clinical implications pointed out by the authors highlight the importance of intervention during the period of cannulation. If possible, the child can be fitted with a pediatric speaking valve. A one-way valve is placed in the stoma, so that the child can channel air upward to the larynx to be used for speech. If this is not feasible, the clinician can help the child to develop a more extensive variety of articulatory movements either without voicing or with an electrolarynx. Of course, when the child is decannulated, intensive speech therapy should be a critical part of the child's medical recovery regime.

Cleft Palate

Individuals with cleft palate form another group of speakers who very commonly have articulation problems. Typically, speakers with cleft palate have velopharyngeal problems that contribute to both distortions of resonance and to misarticulations. Consonants that require a buildup of oral pressure, such as stops, fricatives, and affricates, are particularly challenging for many speakers with cleft palate, since intact hard and soft palates are essential to prevent air from escaping through the nasal cavities.

Speakers with clefts often have compensatory patterns of misarticulation that are unique, such as glottal stops and pharyngeal fricatives. These kinds of maladaptive compensations are often very difficult to eliminate or reduce using traditional auditory stimulation types of therapeutic procedures. Visual feedback has been found to be beneficial for some speakers with cleft palates. For example, Michi et al. (1993) compared the use of visual feedback using an electropalatograph versus purely auditory training with children who had had their palates repaired before age 2, but who had not received speech treatment. The palatograph provided feedback regarding tongue and palate contact and the degree of frication produced by the child for the production of fricatives. The children who received this feedback improved very rapidly to almost 100 percent correct level.

> Articulatory problems are common in individuals with cleft palates, and spectrographic or palatographic feedback can be clinically helpful.

The authors noted that, although there are some disadvantages of this system, including its cost and the necessity of customizing a pseudopalate, the numerous advantages outweigh the disadvantages. The advantages include the visual feedback for the child regarding his or her articulatory movements, the objective documentation of progress, the ease with which even young children can understand the feedback, and the speed and effectiveness with which articulatory gains can be achieved.

Clinical Study

Background

Cindy is an 11-year-old girl with ataxic cerebral palsy. She is ambulatory, but uses crutches to increase her sense of stability. Cognitively, Cindy is functioning within the normal range of intelligence and is attending a regular school where she is performing at grade level. Even though Cindy does have a small group of good friends, she is frustrated because her friends and teachers often ask her to repeat herself. As Cindy will soon be entering middle school, she is concerned that the older children will make fun of her speech.

Clinical Observations

Upon reevaluation at the start of fifth grade, Cindy expressed her concerns to you, the school speech pathologist. Cindy has been receiving speech therapy services since kindergarten, and her speech intelligibility is fairly good. However, she still tends to slur some words due to vowel distortion and consonant imprecision, and her prosody in connected speech is noticeably monotone. Consequently, her speech sounds slow and labored. As part of a thorough diagnostic workup, you think it important to establish baselines for vowel duration, overall articulatory rate, and intonation as reflected by pitch variability. You will obtain these measures using the most current version of the Visi-Pitch, which your school has recently purchased.

Acoustic Measures

You tested Cindy's speech patterns in single words, sentences, and structured conversation. On the word level, spectrographic analysis showed that target formant frequencies were within the normal range. Vowel durations fell at the low end of the normal range. At the sentence level, distortions of all articulatory movements became more evident, with slow transitions between sounds and neutralized formant frequencies for all cardinal vowels. Consonant durations were also longer than normal, and stops were intermittently fricated. In addition, the pitch analysis program demonstrated that Cindy's F_0 range in sentences and in connected speech was limited to an average of 56 Hz, considerably lower than the expected range for her age.

Clinical Questions

1. Based on these findings, generate an age-appropriate F_1/F_2 plot for Cindy that will serve as a baseline against which to measure her progress.
2. Develop three goals related to Cindy's speech intelligibility/prosody and provide a rationale for each goal.

3. How might acoustic instrumentation be used to verify that Cindy is achieving the therapeutic objectives?

summary

- Acoustic analysis can provide information about a speaker's articulatory movements.
- Measures of duration of vowels and consonants can distinguish between normal and dysarthric speakers.
- Charts of vowel space can show changes in the speaker's articulatory patterns before and after treatment or over the course of time.
- The slope index reflects tongue movement and can reveal differences between normal and neurologically disordered speakers.
- Spectral analysis of stops and fricatives can reveal distinctions in speakers' articulatory positions.
- Spectral analysis can show how children with hearing impairment produce consonants and vowels and can suggest a physiologically based starting place for intervention.
- Palatometry and glossometry can be valuable aids in achieving more precise articulatory targets for speakers with hearing impairment.
- Productive knowledge in phonologically disordered children can be determined through acoustic analysis of their productions.
- Acoustic analysis shows reduced vowel space in children who received early tracheotomies.
- Visual feedback using palatometry can be helpful in remediating articulatory problems in children with cleft palate.

review exercises

1. Discuss the relevance of the source-filter theory to problems in speech production. Provide an example of a disorder in which the source is affected and one in which the transfer function of the vocal tract is affected.
2. Compare the kind of information obtained from acoustic analysis of vowels and consonants.
3. Describe the slope index and explain how it can help to understand a person's articulatory functioning.
4. Explain the relationship between spectral analysis of stops and fricatives and articulatory positioning in individuals with neurological disorders.
5. Compare the kind of information obtained from a spectrogram, palatogram, and glossogram.
6. What is productive knowledge, and how is this determined in children with phonological disorders?
7. Explain why an early tracheotomy can have a long-term impact on speech production.

The Auditory System

After reading this chapter, you will

1. Be familiar with the structure and function of the outer, middle, and inner ears.
2. Understand the relationship of the basilar membrane in the cochlea and the traveling wave.
3. Appreciate the segmentation problem in speech perception.
4. Be able to explain the acoustic patterns in the perception of vowels and consonants, such as formants, formant transitions, categorical perception, and multiple cues.
5. Be able to describe immittance audiometry and otoacoustic emissions.
6. Understand cochlear implants and different signal-processing strategies used to transmit speech.

We turn our attention now to the perception of speech, an extraordinarily complex process mediated by the auditory system. The auditory system consists of the outer, middle, and inner parts of the ear and the auditory nerve pathway to the brain. In this chapter we focus on the parts of the ear and the role that each plays in detecting and processing sound waves.

Parts of the Ear

The ear acts as a *transducer*. A transducer is a device that converts energy from one form to another. For example, a microphone transduces sound waves into electrical energy. A loudspeaker converts electrical energy into acoustic pressure waves. The ear converts acoustic pressure waves to mechanical energy in the middle ear and mechanical to electrical energy in the inner ear. The ear in some ways can also be likened to a spectrographic analyzer, because the auditory system detects changes in the frequency and intensity of sound waves over time. To understand the transformations of the acoustic signal that take place in the ear, allowing us to perceive sounds, it is important to gain an understanding of the structures involved, including the outer, middle, and inner ears.

The ear acts as a transducer, converting acoustic to other forms of energy, including mechanical and electrical energy.

Outer Ear

Two parts make up the outer ear, the **pinna** and the **external auditory meatus**, or ear canal. The pinna is the external portion on the side of the head, made of flexible elastic cartilage. The pinna is attached to the side of the cranium by ligaments. Although the pinna does contain some muscles, they are vestigial in humans (Dickson & Maue-Dickson, 1982). The main function of the pinna is to help channel sound waves into the ear. It also helps in the localization of sounds and protects the entrance to the external auditory meatus. However, compared to animals, the pinna in humans does not play a particularly important role in sound detection.

The external auditory meatus acts as a quarter-wave resonator that boosts the amplitude of high-frequency sounds entering the ear.

The external auditory meatus leads from the pinna to the eardrum, or *tympanic membrane* (TM) (see Figure 10.1). This meatus is a tube or channel lined with a layer of epithelium and cilia. A waxy substance, the **cerumen**, is produced by glands in the meatus. The cilia move in a wavelike fashion, which helps to propel the cerumen together with small particles of dust or other substances toward the outside. The ear canal has been described as S-shaped in adults and is about 6 mm in diameter and about 2.5 cm long (Kent, 1997a).

The ear canal has several functions. First, it protects the middle and inner ears. Second, the ear canal plays an important part in terms of sound detection, because it is a quarter-wave resonator, open at the pinna and closed at the tympanic membrane. As with any quarter-wave resonator, the lowest resonant frequency (RF) of the canal has a wavelength that is four times the length of the resonator. The lowest RF of the canal is therefore 3400 Hz: $2.5 \times 4 = 10$ cm; $34,000/10 = 3400$ Hz. Due to this high-frequency resonance, the external auditory meatus resonates and boosts the amplitude of high-frequency sounds

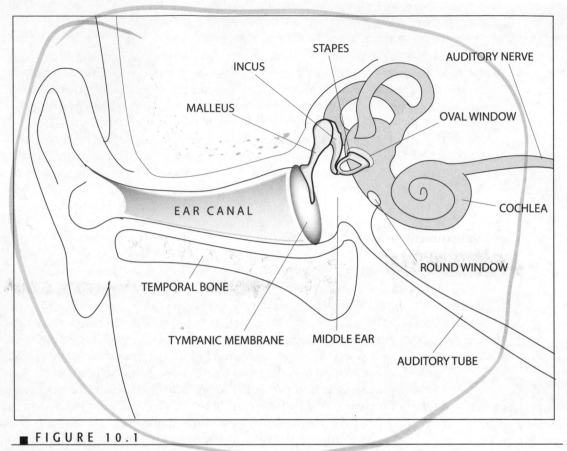

FIGURE 10.1

Outer, middle, and inner ears.

entering the ear. This is helpful for sounds such as /s, z, ʃ, ʒ/, which have much of their acoustic energy in frequencies above 2000 Hz. Together the pinna and ear canal create a broad resonance, resulting in approximately 10 to 15 dB of amplification of the spectrum between 2500 to 5000 Hz (Greenberg, 1996). This increase in high-frequency amplitude enables us to detect sounds that would not otherwise be audible if the TM were located at the surface of the head.

Tympanic Membrane

The tympanic membrane (TM) is a semitransparent, oval-shaped sheet of membrane that acts as a boundary between the outer and middle ears. It is concave on its external surface, giving it a conical shape. The tip of the cone is called the **umbo.** The membrane is held in position by a ligament and is composed of external, middle, and internal layers. The internal layer is mucous

The tympanic membrane is the boundary between the outer and middle ears.

membrane and is continuous with the mucous membrane that lines the cavity of the middle ear. One of the bones of the middle ear, the **malleus**, is embedded in the TM.

The primary function of the tympanic membrane is to vibrate when acoustic pressure waves impinge on it. Because the malleus is embedded within the TM, the vibration of the TM is transmitted to the malleus and to the other two bones in the middle ear. The TM is extremely sensitive to tiny variations in pressure and responds to an extraordinary range of pressures across a wide range of frequencies. Thus, the TM is involved in the process of transducing pressure waves to mechanical vibration.

Middle Ear

Lying directly behind the TM is the middle ear. The middle ear is a tiny space, about 0.6 cm wide and about 0.4 cm deep (Kent, 1997a). This air-filled cavity contains three small bones called the **ossicles**, ligaments holding the ossicles in place, and two muscles.

Ossicles   The three ossicles are the smallest bones in the human body. They are connected to each other, to the TM on one side, and to a part of the ear called the oval window of the inner ear on the other side. The malleus, or hammer, is partly embedded in the TM; the **incus**, or anvil, is connected to the malleus, and the **stapes**, or stirrup, is attached to the incus and to the oval window. The malleus measures about 8 mm in length. It consists of a head and neck and a handle, called the **manubrium**. The manubrium is attached to the TM. The incus is also about 8 mm in length. It has a rounded body from which two processes extend. The stapes has a body, with an anterior and posterior arm converging on it from either side. The oval-shaped footplate of the stapes fits into the oval window of the inner ear. This ossicular chain, as it is sometimes called, is held in place by ligaments and forms the mechanical vibrating element of the auditory system.

Three ossicles in the middle ear cavity connect the tympanic membrane to the oval window of the inner ear.

Muscles   The two muscles of the middle ear are the **stapedius** and the **tensor tympani**. The stapedius muscle is about 6 mm long and runs from the posterior wall of the tympanic cavity to the head of the stapes. The stapedius muscle is involved in a reflex known as the **acoustic** or stapedial **reflex**. This reflex occurs when the stapedius muscle contracts strongly in response to intense sound of 80 dB or more. When the stapedius muscle contracts, it pulls the stapes to one side. This has the effect of reducing the pressure applied to the oval window, which in turn reduces the sound intensity by around 10 dB. The reflex does not occur instantaneously, but takes some fractions of a second to act. Therefore, sounds that occur very suddenly can be transmitted to the inner

The stapedius muscle is involved in the acoustic reflex, which occurs in response to very intense sounds.

ear before the reflex has had time to occur. Also, like any muscle, the stapedius eventually fatigues. Consequently, in a noisy environment, the reflex becomes less effective at damping loud sounds.

The tensor tympani muscle is longer than the stapedius, around 20 mm, and runs parallel to the auditory tube. The tensor tympani originates at the tendon of the tensor veli palatini muscle, passes through a bony canal in the temporal bone of the cranium, emerges into the tympanic cavity, and connects with the manubrium of the malleus. The tensor tympani is involved in auditory tube function. When it pulls on the malleus, the TM is drawn inward. This movement may slightly increase the pressure in the middle ear and auditory tube, which stimulates a contraction of the tensor veli palatini to open the auditory tube.

Auditory Tube   The auditory tube, also called the Eustachian tube, is about 3.5 cm in length. The frontmost two-thirds of the auditory tube lie within a canal made of cartilage, while the posterior one-third lies within a bony canal. The tube runs from the nasopharynx to the middle ear. The pharyngeal opening of the tube is a slit approximately 8 mm in height and 1 mm in width that is usually closed, except when one swallows or yawns, when it opens. The part that connects to the middle ear is normally open. The inside of the tube is lined with epithelium. Where the tube opens into the pharynx, the cartilage is enlarged, creating a bulge in the lateral pharyngeal wall, the **torus tubarius**. The primary muscle that opens the auditory tube is the tensor veli palatini, due to the fact that some of the fibers of this muscle attach to the lateral membranous wall of the auditory tube. When the tensor veli palatini contracts, it pulls the membranous wall laterally, thus opening the tube.

The Eustachian tube acts to drain fluid from the middle ear and to equalize the pressure between the middle ear and the atmosphere.

The auditory tube is extremely important for middle ear function. First, it helps to clear mucus from the middle ear by draining the mucus to the pharynx, where it is swallowed. If mucus is not cleared, it can lead to **otitis media**, that is, middle ear infections. Young children are particularly susceptible to middle ear infections because their auditory tubes run nearly horizontally, so fluids do not drain as easily as they do in adults. Second, the auditory tube acts to equalize the air pressure in the middle ear and in the external atmosphere, because air from the atmosphere enters the middle ear when the tube opens. If anything prevents the tube from opening, this equalization of air pressures becomes difficult or impossible, resulting in middle ear infections.

Functions of the Middle Ear   The middle ear performs several crucial functions in hearing. First, it increases the amount of acoustic energy that gets transmitted into the inner ear by overcoming the **impedance mismatch** between the middle and inner ears. **Impedance** is a measure of how easily signals are transmitted through a medium, such as a gas or liquid. Mediums can offer

The middle ear helps to overcome the impedance mismatch between the middle and inner ears.

Pressure amplification is achieved by the leverage of the ossicles and the difference in surface areas between the tympanic membrane and the oval window.

more or less resistance to sound waves. Liquids have a higher impedance to sound waves than does air. When sound waves traveling through air come to a fluid, the difference in impedance acts as a barrier, and most of the sound energy is therefore reflected, rather than being transmitted. The middle ear is filled with air, whereas the inner ear is filled with fluid. The boundary between these two areas is the oval window. When sound waves propagating through the air in the middle ear come into contact with the fluid in the inner ear, almost all the incident energy is reflected and very little is transmitted to the fluid.

To overcome this impedance mismatch, it is necessary to increase the amplitude of the pressure changes at the oval window. The middle ear achieves this pressure amplification in two ways. First, due to their structure, the ossicles work like a lever that increases the force at the stapes footplate by a factor of about 1.3, or approximately 2 dB, in comparison to the force at the malleus (see Figure 10.2).

The second way in which pressure amplification is achieved relies on the difference in the surface area of the TM compared to the oval window. The area of the TM is about 0.85 cm^2, although only about 0.55 cm^2 is active in vibration. The area of the oval window is about 0.03 cm^2 (Borden et al., 1994). According to Seikel et al. (1997) and Zemlin (1998), this difference in surface area results in a gain of about 17:1. Pressure is equal to force over a surface area, so a given force will exert greater pressure over a smaller area than over a larger one. Therefore, the pressure changes causing vibration of the much larger TM become more intense when they are transmitted by the ossicles to the smaller oval window, yielding an increase of approximately 25 dB (see Figure 10.3). These effects interact, increasing the pressure at the oval window by about 30 dB. This is still not enough to pass along all the acoustic energy arriving at the TM. Only about half the sound energy arriving at the TM is actually transmitted into the inner ear.

The second function of the middle ear is to attenuate loud sounds by the acoustic reflex, mediated by the stapedius muscle. The third function is to keep the air pressure inside the middle ear cavity and in the ear canal equal by means of the auditory tube. For the TM to vibrate properly, the pressure in the middle ear must be equal to that in the canal. Higher pressure within the middle ear pushes out on the TM, causing discomfort and interfering with the transmission of sound.

Inner Ear

The inner ear lies deep within the temporal bone and is composed of the cochlea, the semicircular canals, and a connecting vestibule between them. The cochlea is involved with hearing, whereas the semicircular canals and vestibule are important for balance. We shall focus on the cochlea, with its extraordinary ability to function as a frequency and intensity analyzer.

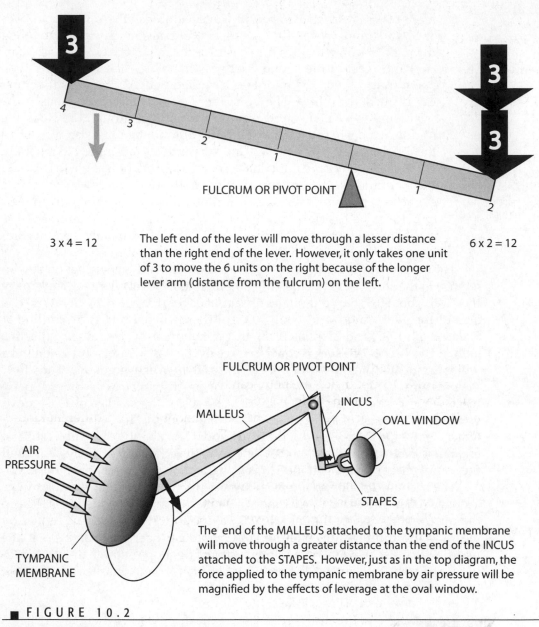

$3 \times 4 = 12$

The left end of the lever will move through a lesser distance than the right end of the lever. However, it only takes one unit of 3 to move the 6 units on the right because of the longer lever arm (distance from the fulcrum) on the left.

$6 \times 2 = 12$

FULCRUM OR PIVOT POINT

INCUS

OVAL WINDOW

MALLEUS

AIR
PRESSURE

STAPES

The end of the MALLEUS attached to the tympanic membrane will move through a greater distance than the end of the INCUS attached to the STAPES. However, just as in the top diagram, the force applied to the tympanic membrane by air pressure will be magnified by the effects of leverage at the oval window.

TYMPANIC
MEMBRANE

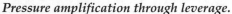

■ F I G U R E 1 0 . 2

Pressure amplification through leverage.

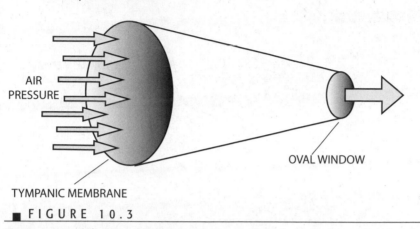

The energy of the air pressure that moves the tympanic membrane is concentrated on the much smaller oval window, creating an amplification effect

AIR PRESSURE

OVAL WINDOW

TYMPANIC MEMBRANE

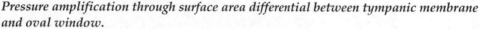

■ FIGURE 10.3

Pressure amplification through surface area differential between tympanic membrane and oval window.

Cochlea   The cochlea (Figure 10.4) is a snail-shaped, bony, spiral canal that makes two- and three-quarter turns. If it were straightened out, it would measure around 3.5 cm. Inside the bony canal is a membrane that takes the same snail shape. Between the bony canal and the membranous canal is fluid, the **perilymph** (peri = around). Within the membranous canal is a different kind of fluid, the **endolymph** (endo = within). The inside of the cochlea is divided along most of its length by the **cochlear duct**, or the *cochlear partition*. The base of this duct is the **basilar membrane** (BM). The roof of the duct is formed by the **vestibular membrane**. The space closest to the vestibular membrane is known as the scala vestibuli, and the space nearest the BM is the scala tympani. Between the scala vestibuli and the middle ear is the oval window, which is covered by the footplate of the stapes. Another opening between the middle and inner ears, the **round window**, is located between the scala tympani and the middle ear. This opening is covered with membrane. The cochlear duct does not completely fill the bony canal, extending almost, but not quite, to the apex of the canal. The apex is that point of the canal farthest from the middle ear. Where the cochlear duct ends, the scala vestibuli and scala tympani meet each other. This point of communication is the **helicotrema**.

Lying within the cochlear duct is the sensory nerve receptor for hearing, the **organ of Corti**. This structure lies on the BM. It consists of rows of thousands of inner and outer hair cells embedded in the **tectorial membrane**. This membrane forms the roof of the organ of Corti and is gellike in composition.

The cochlea is a snail-shaped structure located within the inner ear and contains two different fluids, called perilymph and endolymph.

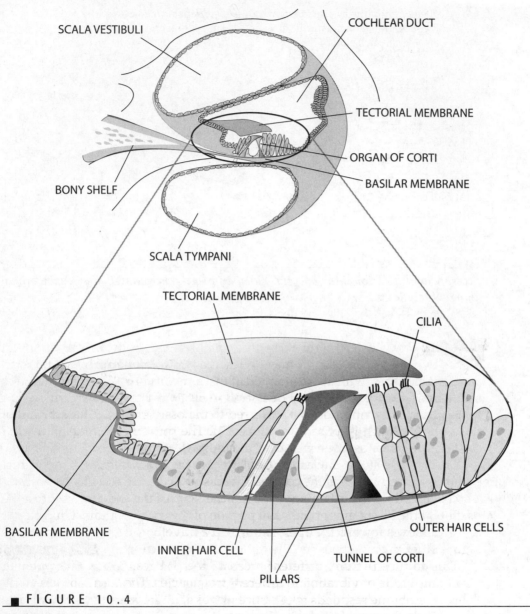

■ FIGURE 10.4

Cochlea.

There are about 3500 inner hair cells and 20,000 outer hair cells, along with other types of supporting cells. The hair cells have cilia sticking out from their tops, and these cilia make contact with the tectorial membrane. The bottom portion of the hair cells contain the endings of the nerve fibers of the auditory nerve. When the BM vibrates, the cilia on the hair cells are bent, which stimulates the auditory nerve to fire. The hair cells thus serve as transducers, transforming fluid vibrations into electrical energy (Rosen & Howell, 1991).

The organ of Corti within the cochlear duct is the sensory nerve receptor for hearing.

Basilar Membrane   The basilar membrane (BM), because of its structure, plays a crucial role in the cochlea's ability to perform a frequency and intensity analysis of all incoming sounds. This membrane is not equally wide along its entire length. At its base, closest to the middle ear, the BM is only about 0.05 mm wide. However, it widens to around 0.5 mm at its apex, farthest from the middle ear. Not only does the width of the BM change from base to apex, but so also does its stiffness. The membrane is stiffest at its narrow basal end and about 100 times more compliant at its wider apical end. These different levels of width and stiffness of the BM are the factors that create the cochlea's capacity to perform a frequency analysis of sounds.

The basilar membrane within the cochlea is involved in frequency analysis of incoming sounds.

Cochlear Function   Events in the cochlea are set into motion through the footplate of the stapes, which is embedded in the oval window. When the TM is set into vibration by increases and decreases in air pressure pushing and pulling at its surface, the vibration is transferred to the ossicles by the manubrium of the malleus, which is embedded in the TM. The movement of the malleus in turn sets the other ossicles, including the footplate of the stapes, into vibration. As the footplate moves inward and outward in the oval window, the vibration disturbs the perilymph in the cochlea. The disturbance in the perilymph causes the cochlear duct to vibrate, in particular the floor of the duct, the BM. The vibration of the BM begins at the basal portion of the cochlea, nearest the middle ear, and moves toward the apex, setting up a traveling wave of vibration (see Figure 10.5).

Due to its structure, different areas of the BM respond with greater or lesser amplitude of vibration to different frequencies. The basal portion of the membrane responds to pressure waves at all frequencies, but due to its high degree of stiffness, it is most responsive to high frequencies. Therefore, at high frequencies the wave motion of the BM reaches a maximum amplitude at the narrow stiff base of the membrane and quickly becomes damped before traveling much farther down the BM. The apex of the membrane, because of its greater width and higher compliance, is most sensitive to low frequencies. At low frequencies, therefore, the maximum displacement of the BM occurs near the apex.

The basal portion of the basilar membrane responds most strongly to high frequencies, whereas the apex is most sensitive to low frequencies.

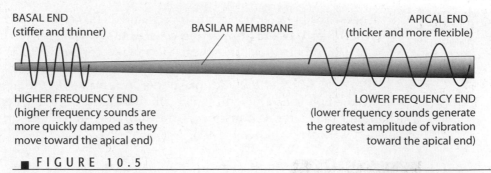

BASAL END
(stiffer and thinner)

BASILAR MEMBRANE

APICAL END
(thicker and more flexible)

HIGHER FREQUENCY END
(higher frequency sounds are
more quickly damped as they
move toward the apical end)

LOWER FREQUENCY END
(lower frequency sounds generate
the greatest amplitude of vibration
toward the apical end)

■ FIGURE 10.5

Schematic representation of the unrolled basilar membrane showing its differential frequency response.

Tonotopic organization refers to the arrangement of frequency sensitivity according to location.

Rosen and Howell (1991) compared the BM to a series of filters, with each point on the BM corresponding to a band-pass filter with a different center frequency. From the base to the apex of the cochlea, the F_c of each band-pass filter becomes lower and therefore resonates to successively lower frequencies in the sound wave. This arrangement of frequency sensitivity according to place is called **tonotopic organization**.

In normal listeners, these filters have a very narrow bandwidth, and there are thousands of them spread across the frequency range of hearing, giving the cochlea an extraordinary degree of frequency resolution. Listeners with only a moderate loss in sensitivity, on the other hand, can show very large increases in auditory filter bandwidth, which contributes to the difficulties they have in understanding speech. Because of the wider bandwidth, the frequency resolution of the sound is less clear. Spectral details tend to be smeared, with more interaction between parts of the speech in different frequency ranges. Rosen and Howell (1991) noted that, whereas a normal auditory system keeps "each frequency in its place," listeners with widened auditory filters have frequencies much more "mixed up." This ties in with the subjective experience of hearing-aid users, who often have little trouble "hearing" sounds, but cannot distinguish them from one another.

The cochlea essentially performs a Fourier analysis of complex sounds into their component frequencies. For example, Borden et al. (1994) showed that the sound of /i/ would result in many traveling waves moving along the basilar membrane with at least two areas of maximum displacement: one near the base of the cochlea for the higher formants and one near the apex for the lower formant. For the word /si/, the high-frequency /s/ would displace the membrane maximally even closer to the base of the cochlea. Also, the traveling waves would be aperiodic during /s/ and become periodic during /i/. These traveling waves are converted into electrical nerve impulses by the organ of Corti. The nerve impulses are transmitted along the auditory pathway to various regions in the cortex of the brain, where the process of speech perception takes place.

■ *Perception of Speech*

Our discussion so far has focused on how we hear. The discussion now turns to how we perceive the sounds that we hear, that is, how we assign meaning to the acoustic sound wave stimulating our auditory system. Speech perception is a very interesting phenomenon, because what we consciously perceive are not the acoustic features that make up the phonemes, such as voicing, place of articulation, manner of articulation, and so on, but linguistic events, such as phonemes, syllables, phrases, and sentences. Speech perception is a search for meaning, which is based on the ability to discriminate between and identify the acoustic–phonetic features of the speech waveform. In fact, a central question in the study of speech perception is how we are able to segment a continuously changing stream of sound into separate units of meaning. This question is deceptively simple, but numerous researchers investigating numerous aspects of perception and many theories are devoted to trying to answer it.

A central issue in speech perception is how people are able to segment a continuously changing stream of sound into separate units of meaning.

Segmentation Problem

When listening to someone talking, an individual perceives a sequence of separate sounds combined in innumerable different ways to form syllables, words, and phrases. These in turn are combined by the perceiver into meaningful ideas and information. However, at the acoustic level, the sound waves carrying the linguistic information are continuous and are not segmented into identifiable units corresponding to each specific phoneme. The problem is even more complicated, because phonemes are extremely variable in their production. Ranges of formant frequencies overlap for vowels produced by different speakers. Phonemes are also influenced, due to coarticulation, by preceding and following sounds. The acoustic waveform for the /k/ phoneme will differ, for example, depending on whether the following vowel is an /i/ or a /u/. Producing sounds at different rates of speech or stressing syllables differently also results in a different acoustic waveform. Rate of speech, patterns of stress and intonation, dialect, and many other factors also contribute to variability in phoneme production. Thus, there is no one-to-one correspondence between individual phonemes and their acoustic underpinnings.

Somehow this continuously changing sound wave is transformed by the listener into the distinct, separate linguistic units of speech. This variability leads to the question of how listeners perceive individual sounds as constant (e.g., an /i/ always sounds like an /i/), even when the acoustic features that underlie the sounds are constantly changing. Some theorists propose that there are invariant and unchanging properties of phonemes that are always present, despite the variability in production, and that this is what listeners use to recognize phonemes. An opposing point of view is that, because of the dynamic and constantly changing nature of speech, phonemes do not possess invariant properties; rather, listeners use the dynamic information in conjunction with contextual clues and their own linguistic knowledge to decode speech. This continues to be a hotly debated question, which has not been resolved to date.

Instrumental Analysis of Vowel and Consonant Perception

Much research has been done since the 1950s to try to understand how the transformation from acoustic to phonemic knowledge occurs. Most of this research has focused on the phonetic level, that is, on the acoustic characteristics that form patterns that we are able to perceive as distinct sounds. Two types of instruments have been particularly valuable in expanding our knowledge in this area. The first is the spectrograph, which provides detailed information about the acoustic structure of speech sounds. The other is an instrument developed in the 1950s, the **Pattern Playback** (PP). The PP works in reverse to the spectrograph: The spectrograph visually displays the acoustic characteristics of individual sounds; the PP takes visual patterns and converts them into sounds. The PP has been extremely useful, because it allows researchers to synthesize speech and to manipulate various acoustic cues in a systematic way.

Researchers continue to investigate how acoustic information is transformed into phonemic knowledge.

Many experiments have been done in which listeners' perceptions of sounds were tested to see how they responded to the manipulations. In these studies the PP was fed spectrogramlike patterns that it scanned with a light beam and then played back the corresponding auditory sound wave. Artificial speech was generated as the PP played back stylized patterns that were painted on a plastic belt. Different patterns were painted to generate many different sounds. Researchers experimented with formants by manipulating the number of formants, their frequencies, and their durations in various ways. Since about 1970, the PP has been replaced by computers, which do essentially the same manipulations, but far more quickly and with much improved sound quality.

Much of the research using the spectrograph and the PP or computerized programs for synthesizing speech has focused on the different classes of speech sounds, such as stops, vowels, and fricatives. These types of sounds have been manipulated in various ways to determine how listeners perceive them and assign them to different classes.

Perception of Vowels and Diphthongs

Vowels Vowels are characterized by distinct patterns of vocal tract resonances, the formants. Vowels are both longer in duration and more intense than consonants. The vowel with the greatest intensity is /a/, which is about 25 dB greater than the weakest consonant, /T/ (Ross, Brackett, & Maxon, 1991). Vowels form the main portion, or nuclei, of syllables. Research has shown that the formants of a particular vowel are not all equal in terms of how much they contribute to a listener's perception of that vowel. When formants are close in frequency, such as F_1 and F_2 are for back vowels and F_2 and F_3 are for front vowels, the listener integrates the two into one perceptual unit, which is the equivalent of an average of the two closely spaced formants. Thus, front vowels are perceived on the basis of the frequency of F_1 and an average of F_2 and F_3, whereas back vowels are perceived on the basis of the average of F_1 and F_2, as well as F_3 (Strange, 1999).

Vowel formant frequencies, however, are variable. Even when a vowel is said by itself, in isolation, formant frequencies differ for the same vowel when it is produced by different speakers. On the other hand, different vowels can overlap considerably in their formant frequencies when produced by the same speaker or by different speakers. Consequently, there is no strict one-to-one correspondence between vowels and their formant frequencies, yet this blurring of the boundaries between vowels is not usually a problem for listeners. Individuals are somehow able to compensate for the differences or similarities in formant frequencies within and between vowels.

> The relatively consistent relationship between formant frequencies for particular vowels may help to explain why differences in absolute formant values do not usually pose a problem for listeners.

Researchers have proposed various theories as to why the lack of consistent formant values for particular vowels is not a problem for listeners. Why should it be possible for an individual to perceive as /i/ a sound with formant values for F_1 F_2, and F_3 of 270, 2290, and 3010 Hz, but perceive equally clearly as /i/ a sound with F_1 of 345 Hz, F_2 of 2470 Hz, and F_3 of 3325 Hz? Shouldn't the different formant frequencies result in the perception of a different sound?

One theory suggests that it is not the absolute frequency values that are important in perception, but the relationships among the formant frequencies. In the preceding example, even though the absolute values are different, each /i/ sound is characterized by a very low F_1 and by very high F_2 and F_3, which are close together in frequency. Thus, when a young child and an adult male say /i/, the formant values for the two productions are very different, because of the differences in vocal tract lengths. Each production, however, is characterized by a similar pattern of formant relationships, and it is the pattern that we perceive, rather than the absolute formant frequency values.

A related theory posits that the ratio of F_2 to F_1 is the important factor in vowel recognition. For instance, high front vowels such as /i/ have very low F_1 and very high F_2; thus, the ratio of F_2 to F_1 is very large, whereas the F_2/F_1 ratio is much smaller for high back vowels such as /u/, which have F_1 and F_2 closer together. For example, F_1 and F_2 for /i/ are around 270 and 2290 Hz for men, 310 and 2790 Hz for women, and 370 and 3200 Hz for children. Based on these figures, the F_2/F_1 ratios would be 8.48, 9.00, and 8.65 for men, women, and children, respectively. These ratios are similar among the three groups. The ratios for /u/ work out to 2.90 for men (F_2 = 870 Hz, F_1 = 300 Hz), 2.57 for women (950/370 Hz), and 2.72 for children (1170/430 Hz). As with /i/, the ratios are similar across the three groups, while the ratios for the two different vowels are quite different.

Table 10.1 shows the ratios for front, back, and central vowels, based on the average formant frequency data reported in Table 8.5. Ratio differences are clearly apparent among the front vowels, but are less clear for the back vowels. Furthermore, you can see that the ratios for /æ/, a low front vowel, overlap considerably with those for /u/ and /U/, the two high back vowels. This overlap between the F_2/F_1 formant ratios also results in ambiguity.

Aside from formant frequencies, listeners also use changing formant patterns to identify vowels in connected speech.

The picture is even more complicated when it comes to understanding how people perceive vowels in connected speech. When vowels are produced in context, the acoustic contrast among them lessens because of coarticulation. The articulators move around constantly, so the formants are very seldom in a steady state, but rather are constantly transitioning. The F_1/F_2 vowel space becomes reduced, resulting in **target undershoot**, in which the formant patterns of different vowels become similar to each other. The amount of undershoot depends on which phonemes precede and follow the particular vowel, as well as on the speaker

■ T A B L E 1 0 . 1

F_2/F_1 Ratios for Men (M), Women (W), and Children (C) for Front, Back, and Central Vowels

	FRONT VOWELS			
	/i/	/I/	/ɛ/	/æ/
M	8.48	5.10	3.47	2.61
W	9.00	5.77	3.82	2.38
C	8.65	5.15	3.78	2.30

	BACK VOWELS			
	/u/	/ʊ/	/ɔ/	/a/
M	2.90	2.32	1.47	1.49
W	2.57	2.47	1.56	1.44
C	2.72	2.52	1.56	1.33

	CENTRAL VOWELS	
	/ə/	/ɚ/
M	1.86	2.76
W	1.84	3.28
C	1.87	3.25

and the speaking style. Some speakers reach vowel targets even when they talk very quickly, while others show less undershoot when they speak more slowly (Strange, 1999).

Even though the formant frequencies of vowels shift and become reduced in connected speech, listeners generally do not have any problem in identifying them. This suggests that listeners use other cues aside from formant frequencies to make judgments about vowel identity in connected speech. Strange (1999) and her colleagues have manipulated aspects of vowels, including vowel duration, formant transitions, and steady-state portions of vowels. Their research has shown that, even when the vowel nucleus of the syllable has been cut out, vowel perception is highly accurate as long as dynamic spectral information, such as the direction and slope of formant transitions, and duration information are present. When duration information was also cut out, this dynamic spectral information was more helpful than the actual formant frequency in identifying the vowel. Thus, the perception of coarticulated vowels appears to be based on dynamic spectrotemporal patterns within the syllable. In other words, it is the changing formant patterns that yield the most important acoustic information for identifying coarticulated vowels.

Listeners use several sources of information to help in identifying vowels. These include not only acoustic information that is present in the vowel itself, such as the F_0 and formants, but also information that is external to the vowel, such as the F_0 and formants of preceding vowels and consonants. That is, listeners use information about the size, age, and gender of the speaker available in the person's speech patterns to interpret ambiguous vowels (Strange, 1999).

However, with both vowels and consonants, it is not only the acoustic features that influence our perception, but also the context of the ongoing speech. The listener's knowledge of the speaker, the social context, the topic, the rules of grammar and environmental conditions (quiet, noisy) all play an important part in speech perception. For example, if two people are having a conversation about their friend Ed, it is unlikely that one of them will perceive the /E/ in *Ed* as /æ/ as in *add*, even though the speaker's formant frequencies for /E/ may be close to or even overlap considerably with his formant frequencies for /æ/. Both participants' knowledge of the topic and their expectations of hearing Ed's name in the conversation reduce the ambiguity of the similar formants of /E/ and /æ/.

The context in which speech occurs provides important cues for perception.

Diphthongs Diphthongs are perceived on the basis of their formant transitions, which change from the steady state of one vowel and transition to the steady state of the second vowel in the diphthong unit. It has been found that it is not the exact formant frequencies that are important in identifying diphthongs; it is how fast the formants change that is the most salient cue. This suggests that listeners are more sensitive to the acoustic consequences of the tongue moving in the appropriate direction, rather than on the final position that the tongue achieves for the sound.

Perception of Consonants

Consonants are produced with much more rapid movements of the articulators than vowels. There is also a much greater variety of consonant types than vowels, and the acoustic cues that enable perception of consonants tend to be more complex than those of vowels.

Categorical Perception   The way that many consonants are perceived is different from how vowels are perceived, because many consonants are perceived categorically. That is, if a series of consonant sounds was heard by a listener, with the sounds differing in one acoustic aspect by small equal steps, the listener would perceive some of the sounds as the same phoneme until a boundary was reached. On the other side of this boundary, known as the **crossover**, the listener would hear the other sounds as a different phoneme (see Figure 10.6). Thus, if there were ten sounds in the series, the listener might group all ten into only two different categories. This has been shown in tests of categorical perception, in which speech sounds are synthesized so as to differ in only one or two acoustic aspects in predetermined steps.

In one early test, for instance, Peter Eimas and his colleagues created a series of /ba/s and /pa/s. The researchers expected that the sounds in the series would be perceived as changing gradually from /ba/ to /pa/, with many sounds in the middle of the series sounding ambiguous. Instead, the listeners reported hearing a series of /ba/s that abruptly changed to a series of /pa/s. Furthermore, when the researchers asked the listeners if they could hear the difference between two adjacent /ba/s or /pa/s in the series, they could not do so, even though the two /ba/s or /pa/s were physically different. Listen-

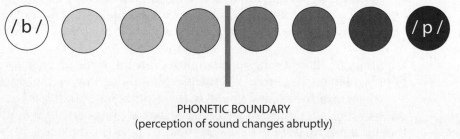

Equal increments of acoustic change from / b / to / p /

PHONETIC BOUNDARY
(perception of sound changes abruptly)

■ F I G U R E   1 0 . 6

Phonetic boundary between /b/ and /p/.

Unlike vowels, many consonants are perceived categorically with the sound changing abruptly from one phoneme to another at a phonetic boundary.

ers could only perceive the difference between adjacent stimuli at the crossover point, when the sound changed abruptly from the phoneme /b/ to the phoneme /p/ (Kuhl, 1991).

It is characteristic of categorical perception that sounds that are perceived as being in the same category are hard to tell apart, whereas it is easy to differentiate those that are perceived as being from different categories. Simply put, it is easy to recognize the difference between /p/ and /b/, whereas it is not easy to distinguish between two /b/ sounds, even if they are acoustically different. The fact that listeners are not able to distinguish among members of the same phoneme class probably facilitates perception, since irrelevant differences can safely be discounted, while only those differences that contribute to the perception of different speech sound categories are taken into account by the listener.

Categorical perception has been shown to occur for VOT and for place of articulation for stops and fricatives. Strange (1999) reported on an investigation in which researchers constructed a continuum of fourteen stop-vowel syllables, in which the syllables differed only in the direction and extent of the F_2 transition of the stop. The F_2 transition changed in small, evenly spaced steps from a low onset frequency and rising transition (typical of a labial stop), through intermediate onset frequencies (typical of an alveolar stop), to a relatively high onset frequency and falling transition (typical of a velar stop). Most listeners reported hearing all stimuli unambiguously as either *bay*, *day*, or *gay*, showing that place of articulation for stops is perceived categorically.

Categorical perception also occurs for other acoustic features, such as duration of transitions, that are important in differentiating stops such as /b/ from glides such as /w/.

Multiple Acoustic Cues in Consonant Perception In natural (not synthetic) speech, listeners use several different acoustic features to categorize a consonant. For example, a listener may use both VOT and onset of F_1 frequency to decide whether a stop is voiced or voiceless. A low F_1 onset frequency and a shorter VOT are characteristic of voiced stops, whereas a higher F_1 onset frequency and a longer VOT are associated with voiceless stops. However, acoustic cues show what are known as *trading relations* between them.

Listeners perceive consonants using multiple acoustic cues that are fused into the perception of a single phoneme.

For instance, one study found that F_1 onset frequency traded with VOT cues for voicing. Stimuli with low F_1 onset, typically associated with voiced stops, could be perceived as a voiceless stop if the VOT was lengthened. Stimuli with a higher F_1 onset, typically associated with voiceless stops, were perceived as voiceless even when accompanied by a shorter than usual VOT (Strange, 1999).

Other acoustic features such as vowel duration, frication noise duration, and F_0 cues to fricative voicing have also been shown to trade off. These multiple acoustic features associated with consonants are somehow fused into the perception of a single phoneme by the listener.

Influence of Coarticulation   It is important to keep in mind that listeners do not just use acoustic information from one specific phoneme to make a decision regarding the identity of that phoneme. Because the articulators move continuously during the production of speech, the shape of the vocal tract is influenced by the shapes for the sounds that occur before and after the target sound. This results in continuously shifting acoustic features that interact with and influence adjacent features. Perceptually, therefore, we integrate information that is spread out over several phonetic segments to make a decision about phoneme identity.

> Perceptual information is obtained from sounds adjacent to the target sound, as well as from the target sound itself.

This was shown in a study in which the researchers synthesized a continuum of fricative sounds (/ʃ/ and /s/) that varied only in the bandwidth of the fricative noise. The noise varied from a wide band for /ʃ/ to a narrow band for /s/ in nine equal steps. Subjects heard the continuum in two different conditions. In one condition the fricative sounds were followed by the /i/ vowel, and in the other condition they were combined with the /u/ vowel (i.e., /si/–/ʃi/; /su/–/ʃu/). The fricative noises that fell in the midrange of bandwidths were heard as /ʃ/ when they were combined with /i/ and as /s/ when they were combined with /u/. Thus, the subjects' perceptions shifted from /ʃ/ to /s/ depending on the vowel context.

Rate of speech also influences a listener's identification of consonants. For example, in continua in which VOT is varied, stimuli with intermediate VOTs are heard as voiceless in fast speech and voiced in slow speech.

Keeping in mind the complex nature of consonants with their multiple acoustic cues and their variability due to coarticulation and context, let us identify the major perceptual features of each class of consonants.

> Liquids and glides are recognized on the basis of their formant transitions.

Liquids   Similar to diphthongs, the liquids /r/ and /l/ are recognized on the basis of their formant transitions. One factor that distinguishes liquids from diphthongs is that the formant transitions in /r/ and /l/ are much more rapid than those in diphthongs. The F_3 frequency is particularly important for differentiating between the liquids. F_3 in /r/ sounds is usually much lower in frequency than the F_3 in /l/ sounds.

Glides   The glides /j/ and /w/ are characterized by transitions that are shorter in duration than those of diphthongs. Experiments have shown that, when the transition duration is shorter than about 40 to 60 ms, listeners tend to hear a stop. When the transition is greater than 40 to 60 ms, but less than 100 to 150 ms, listeners usually judge the sound to be a glide. Finally, when the transition exceeds about 100 ms, listeners hear a vowel plus vowel sequence (Denes & Pinson, 1993).

Nasals   Nasals are recognized on the basis of their internal formant structure, as well as on the basis of the formant transitions of the vowels occurring before and after the nasal sound. F_1, F_2, and F_3 of nasals are weak in intensity because of antiresonances resulting from the structure of the nasal cavities.

Perception of nasal sounds is based on the additional nasal formant as well as on the formant transitions of the preceding and following vowels.

Nasals also have an extra formant, the nasal formant. These two features help listeners to recognize that a sound is a nasal. In synthetic speech it has been found that when the upper formants are cut out the nasal formant by itself is enough to judge a sound as a nasal. Researchers have also found that when a nasal occurs at the end of a syllable, information in the vowel preceding the nasal is enough to identify the nasal. When the researchers cut out the transitions between the vowel and the nasal, as well as the nasal phoneme itself, listeners could still detect nasality in the vowel.

According to Borden et al. (1994), the formant transitions (particularly F_2) between a nasal and a preceding or following vowel are what signal the place of articulation of the nasal. These transitions contain frequency and durational cues. The formant transitions from /m/ are the lowest in frequency and the shortest in duration, those for /n/ are higher in frequency and a bit longer in duration, and those for /ŋ/ are the highest and the most variable in frequency and the longest in duration.

Stops   Stops are perceived on the basis of numerous acoustic cues that are intertwined with the acoustic cues for the vowels and consonants surrounding the phoneme. Part of recognizing a stop involves perceiving the relationships between the stop and its neighboring sounds. Some acoustic cues signal the manner of the stop, some are clues to its place of articulation, and others provide information about voicing status. Cues to manner include a brief interval of silence or attenuation of sound, a transient burst of noise, and rapid formant transitions between the stop and a preceding or following vowel.

Numerous acoustic cues are present in stops, signaling manner, place, and voicing of the sound.

Research has shown that just inserting an interval of silence between two phonemes can cause a stop sound to be heard. For example, in the word *slit*, if a silent interval is inserted between the /s/ and the /l/, the word will be heard as *split*, with a /p/ being perceived rather than just silence. In terms of formant transitions, the duration of the transitions seems to play an important part in identifying manner of articulation.

For example, investigators have synthesized the stop plus vowel combinations of /be/ and /ge/ on the PP using very brief formant transitions of less than 40 ms. Even though release bursts were not included, listeners were able to recognize the sounds without any difficulty. When the researchers extended the duration of the transitions to 40 or 50 ms, listeners heard glides, rather than stops, at the start of the syllables /we/ and /je/. When they lengthened the transitions to 150 ms or more, listeners perceived not a consonant and vowel sequence, but a sequence of two vowel sounds, /ue/ and /ie/ (Borden et al., 1994).

Place of articulation of stops is also signaled by several acoustic cues, including the frequency of the burst in relation to a vowel, the F_2 transition between the stop and the adjacent vowel, and VOT. VOT differs according to place of articulation, with bilabial stops showing the shortest VOTs (or negative VOTs) and velar stops having the longest VOTs. The F_2 transition seems to be a particularly strong cue in recognizing different stops, at least in synthetic speech. It has been shown in experiments using synthetic speech that the F_2 transition for /p/ and /b/ begins at a low frequency, around 600 to 800 Hz. The alveolars /t/ and /d/ have their F_2 transitions beginning in the midfrequency region, at approximately 1800 Hz. The starting position for the F_2 transition for /k/ and /g/ depends on whether the stop is produced in combination with a back or a front vowel. When combined with a front vowel such as /i/, the stop is made farther forward in the oral cavity. Conversely, the stop is made more toward the back of the oral cavity when followed by a back vowel such as /u/. The starting frequencies for the F_2 transition for velar stops, therefore, can be either around 1300 Hz, appropriate for a high back vowel, or much higher, at about 3000 Hz, appropriate for a high front vowel.

However, these starting frequencies for the F_2 transition, which are known as loci (singular: locus), have not been found to be as important in natural speech as they are in synthetic speech. It is currently thought that all the formant shifts (for F_1, as well as F_2 and F_3) are important cues for listeners to identify the place of articulation of a stop (Kent & Read, 1992). In fact, in experiments in which the bursts of the stops are cut out, listeners can recognize the stop based only on the formant information.

Stops also differ from each other in terms of their voicing. As with manner and place of articulation, several acoustic cues help to identify the voicing status of a stop. The presence or absence of phonation and the degree of aspiration noise when the stop is released play an important role. VOT is also a major indicator of voicing, with voiceless stops in English being characterized by longer VOTs and voiced stops being associated with much shorter (and sometimes negative) VOTs. The relationship between the F_1 and F_2 transitions from the stop to the following vowel can also signal whether the stop is voiced or voiceless. A delay of F_1 relative to the beginning of the F_2 transition is referred to as F_1 **cutback** (Figure 10.7). Research has shown that listeners usually report hearing voiceless stops when the F_1 cutback is 30 ms or more.

The cues for voicing, however, depend to some degree on the position of the stop in the syllable. At the beginning of a syllable, cues include VOT, F_1 cutback, and the F_0 of the vowel following the stop. Vowels that follow voiceless stops tend to have a higher F_0 than those that follow voiced stops. For stops that occur in the final position in a syllable, vowel duration is an important cue. Vowels are longer before voiced stops and shorter before voiceless stops. The

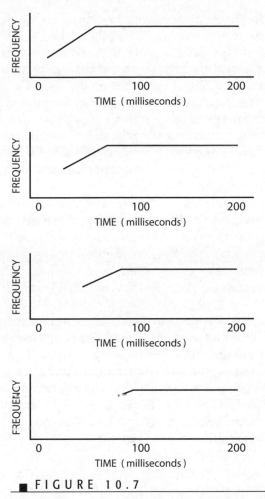

■ FIGURE 10.7

F_1 *cutback.*

duration of the silent interval in a stop can also help to signal its voicing status. Thus, numerous acoustic cues are generated in the production of a stop. Many of these cues are redundant, which helps to make stops easy to perceive for individuals with normal hearing.

Fricatives   Frication noise provides the major cue as to the manner of articulation of fricatives. The noise is longer in duration than that of stops. Sounds tend to be heard as fricatives when the noise is around 130 ms or greater, whereas sounds with noise durations less than around 75 ms are perceived as stops. The frication noise also signals voicing status, being both longer in duration and greater in amplitude for voiceless fricatives than it is for the voiced variety.

The major perceptual cue for fricatives is the duration of the frication noise.

Sibilant fricatives are characterized by high-intensity, high-frequency noise; the spectrum of nonsibilant fricatives is flatter.

Place of articulation of fricatives is perceived on the basis of the spectrum and intensity of the noise. The sibilant fricatives (/s, z, ʃ, and ʒ/) have steep, high-frequency spectral peaks, whereas the nonsibilants (/f, v, T, θ, and ð/) have rather flat spectra. The location of the spectral peaks can also aid in distinguishing between the alveolar and palatal sibilant fricatives. The alveolars /s/ and /z/ have a prominent peak at around 4000 Hz, and the peak for /ʃ/ and /ʒ/ is lower, at around 2500 Hz. The labiodental and linguadental fricatives have very similar spectra, so it is not as easy to tell them apart as are the sibilants. Also, the sibilants have a much more intense spectrum than the nonsibilants. In fact, the /T/ is the sound that has the weakest intensity in English.

Affricates share acoustic features with stops and fricatives.

Aside from these spectral differences, the formant transitions to and from the fricative also play a role in differentiating between the fricatives, although not to as great an extent as for the stops. F_2 transitions to and from adjacent vowels are probably more important for the weaker fricatives than for the sibilants, because the spectral shapes of the weaker fricatives are similar and do not help to distinguish between them.

Affricates   Because affricates are produced as a stop plus a fricative, they share acoustic features with both types of sounds. The **rise time** may be particularly important in recognizing affricates versus fricatives. Rise time refers to how long it takes for the amplitude envelope to reach its highest value. The rise time for affricates has been measured at around 33 ms; that for fricatives is longer, about 76 ms (Kent & Read, 1992). The duration of the frication noise is also different, being longer for the fricatives than for the affricates.

Figure 10.8 shows the frequency and intensity regions for vowels and consonants.

The Role of Context in Speech Perception

Although we have a good idea of the acoustic structure of sounds, experiments with filtered and distorted speech have shown that acoustic cues are not only ambiguous, but that we can actually eliminate many of them and still maintain good speech perception (Denes & Pinson, 1993). The fact that multiple acoustic cues are embedded within single phonemes, as well as information from many phonemes converging on a specific sound, probably helps in perception. What is equally important for decoding speech is that most perception occurs in context. We know from our experience with a language which sounds go together and which do not.

Perception is facilitated by multiple acoustic cues within a single phoneme, information from surrounding phonemes, and contextual and linguistic cues.

When we hear a speaker start to produce the /n/ sound, for example, as English speakers we know that the following sound must be a vowel. We would not expect to hear an /nd/ sequence at the beginning of a word, whereas we might well hear it at the end of a word (e.g., *end*).

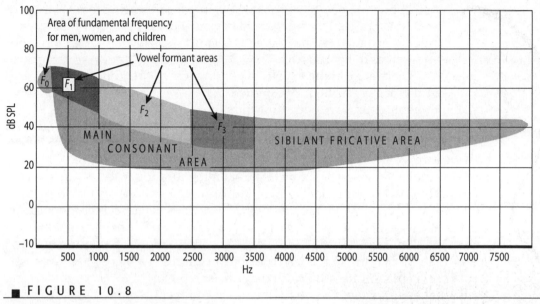

■ **FIGURE 10.8**

Speech frequencies and intensities.

We have similar expectations of other linguistic parameters, such as syntax (word order) and semantics (meaning). Thus, contextual and linguistic information serve to enhance speech perception and the decoding of the acoustic signal into meaningful units.

Indeed, as Denes and Pinson (1993) pointed out, familiarity with the sub ject matter can make speech recognizable even when the acoustic cues alone, because of noise, poor intelligibility, and the like, are ambiguous and not sufficient for accurate perception. According to Denes and Pinson,

> The incoming information is combined with a great deal of information already stored in our brain, such as how our articulators produce speech waves, the words and rules of our language, the subject matter, and much else. Speech perception is the result of interaction between incoming and stored information. When we listen under the most favorable conditions, the cues available are far in excess of what is actually needed for satisfactory perception. (p. 182)

Immittance Audiometry, Otoacoustic Emissions, and Cochlear Implants

Problems in any part of the auditory system may result in subtle problems of auditory processing in which the person's hearing acuity is normal, but

Problems with the middle ear result in a conductive hearing loss; sensorineural hearing loss results from inner ear dysfunction.

perception of speech is problematic, in partial hearing loss, or in deafness. It is unusual for a person to have no hearing at all. Typically, even a deaf person has some degree of residual hearing, although it may be so slight as to be unusable.

There are different types of hearing loss, depending on which part of the ear is affected. A **conductive hearing loss** occurs when something interferes with the transmission of the sound wave on its way to the inner ear. For example, the external auditory meatus might get plugged by a lump of cerumen. This would absorb much of the sound wave before it gets to the TM. Within the middle ear, several conditions can interfere with or prevent the ossicles from being set into vibration, such as otitis media, or **otosclerosis**, a condition in which the formation of bone around the stapes prevents it from being set into vibration. Conditions that affect the inner ear result in a **sensorineural hearing loss**, such as intense noise exposure that damages the hair cells in the cochlea. A combination of conductive and sensorineural hearing loss is also possible, resulting in a **mixed hearing loss**.

Various diagnostic procedures have been developed to assess middle ear and inner ear function. Two instrumental techniques, in particular, have had a large impact on clinical diagnostic practice. These are **immittance audiometry** and **otoacoustic emissions**.

Immittance Audiometry

The current method of choice for diagnosing middle ear problems is based on immittance audiometry. **Immittance** is a measure of how easily a system can be set into vibration by a driving force. The term immittance includes two reciprocal concepts: **admittance** and **impedance**. Admittance refers to how easily energy is transmitted through a system and is measured in units called **siemens** (formerly millimhos). Impedance describes how a system opposes the flow of energy through it and is measured in units of **ohms**. The reciprocal nature of admittance and impedance is also expressed in their units of measurement: note that mho is ohm spelled backward.

If a system can be set into vibration easily, its admittance is high and its impedance is low. Conversely, if it takes a lot of force to set the system into vibration, its admittance is low and its impedance is high. Measuring immittance is important in evaluating conductive hearing loss, which is caused by changes in the transmission characteristics of the middle ear vibratory system (Jerger & Stach, 1994). Immittance is measured and displayed on an instrument called a **tympanometer**, which produces a graph of immittance called a **tympanogram**.

Tympanograms   A tympanogram is a graph that represents changes in the immittance of the middle ear vibratory system as air pressure is varied in the external ear canal. The immittance of the normal middle ear is greatest when the air pressure in the external ear canal and in the middle ear cavity are the same. In this situation the transmission of sound waves occurs with maximum admittance. If the air pressure in the external ear canal becomes either positive or negative in relation to the air pressure in the middle ear space, the admittance of the system decreases, reducing the transmission of vibration. Jerger and Stach (1994) pointed out that in the normal system the effect is quite precipitous. As soon as the air pressure changes even slightly below or above the level that produces maximum immittance, the energy flow through the system drops quickly and steeply to a minimum value.

Tympanograms indicate how the middle ear is functioning in terms of its immittance characteristics.

Tympanometric Procedure   Obtaining a tympanogram is quick, easy, and noninvasive. A small device called a **probe tip** is inserted in the external ear canal. A complete seal is created between the probe tip and the ear canal because the probe tip has a flexible plastic cuff around it that plugs the ear canal, preventing any leakage of air. Four small tubes connect to the probe tip. One tube is connected to a loudspeaker that delivers a tone into the ear canal. This sound is called the probe or probe signal. The second tube is connected to a microphone that measures the probe tone in the ear canal. The third tube is connected to an air pressure pump and manometer and the fourth to another receiver used to present stimuli for testing the acoustic reflex (Gelfand, 1997).

Normal middle ear immittance occurs when the air pressures inside the middle ear and in the external ear canal are the same.

To measure the immittance, a probe signal of 85 dB is transmitted to the ear canal by the probe tip. The intensity of the tone is monitored by the microphone. Changes in the level of this tone reflect the immittance of the system. Typically, in the clinical setting, only a single frequency is used for the probe tone, either 220 or 226 Hz. Occasionally, a higher probe frequency of 660 or 678 Hz is also used. Researchers have found, however, that valuable information can be obtained by testing immittance at many different frequencies, so many tympanometers incorporate multiple probe tone frequencies from 200 to 2000 Hz (Shanks et al., 1988).

During the procedure, different amounts of air pressure are introduced into the air canal by means of the air pressure pump and manometer attached to one of the tubes. The air pressure is measured in relation to the P_{atmos} of the test location in units of decapascals (daPa), or millimeters of water (mm H_2O). One daPa = 1.02 mm H_2O at 20°C (Shanks et al., 1988). Zero daPa reflects an equal relationship between the pressure in the ear canal and P_{atmos}; positive pressure (e.g., +100 daPa) means that the ear canal pressure is greater than P_{atmos}, and negative pressure (e.g., −100 daPa) means that the pressure in the canal is less than P_{atmos}. This information is shown on a diagram called a tympanogram, with admittance on the y-axis and pressure on the x-axis. P_{atmos} (0 daPa) is in the middle, with P_{pos} increasing to the right and P_{neg} increasing to the left (Gelfand, 1997).

Tympanogram Shapes   There are several ways of interpreting tympanograms. In clinical situations, typically, the shape of the tympanogram is used to provide diagnostic information about the functioning of the middle ear. Figure 10.9 shows that in the normal middle ear the tympanogram is similar to a bell-shaped curve. The highest point of the graph, the peak, occurs around 0 daPa of air pressure (i.e., P_{atmos}) and indicates the greatest immittance of the middle ear at that pressure. The slopes of the curve are quite steep, showing that the immittance decreases quickly as the pressure in the canal becomes either positive or negative. This shape, called type A, is typical of normal middle ear function.

Interpretation of tympanograms is based on the shape of the graph, which is classified as type A, B, or C.

      Types B and C are different in shape from type A, reflecting changes in middle ear immittance due to various disorders. The type B tympanogram has a much flatter peak than the type A. This kind of tympanogram is typical of otitis media, in which the middle ear space is filled with fluid. In this condition the ossicles cannot vibrate freely, so acoustic energy is hindered from being transmitted across the ossicular chain.

      The type C tympanogram has a similar peaked shape to the type A, but instead of the peak being at or close to 0 daPa of air pressure, the peak is in the negative pressure region, to the left of 0 daPa. This kind of tympanogram is typical of conditions in which the auditory tube does not function normally, so middle ear pressure is not replenished and equalized with P_{atmos}. The lack of equalization causes a decrease of pressure in the middle ear, because air is continually absorbed by the tissues of the middle ear. When we swallow we open the auditory tube, which allows the air in the middle ear to be reequalized with air from the atmosphere. When the tube does not function normally, the pressure cannot be equalized, so the pressure in the ear canal is higher than that in the middle ear. This difference in pressure causes the TM to be pulled inward. To match the lower middle ear pressure and have acoustic energy flow through the system, the pressure in the ear canal must be decreased as well. Once this happens, energy can be transmitted through the system, resulting in a normal tympanogram peak, but at a negative pressure, usually below −100 daPa. Thus, a type C tympanogram reflects a condition of negative middle ear pressure.

Type A tympanograms indicate normal middle ear function; type B is typical of otitis media; and type C reflects abnormal Eustachian tube function.

      Jerger and Stach (1994) pointed out that anything that causes the ossicular chain to become stiffer, resulting in a reduction in energy flow through the middle ear, will attenuate the peak of the tympanogram. For example, otosclerosis, a disease of the bone surrounding the footplate of the stapes, prevents the ossicles from vibrating. This generates a type A shape, but with a lower peak, and is designated type A_s ("s" represents the stiffness of the ossicles or the shallowness of the tympanometric peak). Conversely, a break or discontinuity in the chain results in a much greater than normal peak, in conjunction with the type A shape. This happens because, with a break in the chain, the

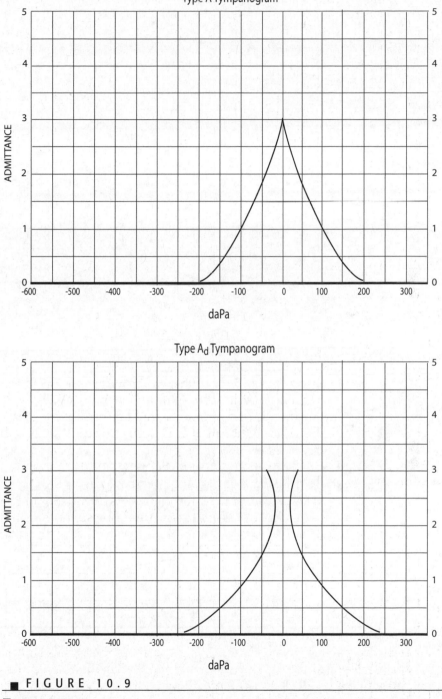

■ FIGURE 10.9

Tympanograms.

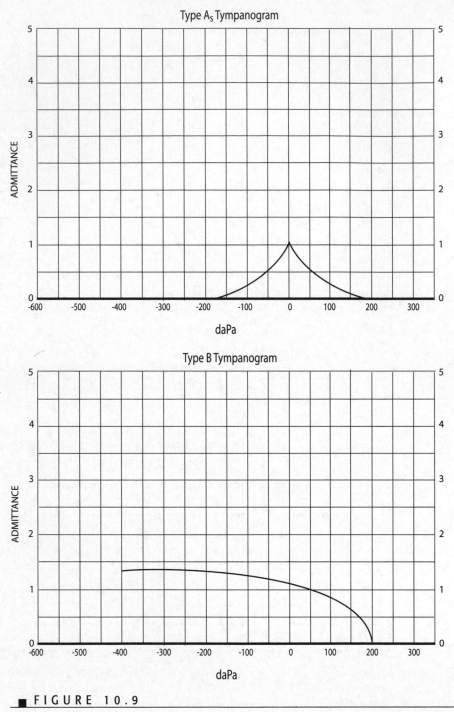

Continued

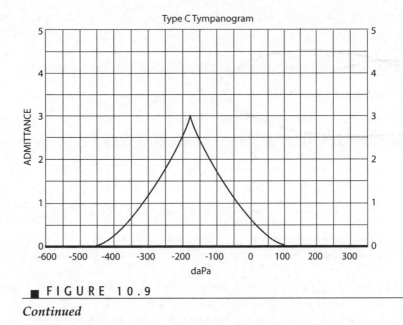

Type C Tympanogram

■ FIGURE 10.9

Continued

middle ear vibratory system is no longer coupled to the cochlear system, allowing the TM to respond with much greater amplitude to changes in air pressure. This is designated type A_d, with "d" referring to the greater depth of the peak or to discontinuity in the ossicular chain.

Advantages of Tympanometry   Acoustic immittance testing is a sensitive diagnostic tool, providing valuable information about the underlying middle ear problem. For example, from this kind of information it is possible to determine whether the problem results from a stiffening of the middle ear structures, whether effusion is present, or whether there is auditory tube dysfunction (Silman & Silverstein, 1991).

Tympanometry is a sensitive and noninvasive diagnostic tool that has become a mainstay of clinical practice in audiology.

Other major advantages of this technique are that it is not time consuming or invasive and is relatively easy to administer. It can therefore be used much more easily with individuals who do not respond well to audiometric or other behavioral tests, such as very young children or people with mental retardation.

Tympanometry has become a mainstay of clinical practice since the 1970s when it was introduced. As with other kinds of instrumental techniques, tympanometry is an excellent way of documenting changes in a patient's middle ear function resulting from surgical and/or medical treatment for middle ear problems. Tympanometry also serves as a quick and easy screening tool to detect the presence of any middle ear pathology in children at all grade levels, including preschool. If a child obtains an abnormal tympanogram, he or she can then be referred to an otolaryngologist or audiologist for a more comprehensive evaluation.

Otoacoustic Emissions

Another recent development that has become a valuable component of the diagnostic process is the measurement of otoacoustic emissions (OAEs). OAEs are extremely low-intensity sounds that originate in the cochlea as the cochlea is processing incoming sound. These cochlear sounds are transmitted in the opposite direction to incoming sounds. That is, they travel back to the footplate of the stapes, across the ossicular chain to the TM, and into the external ear canal, where they can be measured. OAEs reflect the activity of the outer hair cells of the organ of Corti in the cochlea.

Otoacoustic emissions are very low intensity sounds that originate within the cochlea and may be spontaneous or evoked.

Spontaneous and Evoked Otoacoustic Emissions   OAEs have been categorized into several types. The two major categories are spontaneous and evoked OAEs. Spontaneous otoacoustic emissions (SOAEs) occur without any incoming auditory stimulation in around 35 to 60 percent of people (including infants) with normal hearing (DeVries & Newell Decker, 1992; Norton, 1992; Prieve, 1992). They are usually detected at frequencies between 1000 and 5000 Hz. According to Bright (1997), most SOAEs in adult ears fall between 1000 and 2000 Hz, while those of infants range between 3000 and 4000 Hz. Females demonstrate twice as many SOAEs as males, and this also holds true for infants.

Evoked otoacoustic emissions (EOAEs) occur in response to acoustic stimulation to the ear and for virtually everyone with normal hearing. There are several types of EOAEs, depending on the type of stimulus used to evoke them. These OAEs that have been found to be extremely useful in clinical situations. The basic procedure used to generate and record OAEs consists of placing a miniature loudspeaker and sensitive microphone in the person's external ear canal by means of a miniature probe. The loudspeaker generates the sound, and the microphone records the emissions.

Evoked otoacoustic emissions are clinically important because they are absent in people with even mild degrees of sensori-neural hearing loss.

EOAEs are clinically important because nearly everyone with normal ears demonstrates them, whereas they are absent in people with even mild degrees of sensory hearing loss. For instance, Robinette (1992) measured EOAEs in 105 normally hearing men and 160 normally hearing women between 20 and 80 years old. EOAEs were observed in all 265 normal ears, but were absent in all ears with sensory hearing loss. Thus, because EOAEs cannot be detected in people with mild or more severe degrees of hearing loss, testing for their presence or absence can be used as an objective, sensitive way of measuring cochlear function. Also, this kind of test is noninvasive and does not require patients to participate actively in the test, so it is a particularly effective way of evaluating cochlear function in infants and young children. Furthermore, EOAEs can be tested very quickly, and the technology is not very expensive, making this an excellent way of screening infants, babies, and children in clinics and hospitals.

One important point to keep in mind, however, is that for the results to be valid the patient's middle ear status must also be assessed. This is because a conductive loss would interfere with the acoustic signal in both directions, that is, both traveling through the middle ear to the cochlea and traveling back from the cochlea through the middle ear to the external canal. A child who has otitis media, therefore, cannot be evaluated for EOAEs. However, EOAEs can be used to measure recovery of conductive function after treatment.

Evoked otoacoustic emissions are valuable in infant screening to identify hearing problems as early as possible in the child's life.

To date, the most valuable use of EOAEs is in neonatal screening. Early identification of hearing problems is a crucial factor in rehabilitation, because the earlier the problem is detected the sooner the child can be fitted with appropriate amplification or even cochlear implants. According to Culpepper (1997), in the United States, the average age at which children with significant hearing impairment are identified is estimated as being between 18 and 30 months of age. The author noted:

> Until recently, universal detection of hearing loss in all live births was not considered feasible due to the validity, practicality, and cost efficiency of existing techniques. EOAEs may finally provide the health care system in the United States the impetus necessary to reduce the average age of identification of hearing loss to 12 months of age. (p. 258)

Cochlear Implants

A cochlear implant is an electronic device designed to directly stimulate the auditory nerve by bypassing a person's damaged cochlea. Part of the device is surgically implanted in the cochlea, and part is worn externally. The parts of the device include a microphone, a signal processor, an external transmittor, and the implanted electrodes. The microphone receives a sound wave and transmits it to the signal processor. Different types of signal processors use different strategies to represent the sound, which is then sent by the external transmittor to the implanted electrodes. The electrodes in turn trigger the auditory nerve to fire and send a signal to the implant user's brain for interpretation.

A cochlear implant directly stimulates an individual's auditory nerve by bypassing the damaged cochlea.

The speech signal processor works by representing acoustic cues such F_0, F_1, F_2, and other high-frequency peaks of energy in the signal. The signal is

An important component of the device is the speech processor, which represents acoustic cues such as F_0, F_1, and F_2 in the signal.

sampled every few milliseconds to detect changes in the acoustic energy peaks over time. Different types of processors use different strategies to represent the speech signal. How the signal is represented is extremely important in re-creating it in such a way that the implant user can gain the most benefit. For example, the range of frequencies represented is an important factor. Speech frequencies have a wide range, from the F_0 of an adult male's voice, around 100 Hz, to the extremely high-frequency energy present in the sibilant fricatives. An implant therefore must be able to detect and transmit a wide range of frequencies, arranged in frequency bandwidths.

Another consideration is that the signal processor must be able to resolve small frequency differences between sounds. For example, to identify a vowel sound, an implant must be able to resolve the formant frequencies of the vowel (Dorman, 2000), which sometimes differ by only a few hundred hertz. The differences in formant frequencies must then be encoded by the implanted electrode(s) in the person's cochlea.

Information about manner of articulation and voicing is contained in the spectrum of sounds, such as stops, fricatives, and nasals. Spectral shapes, as we know, are different for stops, fricatives, glides, liquids, and nasals. For example, a stop has a short duration of aperiodic sound (the burst), whereas fricatives are characterized by longer duration aperiodic noise. This kind of spectral information can be coded by one electrode. However, information signaling formant frequencies for vowels and place of articulation for consonants is best coded by multiple electrodes (Dorman, 2000). Furthermore, because of the dynamic nature of speech with its rapidly changing frequencies and intensities, an implant must be able to resolve not only the formant frequencies, but where the formant frequencies are at a given moment in time. In other words, the implant works to resolve rapid changes in formant frequencies over time (Dorman, 2000).

Several different types of strategies are implemented by different cochlear implants to transmit the acoustic information in the speech signal. One strategy is the **m-of-n strategy**, or the *SPEAK strategy*. "N" is the overall number of frequency bands, and "m" is the number of channels with the highest energy peaks. This strategy typically divides the acoustic signal into around twenty frequency bands to achieve a satisfactory frequency resolution. The six or so channels with the highest energy are determined in 4 ms processor cycles, and the electrodes associated with these channels are stimulated. The "m" channels thus represent the formants in the speech signal. Dorman (2000) pointed out that the m-of-n strategy is an excellent way to transmit speech because only the formants are transmitted and, as the formant frequencies change, so do the electrodes being stimulated. Early experiments using the Pattern Playback with normally hearing listeners showed that speech can be transmitted with very good intelligibility based only on information about the location of the formant peaks. In effect, the change in location of the stimulated electrode mimics the normal frequency change in location along the basilar membrane (Dorman, 2000).

Another strategy for transmitting speech is a **fixed channel strategy** in which the acoustic signal is divided into a smaller number of frequency bands (e.g., 4 to 12). Unlike the m-of-n strategy, rather than selecting the channels with the highest peaks, the energy in all the bands at each processor cycle is transmitted. In this strategy all the electrodes are stimulated on each cycle, so the location of the formant peaks must be inferred from the different amounts of energy delivered to adjacent electrodes (Dorman, 2000). Similar to the m-of-n strategy, early experiments showed that normally hearing individuals can understand speech with a high degree of accuracy even when only a few fixed channels are used.

Other strategies include the $F_0F_1F_2$ **strategy**, which stimulates only two electrodes, based on estimates of the F_1 and F_2 frequencies. The stimulation occurs at a rate that corresponds to the F_0 of the signal when the stimulus is voiced and to a random rate around F_0 when the stimulus is not voiced. The **MPEAK strategy** stimulates two electrodes representing F_1 and F_2, as well as two or three electrodes that stimulate high-frequency peaks of energy corresponding to the higher formant regions. This strategy extracts F_0, F_1, and F_2 and their amplitudes, as well as energy peaks in the frequency ranges of 2000 to 2800, 2800 to 4000, and 4000 to 6000 Hz (Hedrick & Carney, 1997).

Contextual cues and linguistic structure play an important role in perception with cochlear implants, just as they do in perception of individuals with normal hearing. Dorman (2000) pointed out that the number of channels needed for accurate speech recognition depends on the amount of linguistic and contextual information available to the listener. Normally hearing individuals can recognize sentences with excellent accuracy when they have access to spectral information (burst, frication noise, etc.) plus a small amount of frequency-specific information, as long as they have linguistic context to aid them. When less linguistic information is available, listeners require more channels to recognize speech signals. Synthetic vowels that differ only in formant frequencies, naturally produced vowels from different speakers, and consonant place of articulation, which depends to a large degree on changing formant frequency information, are more difficult to identify. These kinds of sounds are recognized with a high degree of accuracy only when the signals are processed into eight or more channels (Dorman, 2000).

Contextual cues and linguistic structure are equally as important in perception with cochlear implants as they are in normal perception.

s u m m a r y

- The auditory system includes the outer, middle, and inner ears and the auditory nerve pathway.
- The middle ear functions to overcome the impedance mismatch between the middle and inner ears, to attenuate loud sounds by means of the acoustic reflex, and to maintain equal air pressures inside and outside the middle ear using the auditory tube.
- The inner ear transduces the mechanical vibrations of the middle ear to fluid vibrations and to electrical energy using the organ of Corti.
- The structure of the basilar membrane facilitates a frequency analysis of all incoming sounds to the cochlea.
- Speech perception is a search for meaning, which is based on the ability to discriminate and identify the acoustic–phonetic features of the speech waveform.
- Vowels and consonants are perceived in terms of multiple acoustic cues that trade off with each other depending on contextual conditions.
- Immittance audiometry and otoacoustic emissions have become valuable diagnostic tools in the assessment of middle ear and inner ear function.
- Cochlear implants are designed to bypass a diseased or damaged cochlea and directly stimulate the auditory nerve.

r e v i e w   e x e r c i s e s

1. Describe how the structure of the middle ear acts to transmit acoustic pressure waves to the inner ear.
2. Explain the relationship between the organ of Corti and the basilar membrane, and discuss the role of the basilar membrane in the frequency analysis of incoming sounds.
3. Discuss what is meant by the term *segmentation problem* in speech perception.
4. Explain how categorical perception, multiple acoustic cues, coarticulation, and context influence speech perception.
5. Draw a type A_s tympanogram, and explain what it tells us about a patient's middle ear function.
6. Choose two signal-processing strategies used in cochlear implants, and discuss their advantages and disadvantages for speech perception.

Clinical Application

Perceptual Problems in Hearing Impairment, Language and Reading Disability, and Articulation Deficits

chapter objectives | *After reading this chapter, you will*

1. Understand the impact of hearing loss on speech perception.
2. Be able to describe speech perception in cochlear implant users.
3. Appreciate that otitis media is a form of early sensory deprivation and understand its effects on speech perception.
4. Be able to explain the links between speech perception problems and language and reading disability.
5. Understand the impact of speech perception and articulation problems.

Speech perception is an integral part of learning a language and of developing all the numerous bases of language, such as phonology, morphology, syntax, and semantics. Reading and language are also closely related, and speech perception plays an important role in the development of reading skills. Consequently, problems in speech perception can have an adverse effect on many different aspects of language and reading.

■ *Hearing Loss*

Hearing loss has been well researched in terms of speech perception. The topic of speech perception of people with different types and degrees of hearing loss is extremely important clinically, because the development and successful use of hearing aids and of other current technology, such as cochlear implants, depends on benefits that can be gained in speech perception and phoneme and word recognition.

Hearing-impaired children and adults have deficits in discriminating between similar acoustic elements, resulting in difficulty in identifying the acoustic–phonetic features of speech. This kind of perceptual deficiency is often particularly detrimental to children during the early years of language development. Ross et al. (1991) noted that impaired hearing reduces the amount of acoustic information available to the child, who cannot integrate the acoustic fragments into a meaningful message. Unlike normally hearing children, who use audition to extract meaning from an utterance, children with hearing impairment must focus on the acoustic–phonetic elements, rather than on the global understanding of the message. Therefore, hearing-impaired children typically do not develop the level of language of their normally hearing peers.

> Hearing loss results in difficulty identifying the acoustic-phonetic features of speech, which can affect language development in the early childhood years.

It is extremely important to evaluate the speech perception abilities of hearing-impaired individuals to gain a precise understanding of their patterns of perception and production errors. Rehabilitation, in the form of amplification, cochlear implantation, speech–reading training, and the like, can then be targeted toward the underlying perceptual errors.

One way of evaluating how hearing-impaired individuals perceive consonants and vowels is by phonetically transcribing the phonemes that they recognize in terms of the traditional classification system or other phonetic classification systems. For example, phonetic transcription may indicate that an individual consistently omits the /s/ sound in the final position of words, suggesting difficulty in perceiving this phoneme. In the distinctive features system, phonetic cues such as voicing, nasality, and lip rounding are determined to be present or absent in specific phonemes produced by the hearing-impaired person. From these types of systems it is possible to understand the kinds of errors in perception made by the listener, but we cannot determine the actual acoustic and perceptual bases for the errors (Ochs, Humes, Ohde, & Grantham, 1989). By using synthetic speech or by digitally manipulating acoustic features of natural speech, it is possible to determine precisely which acoustic features are important for individuals with hearing loss.

The acoustic structure of vowels and consonants provides many different cues to perception, including formant frequencies, formant transitions, spectral characteristics, and others. Individuals use multiple cues to identify phonemes. People with normal hearing probably do not need all the cues present in a phoneme to judge its identity, because of the redundancy of the acoustic cues. Different acoustic cues usually play more or less of a role in identifying sounds. For instance, young children assign more importance to dynamic information provided by formant transitions and less to more static spectral information, whereas older children and adults seem to be more sensitive to spectral differences between sounds, such as the information contained in the burst of a stop or in the frication noise of a fricative.

Acoustic cues that may be of secondary importance to individuals with normal hearing may be more salient to those with hearing loss.

Some cues that may be of secondary importance to normally hearing listeners may be considerably more salient to people with hearing impairment, as long as they can detect the particular acoustic feature. For example, because the spectral energy of stops and fricatives is greatest in the higher frequencies, spectral cues are often inaudible to a person with a high-frequency hearing loss or to an individual whose hearing aid has a limited high-frequency range. Formant transitions, however, are greatest in intensity in the lower frequencies and may allow the individual to detect the presence of a stop or fricative despite the lack of available spectral information. In addition, duration cues present in phonetic segments may be accessible to hearing-impaired listeners and may act to signal a particular phonetic cue. For instance, vowels are longer when they precede a voiced consonant than when they precede a voiceless one.

Vowel Perception

Listeners with hearing impairment often show impaired frequency resolution. This lack of ability to discriminate between frequencies might be expected to interfere with their perception of vowels, which depends to a large degree on the ability to detect subtle differences in formant frequencies. However, many listeners with hearing loss are able to discriminate vowels without any problems, perhaps due to the redundancy of acoustic cues in the signal (Summers & Leek, 1992). On the other hand, many children with high-frequency hearing losses often confuse vowels, because of poor frequency resolution and poor au-

Many children with high-frequency losses confuse vowels such as /i/ and /u/ because of poor frequency discrimination.

dibility. For instance, one fairly common vowel confusion is /i/ and /u/. The F_1 of /i/ and /u/ are fairly close in frequency (270, 310, and 370 Hz for men, women, and children for /i/; 300, 370, and 430 Hz for /u/). Because F_2 for /i/ is relatively high in frequency (between about 2300 and 3200 Hz), it may not be detected by the hearing-impaired child, so he or she does not have access to the salient acoustic information that would help to discriminate these vowels.

Consonant Perception

Although vowel perception does not seem to pose a great problem for most hearing-impaired speakers, consonant perception is more of a challenge.

Because sibilant frica-
tives contain mostly
high-frequency noise,
perception of these
sounds poses a parti-
cular challenge for
speakers with high-
frequency hearing
losses.

Fricatives in particular are difficult to perceive for many hearing-impaired speakers with high-frequency losses. The cues for fricatives include the duration of the frication noise, the spectrum of the noise, formant transitions, and the amplitude relationship between the fricative and the adjacent vowel in the F_3 region (Hedrick, 1997). The spectral energy of fricatives, particularly the stridents, is extremely high in frequency, with that of /s/ being above 3500 Hz. Consequently, this spectral information is not accessible to many hearing-impaired individuals, even with amplification. Despite recent improvements in hearing aid technology, it is still difficult to make high-frequency phonemes audible to people with high-frequency losses.

The difficulty in perceiving /s/ is particularly disruptive to language, because the /s/ phoneme has many linguistic functions. For example, it acts as a plural (cat–cats), as a possessive (Jack's hat), as a marker for third-person singular (he walks), and as a copula (it is–it's). Clinically, therefore, enhancing a child's auditory perception of this phoneme is a high priority. Amplification may not be too helpful for this problem, because the response curves of hearing aids begin to roll off at around 3000 Hz (Hedrick, 1997). Spectral information, therefore, is not as accessible to hearing-impaired children, even with amplification.

The /s/ phoneme has
many linguistic func-
tions, and difficulty in
perceiving this sound
can be disruptive to
language development.

Adults with normal hearing typically weight the spectral information in the fricative noise more than the formant transitions. Some researchers hypothesized that adults with sensorineural hearing loss would weight the formant transitions more, because these transitions are usually in the frequency band that is amplified by most hearing aids, whereas the spectral information, at least for /s/ and /ʃ/, is not. Despite this, Hedrick (1997) reported that, similar to normally hearing listeners, adults with sensorineural hearing loss weighted spectral information more heavily than formant information, even though the formant information was actually more audible to them than the spectral information.

Audibility and **suprathreshold discriminability** are the two factors that affect speech recognition in hearing-impaired individuals. Audibility refers to whether a specific speech cue is presented at a level that the person can hear. This level is known as a **suprathreshold level**. However, individuals with hearing loss often cannot recognize sounds even when they are audible. In this case there is a loss of suprathreshold discriminability, which may be caused by factors such as deficits in detecting frequency and timing cues present in the sound wave. Zeng and Turner (1990) tested this notion by investigating whether hearing-impaired listeners could identify four fricative vowel syllables (see, fee, thee, and she). When the frication portion was audible to the hearing-impaired speakers, they used it as their primary cue for the fricative, whereas, even when the transition cues were audible, these individuals did not use them for fricative recognition. The normally hearing individuals in this study used transition information to recognize fricatives when the spectral information was experimentally masked and was not audible to them, but the hearing-impaired listeners did not do this. Consequently, it seems that one factor that makes it hard for hearing-impaired people to discriminate fricatives is their lack of ability to use dynamic information from the formant transitions between the fricative and the adjacent vowels.

Zeng and Turner (1990) illustrated this point with a typical case of a person with a moderate to severe hearing impairment wearing a hearing aid. In such a case, when the vowel portion of the syllable has been amplified to the maximum loudness level that the person can tolerate, the frication portion is still not audible, because the fricative noise is typically about 30 dB lower than the vowel in intensity. On the other hand, although the transition portions, which are about 5 to 10 dB less intense than the vowel, are audible to the hearing-impaired person, he or she is unable to make full use of them. Clinically, this means that to improve the person's discrimination it is the frication portions that should somehow be boosted in audibility.

The most common perceptual errors made by hearing-impaired individuals involve place of consonant articulation. Acoustic correlates of stop consonant place of articulation are typically found in the first 20 to 40 ms of a consonant–vowel syllable. Dubno, Dirks, and Schaefer (1987) examined stop consonant (CV) identification ability in hearing-impaired persons using syllable durations ranging from 10 to 100 ms. Normally hearing subjects achieved good identification for CV syllables with 20 to 40 ms durations. Hearing-impaired subjects did much more poorly even at the longest syllable durations. Hearing-impaired listeners seem to assign less weight to F_2 frequencies than normally hearing listeners and more weight to other cues that may be more accessible to them, such as F_1, or vowel duration.

Place-of-articulation errors are very common in speakers with hearing impairment.

Sammeth, Dorman, and Stearns (1999) suggested that another factor that plays a part in speech recognition for people with sensorineural hearing loss is the relationship between the amplitudes of the consonant and the adjacent vowels, known as the **consonant-to-vowel amplitude ratio** (CVR). CVR could be increased in hearing aids by boosting the higher frequencies (where much of the consonant information is located) more than the lower frequencies (where much of the vowel information is located). This may improve speech recognition for some listeners for some consonants. However, the relationship between CVR and speech recognition is complicated and seems to depend on the specific phonemes involved.

We still do not know exactly why some listeners with sensorineural hearing loss (SNHL) have difficulty understanding speech, even when audibility is boosted, but one factor may be the poor frequency selectivity that is common in hearing impairment. When normally hearing listeners are presented with a frequency of 1000 Hz, the nerve fibers respond to a bandwidth of about 100 to

150 Hz around this frequency. This is a percentage of approximately 10 to 15 percent of the center frequency of 1000 Hz. For listeners with SNHL, this filter bandwidth of the auditory nerve fibers could be as much as three to four times larger than normal, with some people's values approaching 50 percent of the center frequency (Turner, Chi, & Flock, 1999). The resulting frequency resolution is very poor, hindering the individual from making the fine frequency discriminations that are so important in the perception of phonemes.

Cochlear Implants

Cochlear implants are becoming increasingly accepted as a viable means of enhancing the speech recognition of children and adults with severe and profound sensorineural hearing loss. Many researchers have examined the resulting phoneme perception in implant users. For example, Meyers, Swirsky, Kirk, and Miyamoto (1998) tested the speech perception of children wearing cochlear implants. They used the Minimal Pairs Test, which assesses vowel height and advancement, consonant voicing, and manner and place of articulation. The authors found that the children's performance depended on how long the implants had been in place. Just prior to implantation, the children's average scores were at chance level. By approximately one year postimplantation, the average consonant perception score reached a level of 65 percent. The authors found that on average children with hearing losses in the 101 to 110 dB HL range received greater speech perception benefits from a cochlear implant than from their hearing aids. This is extremely valuable information, pointing to the possibility of better speech perception for at least some children using cochlear implants.

> Cochlear implants have been shown to improve speech recognition of children and adults with severe and profound sensorineural hearing loss.

In a test of adult cochlear implant users' speech perception, Hedrick and Carney (1997) presented fricative and stop continua varying in relative amplitude to adults with normal hearing and to listeners wearing cochlear implants. The deaf adults were able to label fricative and stop places of articulation, but they seemed to use different acoustic cues for recognition. Normally hearing listeners integrated relative amplitude and formant transition information to arrive at their judgments, whereas, even with the cochlear implants, most of the deaf listeners did not use formant transition information.

Training for Cochlear Implant Users   Training in speech recognition is essential for a person who has received an implant, and visual feedback is crucial for training, at least in the early stages. Electroglottography and spectrography are often used to visualize the phoneme contrasts being trained. As soon as the patient can discriminate the contrast through auditory input alone, the visual feedback is withdrawn.

> Visual feedback is a crucial component of speech recognition training in cochlear implant users.

Training should occur at both segmental and suprasegmental levels. In fact, one of the first discriminations a new cochlear implant user is able to make is the overall temporal structure of the segments, for example, counting the number of sounds heard (Cooper, 1991). Intonation is also an extremely important aspect of rehabilitation, and training involves the user's learning to perceive and produce different F_0 contours. The suprasegmental aspects of speech, such as intonation, stress, duration, and rhythm, are carried in the low frequencies and are often more audible to people with severe and profound losses. Training should capitalize on these aspects so that improved suprasegmental perception becomes a bridge to increased phoneme and word recognition. Visual feedback from spectrograms, electroglottography, instrumental tracking of F_0 and intensity contours, and so on, acts as a powerful clinical tool to facilitate the implant user's suprasegmental and segmental recognition.

Otitis Media

The most common cause of conductive hearing loss is otitis media (OM). Anyone can get OM, but it is particularly prevalent among young children. This

Otitis media is prevalent in young children from causes including upper respiratory infection, allergies, and enlarged adenoids.

happens in part because of the different shape of the auditory tube in children and adults. The adult tube lies at an angle of about 45° to the horizontal, whereas it is almost horizontal in young children (Gelfand, 1997). The horizontal position makes drainage of fluids through the tube less efficient, and thus it is more likely that fluid will build up in the middle ear. Tube dysfunction can also be caused by an upper respiratory infection, in which edema and fluid block the tube, and by allergies, enlarged adenoids, or structural problems such as cleft palate. When the tube does not open properly, the middle ear cannot be ventilated. Some of the air in the middle ear gets absorbed into the tissues of the middle ear. Consequently, the air pressure inside the middle ear becomes lower than in the surrounding atmosphere, including in the ear canal. This causes the tympanic membrane to be drawn inward, or retracted, and the air pressure cannot be equalized because of the blockage of the auditory tube. Because the middle ear cannot be drained properly, fluids often build up within the middle ear. This is known as **otitis media with effusion** (OME).

Episodes of otitis media with effusion cause temporary conductive hearing losses of about 20 to 40 dB.

OME is very prevalent in preschool children and can cause temporary conductive hearing losses of approximately 20 to 40 dB (Groenen, Crul, Maassen, & van Bon, 1996a). Many young children have recurring bouts of OM, called chronic OM. Each episode leads to a temporary conductive loss. These recurring periods of hearing loss have been linked to problems in perception, subtle language deficits, and academic difficulties. Even though the hearing loss is temporary, if the child has recurring periods of loss during the interval in which he or she is acquiring speech and language, the youngster may be at risk for language problems later.

Children with a history of recurring OME in early childhood have been shown to have subtle differences in speech perception from their peers. For instance, some children with early OME show poorer VOT perception, and some show less mature weighting strategies for the perception of synthetic /s/ and /ʃ/ continua. For example, Groenen et al. (1996a) tested the voiced–voiceless distinction using VOT continua varying from /b/ (/bak/) to /p/ (/pak/). Children without OME or language impairment were compared to children with a history of OME only and to children with both OME and language impairment. Children with either early OME or language impairment were not as adept at identifying the sounds. Thus, a history of OME appears to result in poorer phonetic processing, irrespective of language impairment. The authors proposed that recurrent OME may be considered a form of early sensory deprivation. Information that is important to the perception and categorization of speech may therefore be less consistent during the years when the child should be acquiring the sound system of his or her native language.

Recurrent otitis media with effusion may be a form of early sensory deprivation that can result in poorer phonetic processing.

These subtle disturbances in phonetic perception can affect the child's linguistic abilities. Nittrouer (1996a) used synthetic /s/ and /ʃ/ fricatives to test whether children with early OME used similar weighting strategies as their peers without early OME. Children with early OME showed less mature perceptual weighting strategies than children with no OM. Very young children give more weight to dynamic information (e.g., formant transitions) than they do to more static spectral information. As they develop a larger vocabulary, they learn to make more subtle perceptual distinctions between sounds, based more on static spectral cues, and with less reliance on dynamic characteristics. Thus, chronic OM clearly puts children at risk for delays in the development of perceptual weighting strategies and phonemic awareness. In turn, this may lead to difficulties with higher level language functioning and with reading.

Language and Reading Disability

Difficulties with the perceptual processing of acoustic cues have been found to be important in some forms of language-learning disorders and in reading disabilities. Much research has focused on whether these difficulties arise from problems in the perception of phonemes at the phonetic–acoustic level or from a higher level, more linguistically based impairment. Much of the research is based on the hypothesis that difficulty in perceiving the rapidly changing sound waves of speech results in problems in relating the acoustic information contained in the phonemes and syllables to the person's mental representation of phonemes. For reading, this may interfere with the process of transforming written symbols to phonetic units (Watson & Miller, 1993). The distinction between a phonetic processing problem and a higher level linguistic problem is important, because treatment strategies would differ depending on the root cause of the problem.

Often the child with a language and/or reading disorder does not have any obvious problems that are causing it, such as mental or emotional challenges or hearing loss. In fact, **specific language impairment** (SLI) is a disorder in which children show a significant problem with language despite having normal hearing, normal nonverbal intelligence, and no known neurological problems. The cause of SLI is not known, but one theory is that these children have a problem with auditory perception that results in the language difficulties. During connected speech the acoustic signal changes rapidly and continuously in frequency and intensity, and a child who has difficulty perceiving these quick shifts may have difficulty in detecting phoneme changes.

This difficulty in processing rapid acoustic signals is referred to as a **temporal processing problem**. According to Tallal et al. (1996), children who are language-learning impaired often cannot identify fast elements, such as formant transitions or spectral information, that are embedded in ongoing speech. If a child has difficulty in perceiving the phonemes of the language, then the child does not have access to complete language input from the environment. This can interfere with higher order language functions, such as phonological processing skills, morphology, syntax, and semantics.

Research over the past two decades has explored how children with reading difficulties and language problems are able to detect small acoustic differences between sounds. Many of these tests use synthetic speech stimuli, rather than naturally spoken speech. For example, Nittrouer (1999) compared children with language-learning difficulty and those with normal language. The first test examined the children's ability to discriminate between voiced and voiceless sounds (/t/ and /d/). Nittrouer manipulated the duration of the F_1 transition and the spectrum of a 10 ms release burst. The F_1 transitions varied from 40 ms to no transition (0 ms) in equal steps of 5 ms each. Each synthetic item was paired up with a 10 ms burst from a speaker saying /da/ and /ta/. The stimuli thus varied from most /da/-like to most /ta/-like. The children were presented with one item at a time and had to decide if it was a /da/ or a /ta/. In another task, the children listened to sounds on a continuum of /s/ to /ʃ/. These sounds varied in the center frequency of the synthetic fricative noises, from 2200 to 3800 Hz in 200 Hz steps. The /s/ is associated with a very high spectral peak, while the /ʃ/ has a much lower frequency spectral peak. As with the /da–ta/ task, the children were presented with one sound at a time, and had to assign it to an /s/ or /ʃ/ category. These kinds of spectral features are extremely brief, and occur very rapidly.

Some children who have language-learning impairment show difficulty in processing the rapidly changing acoustic signals in speech.

Both groups of children in Nittrouer's (1999) study used these acoustic cues similarly in deciding on the identity of the sound. The children with language-learning difficulties, however, performed more like younger children developing language normally for the fricative task, thus demonstrating subtle delays in perceptual processing of at least some phonemes.

Perceptual processing delays were also reported by Elliott and Hammer (1993), who tested older and younger children in three groups: children with a language-learning problem, children in a regular school placement, and children with moderate intellectual impairment. The test activities involved a place of articulation continuum (/ba–da–ga/) and a VOT continuum (/ba–pa/). The place continuum differed in frequency characteristics, with different starting frequencies for F_2 and F_3. The VOT continuum differed in temporal characteristics, that is, the amount of time between the release burst of the consonant and the onset of vibration for the following vowel. The older children performed better than the younger children on most of the tasks. The younger children with language problems performed more poorly than the younger children in regular school placements on every test measure. For example, the children with language problems required a VOT of 23 ms to differentiate /ba/ from /pa/, whereas the normally developing children required only 17 ms. Performance for the children with intellectual impairment was poorer than for the other two groups.

The authors suggested that the lower the level of a young child's speech and language skills, the greater is the importance of auditory discrimination of small acoustic differences in increasing receptive vocabulary and language skills. The authors proposed a hypothesis that young normally developing children are primarily dependent on auditory stimulation for language learning. As they mature, other influences such as reading become increasingly important; so older children may rely less on audition, and auditory discrimination becomes less important.

Other research confirms that older children do not seem to rely as much on auditory discrimination as younger children. Bernstein and Stark (1985) followed up the speech perception abilities in language-impaired children four years after the children had first been tested, using synthetic /ba/ and /da/ syllables. Of the 29 children in the follow-up study who were identified as language impaired at time 1, 23 were still language impaired at time 2. However, the authors found some perceptual development among the language-impaired children, suggesting that these children beyond the age of 8 years do not have difficulties obtaining perceptual information. The authors suggested that early perceptual deficits do not prevent language development, but language develops more slowly than it does for normal children. These kinds of perceptual deficits have been shown to be highly correlated with children's scores on language tests, such as the *Peabody Picture Vocabulary Test–Revised* and the *Token Test for Chil-*

Younger children have been shown to rely more on auditory discrimination of small acoustic differences than older children.

dren (Stark & Heinz, 1996a). In fact, these kinds of acoustic characteristics can be very accurate in predicting whether schoolchildren will have language-learning disabilities.

Leonard, McGregor, and Allen (1992) provided a specific link between the perceptual processing difficulties of children with SLI and grammatical function. Morphology is often an area of particular difficulty for these children, including inflections such as the third person singular *-s*, as well as function words such as the articles *a* and *the*. Interestingly, the morphological features that seem to pose the most difficulty are consonant segments (e.g., third person singular *-s*) and unstressed syllables (e.g., *the*), which are characterized by shorter duration than adjacent morphemes and often lower F_0 and amplitude.

These children, however, use some of the same phonetic forms in other contexts. For example, Leonard et al. (1992) pointed out that the children used the /d/ in *braid* much more than in *played* and the /s/ in *box* more than in *rocks*. They proposed that the difficulty seems to be not so much in perceiving the sound, but in both perceiving it and treating it as a morpheme. The child must not only perceive the /d/ in *played*, but also relate *played* to *play*, and put *-ed* in the proper place. Because these additional operations are not involved in *braid*, acquisition and use of /d/ will be more advanced in *braid*.

The authors also suggested that the duration of the contrastive portion of the stimulus is important for its perception in children with SLI. When the part of the word to be discriminated is shorter than that of the remaining portion, children with SLI have greater difficulty than normally developing children of the same age. However, when the duration of the contrastive feature is longer than that of the rest of the stimulus, these children perform adequately.

Leonard et al. (1992) suggested two possible sources of the children's difficulty. The first is that their perceptual abilities are extremely fragile. Therefore, when they need to make difficult discriminations between sounds, any additional processing that needs to be done suffers. The second possibility is that these children have some kind of generalized processing problem so that, when they need to use extra resources for a particularly hard task, fewer resources are left for other mental operations.

Other research has found that children with **developmental dyslexia** do not show as clear-cut categorical perception of synthetic continua as normally reading children. Developmental dyslexia is a disorder in which the person's reading ability is significantly lower than what would be predicted on the basis of age and IQ (McAnally, Hansen, Cornelissen, & Stein, 1997). Many of these individuals have difficulty perceiving consonant contrasts and may confuse sounds that are phonetically similar more often than normal. People with dyslexia may have deficits in processing the temporal order of acoustic information. Language and reading are integrally related. Stark and Heinz (1996b) reported that children with language impairment find it difficult to discriminate and

Research suggests that children with developmental dyslexia do not show the same degree of categorical perception as normally reading children.

identify phonemes and also have problems in judging the order in which phonemes are heard. Many of these children, according to Stark and Heinz (1996b), go on to have a reading disability.

It is clear that many children with language and/or reading impairment have difficulties in segmenting, discriminating, and identifying speech sounds (Bishop et al., 1999). The temporal characteristics of auditory stimuli are critical for children with language impairment. When stimuli are either very short in duration or very rapid, this presents a serious challenge to children with language impairment. However, these children seem to have less difficulty in discrimination when the stimuli are lengthened or presented at a slower rate. The question is whether such difficulties have their basis in a more fundamental auditory perceptual deficit that affects the processing of all sounds. It is currently thought that the impairment in discriminating brief or rapid events is not specific to auditory processing, but also occurs in other sensory areas. However, this difficulty in rapid processing is thought to have an especially severe impact on language development, which is crucially dependent on the ability to distinguish and identify brief and rapid auditory events (Bishop et al., 1999).

Articulatory Problems

Researchers and clinicians have long suspected that there may be a link between errors in articulation that do not result from problems such as cleft palate or deafness and perception. However, the nature of this link is far from clear. Some children have been found to have similar abilities in articulation and perception. Some children misarticulate specific sounds, but can perceive the sounds they misarticulate without a problem. Others misarticulate specific sounds and also have difficulty perceiving these sounds.

Some children with misarticulations demonstrate variability and lack of precision in their perception of speech sounds.

Investigators have used synthetic speech sounds to try to clarify this link, because synthetic speech sounds can be manipulated more easily to show precisely which acoustic cues in the signal influence children's perception and production of the sounds. For example, Raaymakers and Crul (1988) tested adults and 5- to 6-year-old children on synthetically generated words ending in /s/ and /ts/. One group of children misarticulated the /s–ts/ contrast. Another group had various other misarticulations. The authors generated a continuum using the Dutch words *moes* to *moets* by adding periods of silence between *oe* and /s/. They found that the poorer the child's articulation skill, the more variable the child was in his or her response.

Other authors have found similar variability and lack of precision in misarticulating children's perception. Hoffman, Daniloff, Bengoa, and Schuckers, (1985) looked at children's abilities to discriminate between the /w/ and /r/ sounds. These sounds are differentiated by their formant frequencies, with /r/

having a much lower F_3 than /w/. Research has shown that 3-year-old children with normal articulation skills can identify synthesized /l/, /r/, and /w/ sounds that differ in the onset frequencies of the first three formants. Many of these children cannot yet produce the /l/ and /r/ sounds accurately, producing them both as /w/. However, 3-year-old children with delayed articulation show a large number of perceptual errors. The authors tested children 6 years to 6 years and 11 months old who substituted /w/ for /r/ and children who produced the sounds correctly, on synthesized /r/–/w/ continua. The misarticulating children's discrimination and identification of these phonemes was less precise than the controls. Approximately two-thirds of the misarticulating children failed to categorize /r/ and /w/ stimuli when they had to rely only on formant trajectories. The remaining third made a categorization that was less well defined than that of the controls. The authors suggested that the /r/-misarticulating children may not be basing their perceptual categorizations on the same acoustic characteristics that are crucial to adult listeners, but may be relying on contextual cues in conversation to help with the perceptual discrimination that they need.

Children learn to produce the phoneme contrasts and sequences of their language gradually during their first years by matching their own productions to an acoustic model. The child who fails to produce speech correctly may omit a target phoneme, produce that phoneme inaccurately, or substitute another phoneme for the intended one. Sometimes a child neutralizes the contrast between the two phonemes. For instance, a child who substitutes /w/ or a /w/-like sound for /r/ neutralizes the contrast between /w/ and /r/. The child may or may not be able to perceptually discriminate between his or her own productions of the error sound and the intended sound. If the child can discriminate the sounds even when the contrast between them cannot be perceived by another listener, the child may be using subphonemic cues to mark the contrast. Such cues are not audible to adults, although often they can be detected with acoustic instrumentation. In some cases a child may maintain a contrast, but misarticulate both phonemes. For example, when a child substitutes /w/ for /r/ and /j/ for /l/, both /l/ and /r/ are misarticulated, but the contrast between them is maintained (Broen, Strange, Doyle, & Heller, 1983).

> Children in their early years learn to produce the phoneme contrasts of their language by matching their own productions to an acoustic model.

Broen et al. (1983) tested the perception of 3-year-olds with misarticulations and normally speaking children who had developmental misarticulations of /l/ and /r/ with the synthetically produced words *wake–rake*, *rake–lake*, and *wake–lake*. They found that, although the majority of children in both groups misarticulated /l/ and/or /r/, the pattern of errors was different. When the normal children misarticulated /l/ or /r/, they produced /w/ or a /w/-like distortion, neutralizing that contrast for the adult listener. However, these developmentally appropriate misarticulations were not accompanied by perceptual problems. All the normal children perceived the three contrasts with no problems. The articulation-delayed children had a much more varied pattern of misarticulations of the /l/, /r/, and /w/ sounds. Some children actually omitted all these sounds. These children also showed problems in the perception of all three contrasts.

Children with articulation problems show similar perceptual difficulties with synthetic /s/–/ʃ/ contrasts. Rvachew and Jamieson (1989) looked at the perception of normally speaking adults, normally speaking 5-year-olds, and articulation-disordered 5-year-olds, in the synthetically generated words *seat* and *sheet*. The adults and the normally speaking children identified fricatives differing in spectral characteristics with equal consistency. The articulation-disordered children, however, were much more variable. More than half of them were unable to classify the stimuli in the continuum reliably. Some children responded *seat* to almost all the stimuli, whereas others responded in an apparently random manner.

Thus, children with a functional articulation disorder can be categorized into at least two subgroups: those with speech perception difficulties and those with normal speech perception skills. It is very important, therefore, to determine children's perceptual skills in the clinic before implementing therapy procedures for articulation problems. Some children may need help in honing their perceptual skills before the production problem is treated, whereas other children with normal perceptual skills may be treated immediately for the articulation problem. The authors also emphasized that children with articulation problems show speech perception difficulties that are not general to all speech sounds, but that are specific to the child's misarticulated sounds. Therefore, speech discrimination tests that cover a wide range of phoneme contrasts might not be sensitive enough to detect the child's very specific perception problem.

> Children with functional articulation disorders can be categorized in terms of those with speech perception difficulties and those with normal speech perception.

■ *Clinical Study*

Background

Mr. Williams, a 69-year-old man, came to your Speech and Hearing Clinic accompanied by his wife of forty-three years. Mrs. Williams reported that her husband does not respond to her conversation at home. She is upset, though, that he seems to have no difficulty in conversing with his male friends at home, and she feels that his problem is with her, and not with his hearing. The Williamses enjoy dining out with friends once or twice per week, and Mr. Williams has lately been having difficulty in following conversations in these situations. Mr. Williams admits that he feels frustrated in these situations, but denies having any difficulty at home. His wife reports that the TV is always on at an uncomfortably high level.

Acoustic Measures

Pure-tone testing revealed normal hearing through 1 kHz dropping to a moderate bilateral high-frequency sensorineural hearing loss. Speech recognition testing indicated only fair recognition of speech. Otoacoustic emission screening showed no emissions bilaterally. Tympanometry was consistent with normal middle ear function.

Clinical Questions

1. Why might Mr. Williams be having difficulty hearing his wife's voice?
2. Why does Mr. Williams have more difficulty in noisy situations?
3. What specific vowels and consonants would you expect him to have particular problems in hearing? Why?
4. With appropriate amplification, do you think he will be better able to perceive his wife's voice? Why or why not?
5. With appropriate amplification, do you think he will be better able to perceive his friends' voices? Why or why not?

summary

- Individuals with hearing impairment do not have access to the multiple acoustic cues used by normally hearing speakers to identify phonemes.
- Hearing-impaired listeners are often able to discriminate vowels, but have problems in identifying consonants, particularly fricatives.
- Training in auditory discrimination using visual feedback is essential for cochlear implant users to receive the greatest benefit from their device.

- Otitis media is a form of early sensory deprivation that has been linked to subtle speech perception and linguistic problems.
- Children with language and/or reading disabilities may have a temporal processing problem that hinders them from perceiving the phonemes of their language.
- Children with articulation problems may or may not have speech perception difficulties related to their specific misarticulations.

review exercises

1. Explain why individuals with high-frequency hearing losses have particular difficulty in perceiving fricatives.
2. Discuss the relationship between phoneme perception and morphological markers in children with hearing impairment and those with language disability.
3. Elaborate on the concept of frequency selectivity, and explain its link to normal hearing and to hearing impairment.

4. Why is otitis media considered to be a form of sensory deprivation, and what is its effect on language?

5. Explain the term *temporal processing problem,* and describe its impact on children with language and/or reading disability.

6. Describe the relationships between phoneme perception and articulation ability in young children.

chapter **12**

The Nervous System

chapter objectives

After reading this chapter, you will

1. Understand the structure and function of neurons.
2. Be familiar with the functional components of the central nervous system and their influence in speech production.
3. Know the origin and target structures of the cranial nerves important in speech and hearing.
4. Appreciate the importance of a steady blood supply to the brain.
5. Understand the structure and function of the upper and lower motor neurons involved in speech production.
6. Be aware of the importance of feedback and feedforward systems in speech motor control.

The nervous system (NS) is the most important regulator and controller of movement, including movement involved in all aspects of speech production: respiration, phonation, and articulation. A normally functioning NS is crucial for normal speech. Disruptions to the NS at any point or location can have devastating effects on speech motor control, as is seen with neurological disorders such as cerebral palsy, stroke, Parkinson's disease, multiple sclerosis, and traumatic brain injury.

The NS is hugely complex in its structure and function and can be examined from many different anatomical and physiological viewpoints. In this chapter we will begin by describing the basic structure of the NS in terms of the neurons that constitute the brain and spinal cord. The electrochemical nature of nerve impulses will be explained. Different functional portions of the NS will be highlighted, and their relationship to speech motor control will be emphasized. The nerve pathways or tracts that are formed by bundles of neurons will then be discussed in terms of their function related to speech production. The chapter closes by exploring various mechanisms used in motor control of the speech subsystems.

The CNS consists of the brain and spinal cord; the PNS includes the cranial and spinal nerves.

The NS is divided into the central nervous system (CNS) and peripheral nervous system (PNS). The CNS consists of the brain itself as well as the spinal cord. The PNS consists of the cranial and spinal nerves that transmit and receive nerve impulses to and from all the muscles and glands of the body. The PNS is further divided into the somatic system and the autonomic system.

Brain Tissue

The mature adult human brain weighs approximately 1400 g.

The brain itself is a small organ, weighing approximately 1400 g in the mature adult, although individual brains range anywhere from 1100 to 1700 g (Nolte, 2002). Two major types of tissue make up the brain: glial cells and neurons.

Glial Cells

Glial cells are a type of connective tissue and, like all connective tissues, perform a variety of functions, including metabolic support, secretion of cerebrospinal fluid, response to injury, and insulation.

Glial cells bring nutrients from the blood vessels to each neuron and remove the waste products of metabolism. Different types of glial cells are located in different areas of the NS. The most common glial cells are called **astrocytes** (Figure 12.1), which are located throughout the system of nerve cells in the brain. These cells have numerous projections that connect to blood capillaries and thereby assist in transporting substances from the blood to the nerve cell.

Glial cells form a support system for neurons, performing functions such as destroying harmful organisms and forming layers of insulation around nerve cells.

Oligodendrocytes in the CNS, and **Schwann cells** in the PNS, form layers of insulation, called myelin, around nerve cells. Other cells called **microglia** help to destroy harmful organisms by engulfing them. Unlike nerve cells, glial cells are able to divide and reproduce throughout their lives. Therefore, if nerve tissue dies, the space previously occupied by the neurons tends to be filled by this connective tissue. When this occurs, the site can become a focal point of epileptic seizures.

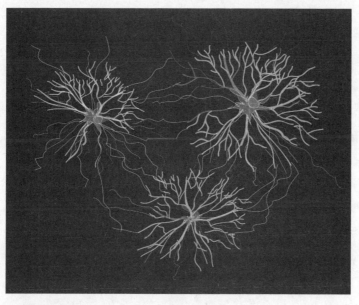

■ FIGURE 12.1

Astrocytes.

Neurons

Neurons are the structures that receive, process, and transmit information to, from, and within the NS. There are about 100 billion neurons in the CNS. All neurons have essentially the same structure, although some have modifications depending on their specific function. The basic structure consists of a **soma** or cell body, dendrites, and an axon, all bounded by a cell membrane (see Figure 12.2).

The soma is formed by a nucleus surrounded by a mass of cytoplasm. Within the cytoplasm are organelles, which are specialized microstructures involved in various cell functions. For example, **Nissl bodies** synthesize proteins that keep the neuron healthy, while **mitochondria** are involved in cell respiration and the production of energy (Clayman, 1995). Other organelles called **Golgi apparatus** secrete proteins and sugars. It is within the soma, thus, that the major metabolic activity of the neuron takes place. Branching off the cell body are numerous short projections called dendrites, which serve to transmit nerve impulses toward the cell body. Also extending from the cell body is an **axon**, which is a projection that transmits nerve impulses away from the cell body. Axons form at a small bump at the cell body called the axon hillock. They vary in length from less than one millimeter (mm) to more than one meter (Hutchins, Naftel, & Arel, 2002; Webster, 1999). Most axons within the CNS are wrapped in myelin. Much like the insulation around a wire, the myelin

Neurons receive, process, and transmit information to, from, and within the nervous system.

The cell body of the neuron contains organelles that are involved in all aspects of cell metabolism.

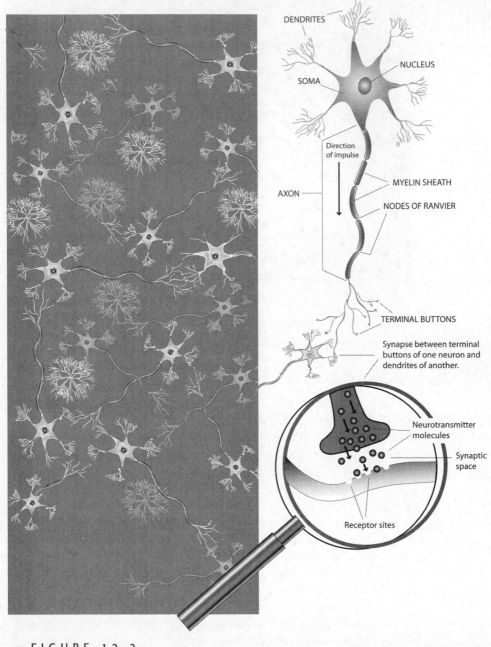

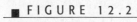

■ FIGURE 12.2

Neurons.

sheath serves to insulate and protect the axon and also helps to increase the speed of nerve conduction along the axon. The myelin sheath is not continuous along the axon, but is interrupted by breaks known as **nodes of Ranvier**. These nodes are involved in speeding up the rate of nerve transmission, as the nerve impulse jumps from one node to the next.

At its end point the axon divides into numerous **terminal branches** (also called *telodendria*), which in turn end in small swellings or bumps, the **terminal buttons**. The number of buttons per axon varies tremendously, from few to many thousands. Within the terminal buttons are tiny containers called vesicles, filled with chemicals known as neurotransmitters. This end point is the site of communication with other nerve cells. Between nerve cells is a tiny gap or cleft, called the **synapse**. A synapse may occur between the axon of one nerve and the dendrites, cell body, or axon of another nerve or nerves, of a muscle fiber, or of a glandular cell. A synapse between an axon and another axon is called an axo-axonal synapse. One between an axon and a soma is an axo-somatic synapse; an axo-dendritic synapse occurs between an axon and a dendrite. An axon that synapses with a skeletal muscle fiber is called the **neuromuscular junction** or the *neuromuscular end plate*. A single neuron may synapse with thousands of other neurons and in return may receive axonal input from many other neurons. This results in extraordinarily complex networks of neuronal connections throughout the NS.

Neurons function in groups. Specifically, axons do not extend to structures as individual projections, but are wrapped together in bundles that form nerve pathways or tracts. Pathways are either *sensory* (**afferent**), transmitting information from sensory receptors toward the CNS, or *motor* (**efferent**), transmitting information from the CNS toward muscles and glands. Mixed nerve pathways contain both sensory and motor components.

Types of Neurons   Neurons vary in their size and shape, as well as in the total number of their receiving and transmitting processes. One way of classifying neurons is according to their number of processes. Unipolar neurons have a single process, while bipolar neurons have two processes. Most neurons in the human nervous system are multipolar, with multiple dendrites and an axon. Multipolar neurons are further divided into Golgi Type I and Golgi Type II. Golgi Type I, also called projection neurons, have long axons that extend to the PNS and synapse with nerves that innervate muscles or glands. Golgi Type II are local circuit neurons with short axons that synapse on nearby neurons within the CNS. Golgi Type I axons are typically myelinated, while Golgi Type II tend to be unmyelinated (Webster, 1999).

Sidebar notes:

Projections off the cell body include dendrites, which transmit nerve impulses toward the cell body, and an axon, which transmits nerve impulses away from the cell body.

Terminal buttons at the terminal branches of axons contain vesicles filled with neurotransmitter chemicals.

Most neurons in the human NS are multipolar, with multiple dendrites and an axon, and are divided into Golgi Type I and Golgi Type II.

■ **TABLE 12.1**

Ways of Classifying Neurons

Number of processes	Unipolar
	Bipolar
	Multipolar
	Golgi Type I
	Golgi Type II
Function	Efferent (motor): Toward periphery
	Afferent (sensory): Toward NS
	Interneurons: Within NS
Neurotransmitter	Dopaminergic
	Cholinergic
	Serotonergic

Neurons can also be classified according to their function. Motor or efferent neurons are those that travel away from the NS and cause a movement to occur, either of a muscle or a gland. Sensory or afferent neurons carry information toward the CNS from peripheral structures such as specialized receptors in the skin, sense organs (eye, ear, etc.), and viscera. **Interneurons**, as the name suggests, connect neurons to each other, either locally—that is, within a small area of the CNS—or over longer distances (projection neurons). Most neurons within the human NS are interneurons.

A third way of classifying neurons is based on the type of neurotransmitter contained within its vesicles. For example, neurons containing the neurotransmitter dopamine are referred to as dopaminergic; those containing serotonin are serotonergic, acetylcholine-carrying neurons are cholinergic, and so on. Table 12.1 summarizes these classifications.

■ *Sensory Receptors*

Receptors are specialized nerve cells that respond to stimuli occurring within or outside of the individual and transmit these responses to the NS.

In order to process information from an individual's external and internal environment, the body is richly supplied with different types of receptors. Receptors are specialized nerve cells that respond to certain changes in the organism or its environment and transmit these responses to the NS. Receptors respond to specific stimuli. For example, receptors in the retina of the eye (rods and cones) respond to light. Receptors of the ear (inner hair cells) respond to sound waves. Receptors in the skin are differentially sensitive to touch, pressure, pain, and temperature. Table 12.2 identifies some different types of receptors.

■ TABLE 12.2

Types of Sensory Receptors

TYPE OF RECEPTOR	SENSORY INFORMATION	ORGAN
Teleceptors	Distant environment	Fye, ear
Exteroceptors	Immediate environment	Skin
Proprioceptors	Position of body structures in space	Inner ear, muscles, tendons, joints
Visceroceptors/Interoceptors	Visceral structures	
Mechanoreceptors	Pressure/deformation	Tissue
Thermoreceptors	Changes in temperature	
Nocioreceptors	Tissue damage	
Photoreceptors	Light	Retina
Chemoreceptors	Taste and smell	Tongue, nose
Baroreceptors	Air pressure	Trachea, bronchi

■ *Neuronal Function*

Nerves work through a complex electrochemical process. Because of their chemical composition, the inside of a neuron and the extracellular fluid that surrounds it are electrically charged. Whether the charge is positive or negative depends on the concentration of **ions**. An ion is an atom or group of atoms that carries an electrical charge (either positive or negative) due to gaining or losing electrons. When the neuron is at rest, there is a higher concentration of positive ions (sodium, Na+, and potassium, K+) outside the cell and a higher proportion of negative ions (chlorine, Cl−) within the cell. In fact, the sodium concentration within the neuron at rest is around one-tenth of the amount outside the cell (Zemlin, 1998). This imbalance creates a voltage across the cell membrane, called the **resting membrane potential** (RMP). At rest the interior of the neuron has a voltage of approximately −70 millivolts (mV), while the extracellular space is positively charged. The RMP is maintained by a process called the sodium-potassium pump. During this process excessive sodium ions inside the cell are pumped out of the neuron as fast as they enter, and K+ ions that may have left the cell are brought back within.

At rest, the interior of a neuron is negatively charged, while the extracellular fluid outside the neuron is positively charged.

The voltage differential between the inside and outside of the neuron causes the cell membrane, in its resting state, to be polarized. In order to generate a nerve impulse, the RMP must be disturbed, or **depolarized**. The neuron is depolarized when the electrical charges within and outside the cell briefly reverse, with the inside becoming positively charged relative to the extracellular fluid and going from − 70 mV to around +30 mV, as shown in Figure 12.3.

Depolarization occurs when the charges inside and outside the nerve cell briefly reverse, with the interior becoming positively charged relative to the extracellular fluid.

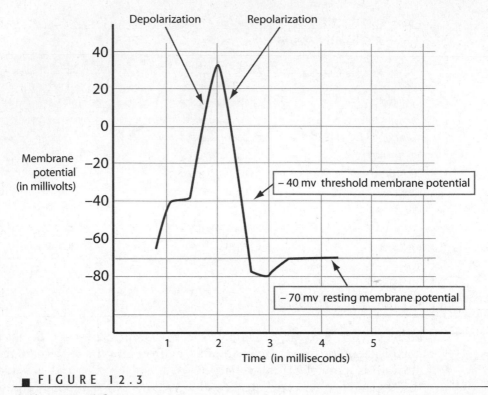

Depolarization   Repolarization

Membrane potential (in millivolts)

– 40 mv threshold membrane potential

– 70 mv resting membrane potential

Time (in milliseconds)

■ FIGURE 12.3

Action potential.

The depolarization occurs when channels in the cell membrane that regulate sodium ions open, allowing sodium ions to enter into the intracellular fluid. The depolarization affects only a tiny portion of the cell membrane and lasts for a very short time. Then potassium channels in the cell membrane are opened and potassium ions escape into the extracellular fluid. Consequently, the cell membrane once again reverts to the negatively charged state. This reverse process is called **repolarization**. As one portion of the cell membrane reverses its voltage and depolarizes, it causes the adjacent portion of the membrane to depolarize. In turn, successive portions of the nerve fiber are stimulated to depolarize, and the depolarization is propagated along the entire length of the nerve. This wave of depolarization is called the **action potential** (AP). When an AP occurs, the neuron is said to have "fired," and a nerve impulse is generated. As each portion of the axon is depolarized, it is followed by the repolarization.

A nerve, however, even when stimulated, may not generate an AP. In order for the neuron to fire and undergo the voltage reversal, the cell membrane of the neuron must reach a critical threshold of approxi-

The depolarization is the action potential, which travels along the length of the axon, and is followed by a repolarization.

In order for a nerve to fire and generate an action potential, a critical threshold must be achieved at the axon hillock.

mately −40 mV at the axon hillock. The initial impulse traveling toward the cell body is known as the graded potential. If the graded potential reaches the critical threshold, the AP will be generated, and the nerve will fire. The AP travels in only one direction, away from the cell body, and it travels in an all-or-none fashion. That is, a neuron either discharges completely or not at all. Once an AP begins, it travels with the same strength along the entire axon. If the threshold is not reached, there will not be an action potential. Not all inputs to the neuron are strong enough to reach the critical threshold. Typically, neurons receive electrical input from many other neurons, and these separate inputs are summed together. The addition of separate neural inputs can increase the strength of the stimulation and reach the membrane threshold. There are two types of summation of impulses: temporal and spatial. **Temporal summation** occurs when separate inputs reach the cell membrane with slight time differences. As long as the differences fall within some brief amount of time, they may add together. **Spatial summation** refers to the addition of impulses arriving at slightly different locations on the cell body or dendrites. Again, as long as the impulses arrive not too far apart from each other, they will combine and increase the strength of the resulting input. Once a nerve has fired, there is a brief period of time (about 0.5 ms) during which it cannot be stimulated, no matter how strong the incoming impulse. During this period, potassium ions flow into the neuron. This is called the **absolute refractory period**. After this brief interval the neuron undergoes a **relative refractory period** during which it can be stimulated but only by a stronger-than-usual stimulus. This whole cycle from RMP to AP and back again to RMP takes about 1 ms in most neurons. In other words, most neurons can fire around 1,000 times per second (Seikel, Drumright, & Seikel, 2004).

So far we have been focusing on the generation of an AP in just one nerve. However, in order to transmit information to and from the brain and spinal cord, nerves must somehow communicate with each other. This communication occurs at the synapse. A nerve signal travels along one nerve, finally reaching the terminal buttons of the axon. The vesicles within the buttons are stimulated to release their neurotransmitter into the synapse between the activated neuron (the presynaptic neuron) and the next neuron in line (the postsynaptic neuron). The neurotransmitter can have one of two actions. It can either lower the threshold of the post-synaptic neuron and make it easier for it to fire, called an **excitatory post-synaptic potential** (EPSP), or it can make it more difficult for the post-synaptic neuron to fire by raising its threshold, called an **inhibitory post-synaptic potential** (IPSP). The neurotransmitter acts like a key to a lock. On the membrane of the post-synaptic neuron are receptors that are selectively responsive to different neurotransmitters. Much as a specific key will only open a specific lock, receptor sites on the membrane will only respond to specific neurotransmitters, as illustrated in Figure 12.4.

Impulses may combine (summate) and increase the strength of the stimulation to the nerve cell; summation can be spatial or temporal.

Neurons are selectively responsive to different neurotransmitters, depending on the specific receptor sites on the neuron.

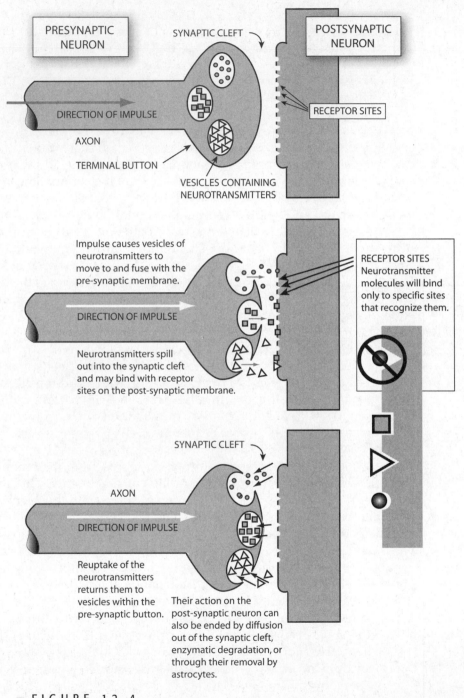

PRESYNAPTIC NEURON

SYNAPTIC CLEFT

POSTSYNAPTIC NEURON

DIRECTION OF IMPULSE

RECEPTOR SITES

AXON

TERMINAL BUTTON

VESICLES CONTAINING NEUROTRANSMITTERS

Impulse causes vesicles of neurotransmitters to move to and fuse with the pre-synaptic membrane.

DIRECTION OF IMPULSE

Neurotransmitters spill out into the synaptic cleft and may bind with receptor sites on the post-synaptic membrane.

RECEPTOR SITES
Neurotransmitter molecules will bind only to specific sites that recognize them.

SYNAPTIC CLEFT

AXON

DIRECTION OF IMPULSE

Reuptake of the neurotransmitters returns them to vesicles within the pre-synaptic button.

Their action on the post-synaptic neuron can also be ended by diffusion out of the synaptic cleft, enzymatic degradation, or through their removal by astrocytes.

■ F I G U R E   1 2 . 4

Nerve synapse.

When the key fits the lock, the neurotransmitter causes either sodium or potassium ion channels to open in the post-synaptic membrane. An inflow of sodium ions lowers the threshold of the cell membrane and makes it easier for an EPSP to occur. An inflow of potassium ions results in an IPSP. Once the critical threshold of the post-synaptic neuron is reached, the nerve fires and the AP travels along the axon. In this manner neural information is transmitted among billions of nerve cells.

There are numerous different neurotransmitters in the NS, including acetylcholine, norepinephrine, serotonin, gamma-amino-butyric acid (GABA), glycerine, glutamic acid, dopamine, adenosine, nitric oxide, and even carbon monoxide (Hutchins et al., 2002). As mentioned above, neurotransmitters can be excitatory or inhibitory, either lowering or raising the cell threshold. However, according to Nolte (2002), there is nothing intrinsically excitatory or inhibitory about any neurotransmitter. The effect of a transmitter at any given synapse is determined by the nature of the receptor to which it binds. There are many different types of receptors for most neurotransmitters, which can therefore have more than one effect. For example, acetylcholine causes EPSPs at the junction between an axon and a voluntary muscle, but IPSPs in cardiac muscle (Nolte, 2002).

Conduction Velocity

Nerve fibers transmit impulses at different rates, depending on the size of the nerve and its degree of myelinization. The larger the nerve, and the more heavily it is myelinated, the faster its conduction rate, and vice versa (see Table 12.3). On this basis nerves are divided into three categories. Type A nerves are large myelinated fibers, both sensory and motor, with conduction rates of up to 120 meters per second (Zemlin, 1998). Type B are myelinated but with smaller diameters than Type A. They conduct at around 3 to 14 meters per second. The slowest conducting nerves, Type C, are very fine fibers, without a myelin covering. They have a rate of 0.2 to 2.0 meters per second (Zemlin, 1998).

Nerves conduct impulses at different rates, depending on the diameter of the nerve and its degree of myelinization.

■ TABLE 12.3

Nerve Types Based on Conduction Rates

TYPE	CONDUCTION RATE	CHARACTERISTICS
A	Up to 120 meters/sec	Large diameter, motor and sensory, heavily myelinated, branches (collaterals) further divided into alpha, beta, and gamma with smaller diameters and slower rates
B	3 to 14 meters/sec	Smaller diameter, myelinated
C	0.2 to 2.0 meters/sec	Very fine fibers, unmyelinated

Functional Anatomy of the Nervous System

The major components of the NS are the central nervous system (CNS) and peripheral nervous system (PNS). The CNS is comprised of the brain itself plus the spinal cord. The somatic portion of the PNS is made up of 12 pairs of cranial and 31 pairs of spinal nerves. The CNS is involved in all aspects of information processing, including interpretation of all incoming sensations; integration of sensory information across modalities; and planning, organization, and monitoring of goal-directed behavior, including motor behavior; as well as memory, language, and abstract functioning in general. The PNS transmits information to and from the CNS. The cranial and spinal nerves fan out to all muscles and glands in the body, thus constituting what is called the "**final common pathway**" to all body structures. Sensory information from these structures travels by way of the spinal and cranial nerves to the CNS for further processing.

We will focus on the primary components of the CNS and PNS that are important for speech and hearing, including the meninges and ventricular system, the cortex and subcortical structures, the brainstem and cerebellum, the spinal cord, and selected cranial nerves.

Central Nervous System

The brain and spinal cord are housed within the skull and the spinal column: These bony structures form an important layer of protection for nervous tissue. The CNS is additionally protected by three layers of non-nervous tissue, the meninges.

The meninges are composed of three layers of connective tissue that surround the brain and spinal cord.

Meninges   The **meninges** form a protective system of tissue and fluid surrounding the brain and the spinal cord. Figure 12.5 shows that immediately deep to the inner surface of the skull is the outermost meningeal layer, the **dura mater**. This is a tough, membranous connective tissue that has two parts, the periosteal layer that attaches to the cranium, and the meningeal layer. The dura is well supplied with blood vessels and nerves. Deep to this membrane is the **arachnoid mater**, so called because it has a delicate weblike appearance. This layer has no blood vessels. The innermost layer is the **pia mater**, which is a thin, delicate, highly vascular tissue that closely follows the grooves and convolutions of the brain matter itself. In between each of these layers is a space. Between the dura mater and the arachnoid lies the **subdural space**; between the arachnoid and the pia mater is the **subarachnoid space**. The subarachnoid space is filled with **cerebrospinal fluid** (CSF). The CSF is produced by specialized cells within four cavities (ventricles) of the brain. This clear fluid contains proteins, glucose that is necessary

The subdural space is located between the dura mater and the arachnoid; the subarachnoid space is between the arachnoid and the pia mater and contains cerebrospinal fluid.

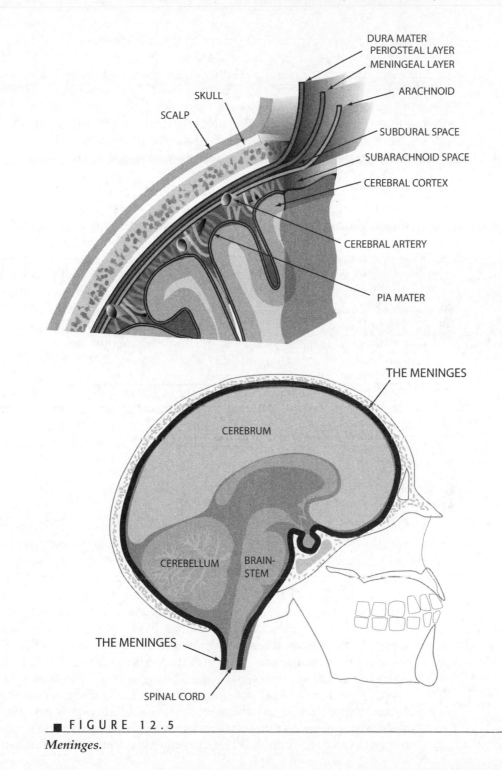

■ FIGURE 12.5

Meninges.

to provide energy for cell function in the brain and spinal cord, and lymphocytes that help to prevent infection (Clayman, 1995).

The CSF circulates around the entire meningeal system, so that the brain and spinal cord are protected by a buoyant fluid shock-absorbing system. Indeed, the buoyancy of the CSF actually reduces the weight of the brain from about 1400 g in air to around 45 g when suspended in the fluid (Corbett, Haines, & Ard, 2002). This prevents the weight of the brain from crushing nerve roots and blood vessels against the internal surface of the skull.

Ventricles   Four ventricles, or cavities, are located within the brain: two lateral ventricles, one in each hemisphere, the third ventricle, and the fourth ventricle. The two lateral ventricles both connect to the third ventricle by way of the interventricular foramen, and the third and fourth ventricles are connected by the cerebral aqueduct (see Figure 12.6).

> There are four ventricles within the brain: two lateral, the third ventricle, and the fourth ventricle.

CSF is manufactured by specialized cells called **choroid plexus cells** within the ventricles, particularly the lateral ventricles. The fluid flows through the ventricles and their connecting areas to escape through median and lateral apertures into the subarachnoid space. It eventually drains out of the subarachnoid space into the venous portion of the circulatory system. Adults produce around 450 to 500 ml of CSF per day, of which approximately 330 to 380 ml drains into the veins. Thus the average volume of CSF is about 120 ml in adults (Corbett et al., 2002). Any obstruction within this system that prevents the fluid from flowing freely and/or draining properly or any kind of problem that results in an excessive amount of CSF can cause serious neurological problems.

> Choroid plexus cells within the ventricles manufacture cerebrospinal fluid, which travels around the brain and spinal cord and eventually drains into the veins.

Overview of Functional Brain Anatomy

The brain is divided into two hemispheres, right and left. These hemispheres are connected by means of nerve pathways. In turn, each hemisphere is divided into lobes. The outermost layer of the brain is made up of cortex, which is tissue formed by the cell bodies of neurons. The cortex is commonly known as "grey matter." The inner mass of the brain is the cerebrum and is primarily made of nerve axons bundled into pathways and covered with myelin. Because myelin is whitish in color, the inner mass is referred to as "white matter." Deep within the white matter of the brain are circumscribed areas of grey matter, known as subcortical areas. These areas include the basal nuclei or basal ganglia, the thalamus, and the hypothalamus. Located immediately behind the cerebrum is the cerebellum, connected to the cerebrum by various pathways. Immediately under the cerebrum is the brainstem, consisting of the midbrain, the pons, and the medulla. The medulla is continuous with the spinal

> Cortical and subcortical areas of the brain are composed of nerve cell bodies (grey matter) while the inner mass of the brain is made up of myelinated nerve pathways (white matter).

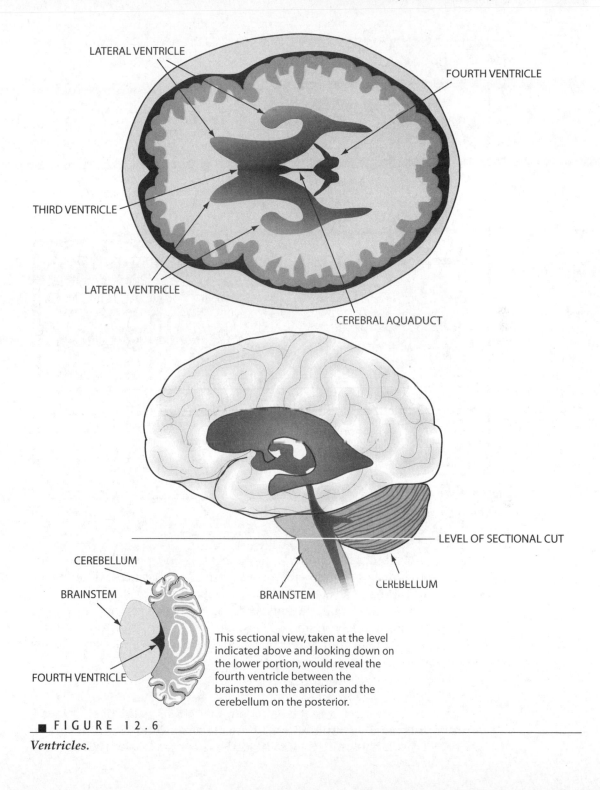

LATERAL VENTRICLE

FOURTH VENTRICLE

THIRD VENTRICLE

LATERAL VENTRICLE

CEREBRAL AQUADUCT

LEVEL OF SECTIONAL CUT

BRAINSTEM

CEREBELLUM

CEREBELLUM

BRAINSTEM

FOURTH VENTRICLE

This sectional view, taken at the level indicated above and looking down on the lower portion, would reveal the fourth ventricle between the brainstem on the anterior and the cerebellum on the posterior.

■ FIGURE 12.6

Ventricles.

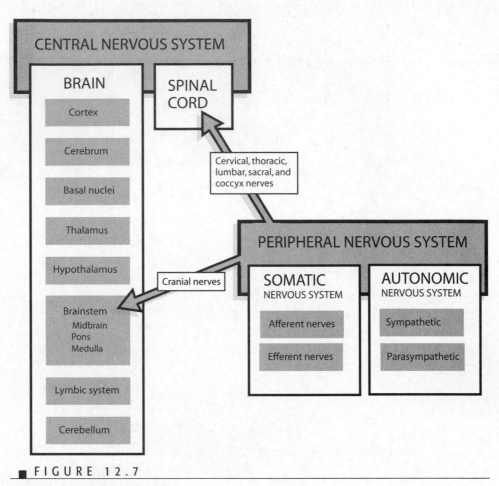

■ FIGURE 12.7

Schematic of nervous system.

cord. Figure 12.7 shows a schematic of the central and peripheral nervous systems with their major components, and Figure 12.8 illustrates relationships among some of the major structures in the central nervous system.

Cranial nerves originate in various areas of the brainstem and extend to muscles and glands in the head and neck areas. Spinal nerves originate at different levels of the spinal cord and travel to all the muscles and glands in the rest of the body.

Cortex

The cortex is the outer covering of the brain, and it is extremely convoluted; that is, rather than being a flat, smooth surface, the cortex is irregular and

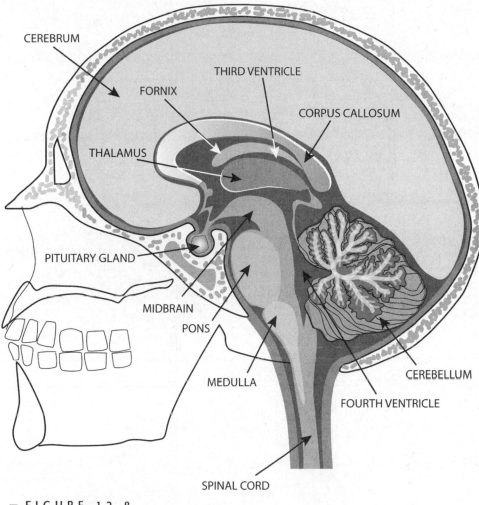

CEREBRUM

THIRD VENTRICLE

FORNIX

CORPUS CALLOSUM

THALAMUS

PITUITARY GLAND

MIDBRAIN

PONS

MEDULLA

CEREBELLUM

FOURTH VENTRICLE

SPINAL CORD

■ **FIGURE 12.8**

Sagittal view of selected major brain structures.

The cortex contains gyri, which are raised surfaces; sulci, which are shallow depressions; and fissures, which are deeper grooves.

bumpy. There are numerous folds on the cortex where the tissue forms raised surfaces called **gyri** (singular: gyrus), shallow depressions called **sulci** (singular: sulcus), and deeper grooves called fissures. These convolutions serve an important purpose by increasing the surface area of the cortex without increasing the space needed to house it. It is certain of these sulci and fissures that divide the brain into hemispheres and lobes. As shown in Figure 12.9, the **longitudinal cerebral fissure** divides the brain into two hemispheres. The **central sulcus** roughly separates the brain into anterior and posterior portions. The **lateral fissure**

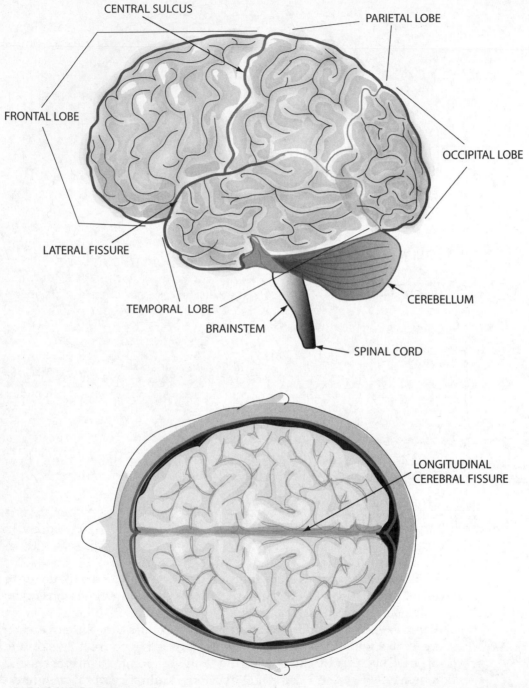

CENTRAL SULCUS

PARIETAL LOBE

FRONTAL LOBE

OCCIPITAL LOBE

LATERAL FISSURE

CEREBELLUM

TEMPORAL LOBE

BRAINSTEM

SPINAL CORD

LONGITUDINAL CEREBRAL FISSURE

■ FIGURE 12.9

Major cortical landmarks and lobes.

The brain is divided into two hemispheres by the longitudinal cerebral fissure, into anterior and posterior portions by the central sulcus, and into superior and inferior sections by the lateral fissure.

delineates the superior and inferior regions of the brain. It is the central sulcus and lateral fissure that demarcate the brain into four major lobes: frontal, parietal, temporal, and occipital. These lobes are visible on the surface of the brain, but there is another lobe that cannot be seen because it lies deeper within the brain. This lobe, called the insula, is located at the bottom of the lateral fissure but can only be seen when the fissure is opened. Some anatomists also include a sixth lobe, the limbic lobe, which is also not visible on the surface of the brain.

The cortex is made up of primary sensory areas, primary motor areas, association areas, and limbic areas.

The cortex is composed of three to six layers of nerve cells and varies in thickness from about 1.5 to 4.5 mm (Zemlin, 1998). The nerve cell bodies that make up the cortex vary in their sizes and shapes. The most numerous neurons of the cortex are called pyramidal cells. They range in size from 10 microns (millionths of a mm) in size up to the 70 to 100 micron giant pyramidal cells, called Betz cells. Betz cells are located primarily the motor cortex. Most of the cortex in the human brain (roughly 95%) is of a type known as **neocortex**. In evolutionary terms, this is the part of the brain that appeared late in human development, and it is greatly expanded compared to other primates. It is the neocortex that allows us to talk, to think abstractly, to plan and organize, and to use different types of symbolic functions, including those involved in language and mathematics.

The cortex receives input and provides output from many other regions in the NS, including subcortical structures. Different cortical areas also connect to each other by means of association fibers. Traditionally, the cortex is considered to be made up of primary sensory areas, primary motor areas, association areas, and limbic areas. Different areas of the cerebral cortex are associated with different functions, such as processing of incoming sensory information, planning and sequencing of motor activity, memory storage and retrieval, and emotional functioning.

Lobes of the Brain   Recall that the sulci and fissures separate the brain into lobes. Areas within each lobe have been associated with various functions. In 1914 Brodmann did extensive work on mapping specific cortical areas with associated functions, and the numbering system he devised is still in use today. Brodmann identified around fifty functional areas of human cerebral cortex, and selected areas important for speech and hearing are presented in Figure 12.10.

In discussing these areas, several caveats are important to keep in mind. First, these areas are not completely separated, and their boundaries are not precise. Second, the identified areas are not the only brain sites for a particular function, as most human behaviors are extremely complex, involving numerous brain areas that work together synergistically. Third, lobes in the left and right hemisphere are not mirror images of each other in either structure or

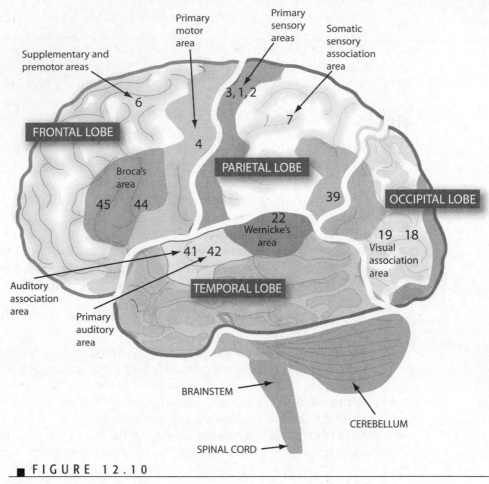

Supplementary and premotor areas

Primary motor area

Primary sensory areas

Somatic sensory association area

FRONTAL LOBE

6

3, 1, 2

4

7

Broca's area

PARIETAL LOBE

45   44

39

OCCIPITAL LOBE

22
Wernicke's area

19   18
Visual association area

41   42

Auditory association area

TEMPORAL LOBE

Primary auditory area

BRAINSTEM

CEREBELLUM

SPINAL CORD

■ FIGURE 12.10

Major cortical areas.

function. In general, the left hemisphere performs functions that are more linear in nature, while the right hemisphere performs functions that are more holistic in nature. In most people, the left hemisphere is the one that is dominant for language processing, while the right is more involved in the emotional expression of language, including intonational patterns of speech. Nonetheless, as Nolte (2002) pointed out, many years of clinical experience have shown that reasonably predictable deficits are associated with damage at specific cortical sites, so the Brodmann system is useful for diagnostic and clinical purposes. Table 12.4 provides selected Brodmann's areas and numbers important for the understanding and expression of language.

■ TABLE 12.4

Selected Brodmann's Areas Important for Speech and Hearing

LOBE	BRODMANN'S NUMBER	NAME(S) OF AREA
Frontal	4	Primary motor area, M1
	6	Premotor area and supplementary motor area
	44, 45	Broca's area (only in dominant hemisphere)
Parietal	3, 1, 2	Primary somatosensory area, S1
	5, 7	Somatosensory association area
	39	Angular gyrus
	40	Supramarginal gyrus
Occipital	17	Primary visual area, V1
	18, 19	Visual association area
Temporal	41	Primary auditory area, A1
	42	Auditory association area
	22	Wernicke's area

The frontal lobe contains important motor areas, including the primary motor cortex in which Broca's area is located, the premotor area, and the supplementary motor area.

Frontal Lobe   The frontal lobe makes up one-third of the cortex (Seikel et al., 2004) and is located anterior to the central sulcus and superior to the lateral sulcus. This is the part of the neocortex that contains areas devoted to language and speech, as well as abstract functions including reasoning, problem solving, personality, and symbolic function. Most motor activity is controlled by the frontal lobe, including primary motor cortex, or M1 (area 4), also known as the motor strip, premotor area (area 6), and supplementary motor area (area 6). Broca's area is located in the lateral portion of the inferior region of area 4 and is numbered areas 44 and 45. The primary motor cortex, M1, is situated on the **precentral gyrus**, immediately anterior to the central sulcus.

The motor strip is organized so that motor control of different body structures is located within specific portions of the tissue. In other words, rather than the entire motor strip's participating in controlling movements of all muscles, specific portions of the motor strip control specific muscles and structures. Furthermore, the organization of control occurs in a particular pattern. Starting at the top of the motor strip and progressing inferiorly toward the lateral fissure are portions of cortex responsible for movement of the hip, trunk (thorax and abdomen), arms, hands, neck, and face. Broca's area, numbers 44 and 45, is located at the most inferior portion of the motor strip and is responsible for sequencing and controlling the motor movements required for the production of speech.

This organization of motor control according to body part is called **somatotopic**. However, the body structures are not represented equally in terms of the amount of cortical tissue devoted to their function. Those structures that require fine levels of motor control for skilled and precise movements have much greater representation on the motor strip than others. The differing amount of neural tissue allocated to motor control of different bodily structures is often represented in a caricature called the **homunculus** (see Figure 12.11).

A caricature known as the homunculus depicts the amount of motor area devoted to specific bodily structures and shows that the articulators have a disproportionately large amount of cortex involved in their control.

This representation shows that the hands and fingers have a much larger area devoted to their control than does the trunk. The structures involved in speech—i.e., the larynx, velum, tongue, and lips—have disproportionately large areas dedicated to them, indicating the extremely fine motor control required for speech production. The premotor and supplementary motor areas are also somatotopically organized, although in a less precise fashion than the motor strip.

The prefrontal cortex is located anterior to the primary motor and premotor areas and has been associated with intellectual traits such as judgment, foresight, a sense of purpose, a sense of responsibility, and a sense of social propriety (Lynch, 2002).

Parietal Lobes   The parietal lobes are found on the **postcentral gyrus**, immediately posterior to the central sulcus. These lobes deal with bodily sensation including touch, pressure, pain, proprioception, and temperature. The primary somatosensory areas (S1) are 3, 1, and 2 and are represented somatotopically, similar to the motor cortex (see Figure 12.11). These areas receive information from many nerve pathways and react to slightly different types of sensory input (Nolte, 2002). For example, area 3a receives input from muscle receptors (Nolte, 2002). The bottom portion of the parietal lobe contains two important areas: the supramarginal gyrus, area 40, and the angular gyrus, area 39. These two areas are composed of association cortex and are important in integrating various sensory modalities including vision, touch, and hearing (Webster, 1999). The angular gyrus is involved in the comprehension of written material, and the supramarginal gyrus is associated with planning of motor activities for speech production (Seikel et al., 2004).

Temporal Lobes   The temporal lobes are important for understanding. Areas 41 and 42 make up the primary auditory cortex (A1) receiving information from the ear and auditory nerve, while area 22 is called Wernicke's area (see Figure 12.10). Area 41 is mapped tonotopically. In other words, specific regions of this cortical area respond selectively to specific frequencies. Wernicke's area is part of the receptive speech association cortex (Webster, 1999), essential for the decoding and comprehension of speech. Broca's area and Wernicke's area are connected by way of an association pathway called the arcuate fasciculus, thus demonstrating the close neuroanatomical relationship between understanding and production of speech.

Wernicke's area is located on the temporal lobe and is crucial for understanding speech.

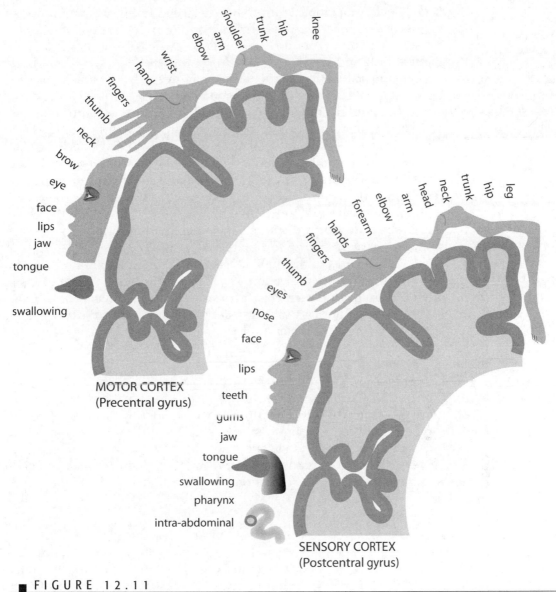

■ FIGURE 12.11

Motor and sensory homunculus.

Occipital Lobe The occipital lobe is situated at the posterior of the brain and is dedicated to the reception and processing of visual information. Area 17 forms the primary visual cortex (V1), and areas 18 and 19 form the visual association cortex (see Figure 12.10). The association cortex responds differentially to different types of visual input, such as movement, color, and shape.

The limbic system comprises the limbic lobe as well as the amygdala, hippocampus, and other structures; it is involved in emotional and sexual function.

The limbic lobe is not an anatomically separate lobe but is made up of the medial margins of the frontal, parietal, and temporal lobes.

Limbic Lobe   The limbic lobe is part of a larger **limbic system**, comprising several brain structures, including the hippocampus, amygdala, septal, mammillary bodies, and anterior nuclei of the thalamus (see Figures 12.12 and 12.15).

The limbic lobe itself is actually made up of the most medial margins of the frontal, parietal, and temporal lobes. The limbic lobe and the other structures making up the limbic system are involved in emotional and sexual function, feeding behavior, and temperature regulation. This system is more primitive than the neocortex. It is connected to the brainstem and hypothalamus, as well as to the prefrontal cortex of the frontal lobe. The brainstem and hypothalamus are important in bodily regulation. The prefrontal cortex, as previously noted, is associated with higher intellectual functions and personality characteristics. Thus, limbic structures form a bridge between autonomic and voluntary responses to changes in the environment (Nolte, 2002).

Two structures of the limbic system are particularly noteworthy in terms of human communication. The **hippocampus** (see Figure 12.15) is involved with learning and memory. It is this structure that enables an individual to form new memories and to transfer these memories from short-term to longer term memory. This is clearly crucial for communication, in which the person must remember what has been said in order to continue the conversation in an appropriate manner.

The **amygdala** (see Figure 12.12) is involved in ascribing emotion to events and behaviors. This structure also participates in memory building, in the sense that it facilitates decisions about which facts and events are important enough to be committed to long-term memory. To illustrate, if one meets a friend and chats about this and that, one is not likely to remember for very long the specific details of the conversation. However, if the friend reveals a shocking or exciting piece of news, information that generates emotion, that is much more likely to be remembered.

Cortical Connections   The cortex, as we have seen, is the prime information processor of the NS. The pathways of the NS are involved in facilitating the flow of information between different areas. As mentioned previously, some pathways deliver information from the various sensory receptors to the NS and are called afferent or sensory pathways. Others, the efferent or motor pathways, transport impulses from the NS to the muscles and glands of the body. Many nerve fibers interconnect various regions of the NS to each other. There are three main types of interconnecting pathways: commissural, association, and projection.

Commissural Fibers   Commissural fibers link two corresponding areas in the right and left hemispheres. The major commissural pathway is the **corpus cal-**

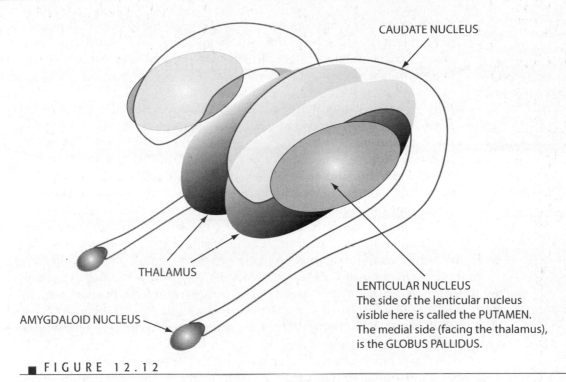

CAUDATE NUCLEUS

THALAMUS

AMYGDALOID NUCLEUS

LENTICULAR NUCLEUS
The side of the lenticular nucleus
visible here is called the PUTAMEN.
The medial side (facing the thalamus),
is the GLOBUS PALLIDUS.

■ FIGURE 12.12

Subcortical structures.

The major pathway
linking the two hemi-
spheres of the brain is
the corpus callosum.

losum, a thick band of white matter that extensively connects the right
and left hemispheres (see Figures 12.13 and 12.14). This pathway has a
fan-like structure, with fibers radiating extensively between many areas
of the two hemispheres, and is the means by which each hemisphere is
constantly updated as to the moment-by-moment functioning of the
other.

Fibers of the corpus callosum are found in the medial parts of the brain and
are arranged longitudinally, so that the pathway runs from anterior to posterior regions of the brain. This pathway is sometimes cut in individuals with
severe epilepsy. Interestingly, in such cases, the individual can function normally, but literally, the right hemisphere does not know what the left is doing,
and vice versa. There are other smaller commissures that link the two hemispheres including the anterior, middle, and posterior commissures, but the
corpus callosum is by far the largest and most important.

Association Fibers   Association fibers can connect different cortical regions
within the same hemisphere or link adjacent areas of cortex. Fibers that connect
different cortical regions are, of course, longer than those connecting adjacent
areas. The pathways formed by the long fibers are called **fasciculi** (singular:

fasciculus). Some important pathways include the superior longitudinal fasciculus, which links the four major lobes, and the arcuate fasciculus, which connects parts of the frontal, parietal, and temporal lobes to each other.

Projection Fibers   Recall that projection fibers, particularly Golgi Type I fibers, have long axons that extend to relatively distant neural structures and to the spinal cord. Two major bundles of nerve fibers, the **internal capsule** and the **corona radiata**, form the primary links between the cortex and other regions of the CNS. Figures 12.13 and 12.14 show that the internal capsule is formed by a large mass of myelinated fibers that runs mainly between the thalamus and the cerebral cortex. This structure forms the main pathway by which most nerve impulses are transmitted to and from the cerebral cortex. The fibers traveling from the cortex to the thalamus are called corticothalamic; those projecting from the thalamus to the cortex are thalamocortical. Some pathways making up the internal capsule also transmit neural information from the cortex to the brainstem (corticonuclear or corticobulbar fibers) and from the cortex to the spinal cord (corticospinal fibers). These specific motor pathways will be discussed in more detail in a later section.

As the fibers of the internal capsule travel from the basal nuclei, thalamus, brainstem, and spinal cord toward the cerebral cortex, they diverge and flare out in a fan-shaped manner, reaching many areas within the cerebrum and cerebral cortex and joining with other pathways that interconnect different cortical areas. This fan-shaped area is referred to as the corona radiata.

Subcortical Areas of the Brain

The cortex, as we have discussed, is composed of grey matter and is involved in various types of information processing. The main mass of the brain, the cerebrum, is made up of white matter, the mostly myelinated nerve fibers that are involved in the transmission of information. Deep within the cerebrum are various circumscribed areas of grey matter: the basal nuclei, the thalamus, and the hypothalamus. These collections of nerve cell bodies are important in the control and regulation of movement, including movement for speech production. Figure 12.14 illustrates the major subcortical regions.

Basal Nuclei   The basal nuclei, also called basal ganglia, are comprised of several areas of grey matter adjacent to each other, in each hemisphere, and include the **caudate**, the **globus pallidus**, the **putamen**, and the **substantia nigra**. These nuclei are often grouped in different ways; thus, the putamen and globus pallidus together are known as the lenticular nucleus, while the caudate and putamen together form the **striatum**.

Association fibers link areas of cortex within the same hemisphere or in adjacent areas and can be short or long.

The internal capsule and the corona radiata form the primary links between the cortex and other regions of central nervous system.

The basal nuclei contain several relatively large clusters of nerve cell bodies, including the caudate, globus pallidus, putamen, and substantia nigra.

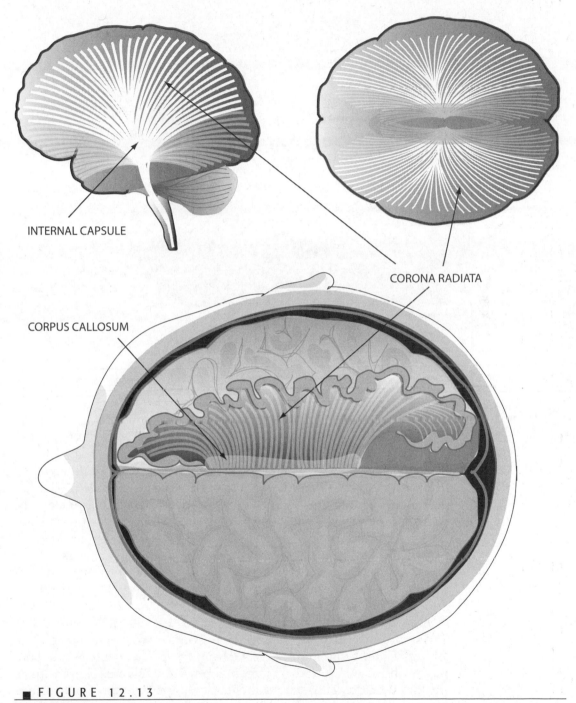

Corona radiata and internal capsule.

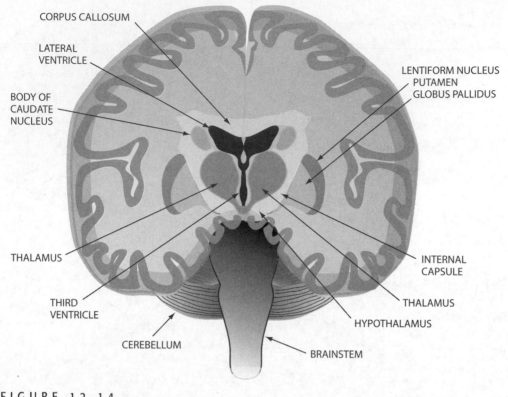

■ FIGURE 12.14

Coronal section of the cerebrum showing subcortical structures.

The basal nuclei connect with many other structures and pathways, receiving input from the motor and other areas of the cortex and the thalamus, as well as making connections with each other and various other nuclei. The pathways running to, from, and among the various components of the basal nuclei form a series of complex circuits between the cerebral cortex, basal nuclei, and thalamus, one of the major ones of which is the motor circuit. Fibers from the primary motor area, premotor area, and supplementary motor area project to the striatum (corticostriatal fibers), which also receives input from somatosensory cortex (Ma, 2002), substantia nigra, limbic lobe, hippocampus, and amygdala (Nolte, 2002). The striatum is, thus, the major receiving center of the basal nuclei. Projections from the basal nuclei leave from the globus pallidus and substantia nigra and travel to the thalamus. From the thalamus, nerve fibers project back to the cerebral cortex via the internal capsule and corona radiata, thus completing the loop. Because of these interconnections, the basal nuclei are constantly informed about most aspects of cortical function.

The basal nuclei form part of multiple neural circuits that run between various regions of the cerebral cortex and thalamus.

One of the primary functions of the basal nuclei is regulating aspects of motor control such as posture, balance, background muscle tone, and coordination of muscle groups. The basal nuclei are also critically important in the indirect control of precise voluntary movements, including those for speech production, through a neural mechanism called inhibition. Recall in our discussion of neuronal function that a post-synaptic neuron can undergo an excitatory or an inhibitory post-synaptic potential (EPSP or IPSP). With an IPSP, the neuron membrane is hyperpolarized, making it more difficult for an action potential to be triggered. One of the neurotransmitters used in the basal nuclei is dopamine, which has an inhibitory effect. Thus the outflow from the basal nuclei to the thalamus and back to the motor cortex is inhibitory, which serves to refine and smooth the initial neuromuscular output from the cortex. Due to this inhibitory feedback system, damage to the basal nuclei typically results in excessive involuntary movements such as tics and tremors, increased muscle tone and rigidity, and other disruptions of movement control. Parkinson's disease is an example of this kind of disinhibition, in which the patient suffers from rigidity and tremors resulting from destruction or damage to the substantia nigra and/or the pathways between the substantia nigra and striatum (nigrostriatal fibers).

The basal nuclei regulate posture, balance, background muscle tone, and coordination of muscle groups.

Damage to the basal nuclei typically results in excessive involuntary and uncontrollable movements such as tics and tremors.

The thalamus contains many nuclei, which process and transmit information to and from many cortical locations.

Thalamus   Similar to the basal nuclei, the thalamus comprises numerous nuclei, some of which are involved with motor function and some with sensory function. Nuclei that receive and transmit nerve impulses to and from specific cortical areas are known as **relay nuclei**. Other nuclei called **association nuclei** receive and transmit to broader cortical areas. Figure 12.15 shows the thalamus in relation to other subcortical and limbic structures.

The thalamus is sometimes called the "gateway to consciousness" because all information traveling to the cerebral cortex, aside from olfaction, passes through the thalamus. The thalamus sorts and interprets neural information and "decides" which signals should be transmitted to the cerebral cortex. This structure can be likened to a relay station that collects inputs from many different locations and structures and relays them to many other locations and structures. The nuclei of the thalamus send information to and receive information from the cerebral cortex via the pathways of the internal capsule. The neuron pools participate in motor, sensory, and limbic functions. Each nucleus projects to a different part of the cerebral cortex (thalamocortical fibers), and that portion of the cortex reciprocally projects to the originating thalamic nucleus (corticothalamic fibers).

The thalamic nuclei that are most important for speech and hearing are relay nuclei, including the **ventral anterior nuclei** (VA), **ventral lateral nuclei** (VL), **medial geniculate body**, and **lateral geniculate body**. The VA and VL

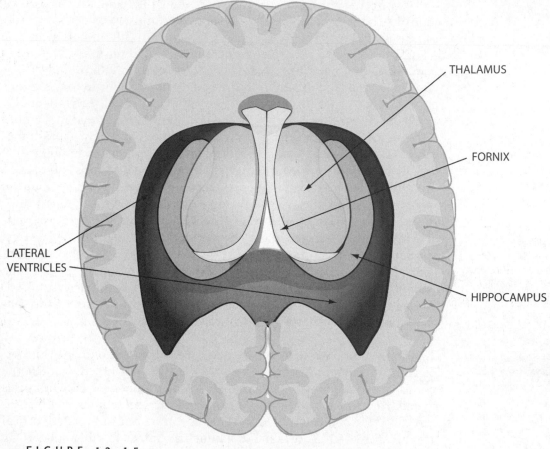

THALAMUS

FORNIX

LATERAL
VENTRICLES

HIPPOCAMPUS

■ **FIGURE   12.15**

Superior sectional view of selected subcortical and limbic structures.

nuclei receive input from the basal nuclei and cerebellum and project to the motor areas of the cerebral cortex. These two nuclei are directly involved in motor function. The medial geniculate body processes auditory information and relays it to the auditory cortex in the temporal lobe. The lateral geniculate body processes visual information and transmits it to the visual cortex in the occipital lobe.

The ventral anterior, ventral lateral, and medial and lateral geniculate bodies are the most important thalamic nuclei involved in speech and hearing.

Hypothalamus   The hypothalamus is another subcortical grey matter structure, containing nuclei that are involved in sensory and motor control of visceral functions. The hypothalamus, like the thalamus, is also strongly linked to the limbic system. In addition, this structure regulates hormonal function, body temperature, hunger, sleep-wake cycles,

The hypothalamus regulates visceral and emotional behavior and is not under conscious control.

sexual drive, blood pressure, and other functions designed to keep the body's internal environment in a state of equilibrium, a condition called homeostasis (see Figure 12.14).

The hypothalamus connects with the limbic system, pituitary gland, and brainstem, allowing widespread control of the visceral and emotional behavior that influence how we react to our internal and external environments (Hardy, Chronister, & Parent, 2002). However, hypothalamic functioning is not under our conscious control.

Brainstem

The brainstem is a collective term for three separate but tightly linked structures: the midbrain, the pons, and the medulla. The brainstem is crucially important, as it is the site of many reflexes involved in respiration, body temperature, swallowing, and digestion. It is also the site of origin of the cranial nerves. As shown in Figure 12.16, the topmost portion, the midbrain, is located directly underneath the cerebrum. The lowermost part, the medulla, connects with the spinal cord. The pons forms a bridge not only between the midbrain and medulla, but also with the cerebellum.

The core of the brainstem is composed of the reticular formation, which controls complex patterns of movement involved in visceral functions.

At the core of the brainstem is the **reticular formation**, a loose and diffuse network of nuclei controlling complex patterns of movement involved in breathing, cardiac function, and swallowing. The **reticular activating system** is part of the network, and the nuclei forming this portion of the brainstem control our state of alertness and level of consciousness. Damage to this neural system results in coma.

Midbrain   The midbrain is a short structure consisting of the two cerebral peduncles and the superior and inferior colliculi (singular: colliculus).

The **cerebral peduncles** are continuations of the internal capsule. They are large bundles of nerve pathways including corticospinal, corticonuclear (corticobulbar), and corticopontine fibers traveling via the cerebrum and midbrain to their respective targets. The paired **inferior colliculi** are masses of grey matter that are linked to different parts of the auditory system and that ultimately project to the medial geniculate nucleus of the thalamus. They also project

Numerous pathways travel through the midbrain, facilitating the flow and integration of information from different areas of the nervous system.

fibers to the **superior colliculi**, which are involved in visual processing, as well as to the cerebellum and spinal cord. These numerous connections facilitate the integration of information from various areas within the nervous system and play an important role in higher level reflexes such as turning one's eyes to the source of a sound and startle responses to unexpected noises. The cerebral aqueduct, linking the third and fourth ventricles, is located within the midbrain. The midbrain is the point of origin for two cranial nerves: CN III (oculomotor) and IV (trochlear).

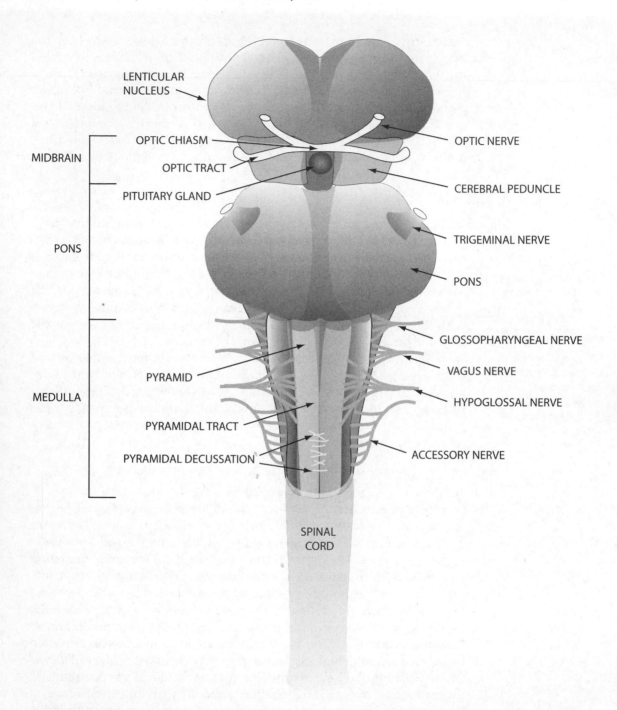

Anterior view of the brainstem.

Pons   The pons is located inferior to the midbrain and anterior to the cerebellum. Pons in Latin means bridge, and this portion of the brainstem includes nerve pathways (superior and middle cerebellar peduncles) that act as a bridge between the cerebellum and the rest of the nervous system. In addition, there are nuclei within the pons that process information arriving from the cerebrum on its way to the cerebellum. Four of the cranial nerves originate at the pontine level: CN V (trigeminal), VI (abducent), VII (facial), VIII (vestibulocochlear).

Medulla   The medulla is the most inferior portion of the brainstem, continuous with the pons above and the spinal cord below. The medulla is around 2.5 cm long and about 1 cm in diameter (Seikel et al., 2004). This is an important structure, because this is where a large percentage of nerve fibers (80 to 90%) originating at the cerebral cortex cross over (decussate) and continue down the opposite (contralateral) side of the body. Thus, it is the left hemisphere of the brain that controls the right side of the body, and vice versa. The decussation occurs at a site on the medulla called the pyramids (see Figure 12.16). These are two pyramid-shaped ridges running from the pons to the inferior border of the medulla. Most of the fibers that form the pyramids arise in the motor cortex as corticospinal fibers (Haines & Mihailoff, 2002). Cranial nerve nuclei in the medulla include CN IX (glossopharyngeal), X (vagus), XI (spinal accessory), and XII (hypoglossal). The medulla also connects to the cerebellum by way of the inferior cerebellar peduncles. The medulla mediates many reflexes such as coughing, sneezing, and vomiting.

> The medulla is the point of decussation where most nerve fibers from the motor cortex cross over and continue down the opposite side of the body.

Cerebellum

The cerebellum is located posterior to the brainstem and inferior to the cerebrum. It connects to the brainstem by way of the inferior, middle, and superior **cerebellar peduncles**. The cerebellum is a relatively large structure, accounting for around 10 percent of the weight of the entire CNS. The cerebellum has some interesting similarities to the cerebrum. Like the cerebrum, it is composed of a mass of white matter overlaid by an outer cortex. Also like the cerebrum, deep within the cerebellar white matter are concentrations of subcortical cell bodies. Similar to the cerebral cortex, the cerebellum has two hemispheres that are connected by a thick nerve fiber bundle. In addition, the cerebellum is divided into lobes. However, unlike the cerebral cortex, which exerts contralateral control of movement, the cerebellum works ipsilaterally.

> Similar to the cerebrum, the cerebellum is composed of a mass of white matter with an outer layer of cortex and concentrations of subcortical cell bodies.

> Unlike the cerebral cortex, the cerebellum projects its fibers ipsilaterally down the same side of the body.

The cerebellar cortex has a different appearance to that of the cerebral cortex. While the cerebral cortex, as we have seen, is irregularly convoluted, the cerebellar cortex is more regular in appearance, with a surface that looks almost like segments of a peeled orange. This characteristic appearance is created by deep straight grooves on the cortex, with smaller indentations within the deeper fissures. This results in a series of ridges on the surface called folia (Nolte, 2002). The inner mass of the cerebellum is composed of white matter that is sometimes called "arbor vitae" (tree of life) due to its branching pattern, as can be seen in Figure 12.17. The nerve pathways that make up this inner mass contain fibers projecting to and from the cerebellar cortex. Deep within the inner mass are four clusters of deep nuclei. These nuclei receive input from and project back to specific portions of the cerebellar cortex, and project as well to the brainstem and thalamus via the cerebellar peduncles.

The various parts of the cerebellum can be identified in an anterior-posterior direction as well as a medial-lateral direction. In terms of anterior-posterior the cerebellum has three lobes: a small anterior lobe, a large posterior lobe, and a very small inferior lobe called the **flocculonodular lobe**. In the medial-lateral direction there are likewise three sections: the midline section called the **vermis** that connects the cerebellar hemispheres and the lateral structures on either side.

The cerebellum receives various types of information from many sources. It receives sensory information via the inferior and middle cerebellar peduncles, including proprioceptive and vestibular (balance) information from spinal and vestibular pathways. It also sends motor information from the deep nuclei to the cerebral cortex, traveling via the superior cerebellar peduncles to the thalamus and ending at the motor areas of the cerebral cortex. Thus the cerebral cortex, subcortical areas, and cerebellum are indirectly linked, allowing for information sharing that is vital to motor function.

The cerebellum is involved in balance, posture, background muscle tone, and also, importantly, the coordination of voluntary movements. With its extensive connections to other motor centers as well as its extensive sensory input, it is well suited to its central role in motor control and coordination. The cerebellum coordinates movements in terms of the direction of the movement, the force and speed with which the movement is executed, and the amount of displacement of the structure that is moving. It also ensures that complex movements are carried out with appropriate timing so that smooth synergistic muscular patterns are maintained. As an example, think of the coordination that is involved in a simple task such as picking up a pen from a table. You first have to move your entire arm toward the pen, which also involves the correct degree and displacement of shoulder, upper arm, and forearm movement. As your arm approaches the pen, your fingers must start to close. The force and speed of the arm and finger movements must be precisely regulated: Too much or too little force and speed will result in overshooting or undershooting the target. Similarly, the direction of your arm and fingers must be correct in order to

The inferior and middle cerebellar peduncles receive sensory information; the superior cerebellar peduncle transmits motor information to the thalamus and ultimately the cerebral cortex.

The cerebellum coordinates movements in terms of direction, force, speed, timing, and degree of displacement.

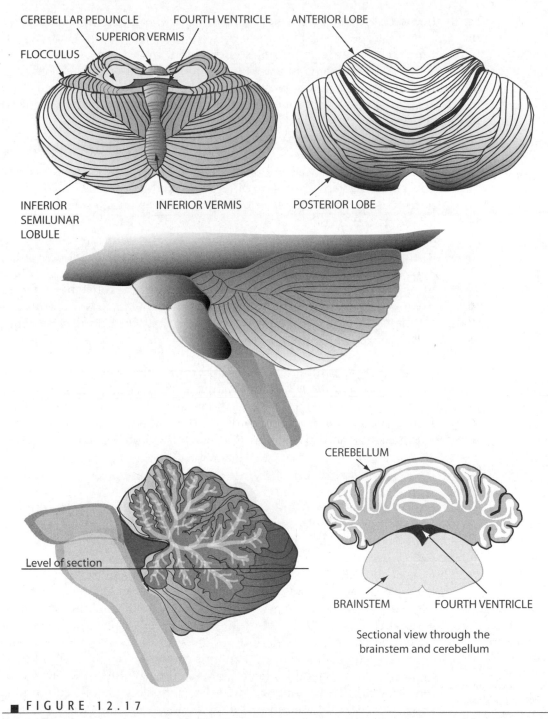

CEREBELLAR PEDUNCLE
FOURTH VENTRICLE
ANTERIOR LOBE
SUPERIOR VERMIS
FLOCCULUS
INFERIOR SEMILUNAR LOBULE
INFERIOR VERMIS
POSTERIOR LOBE

Level of section

CEREBELLUM
BRAINSTEM
FOURTH VENTRICLE

Sectional view through the
brainstem and cerebellum

■ FIGURE 12.17

Cerebellum.

reach the pen. As your fingers close around the pen, their muscular force must be finely graded in order to successfully complete the task. Individuals with cerebellar damage lack this fine coordination, and their movements tend to be jerky due to problems in their timing, force, direction, and speed. Another problem often seen in such an individual is that movements take longer to begin, and the person cannot easily stop the movement or change it once it has been initiated.

One way in which the cerebellum performs this type of precise coordination is by comparing a person's intended movement with the actual neuromuscular command issued by the motor areas of the cerebral cortex and correcting any errors or differences that are detected. The comparison is performed in terms of the status of the muscles (e.g., tension, length, force) involved in the movement, proprioceptive information about the position of relevant structures, and information arriving from the spinal cord, from the basal nuclei, from the vestibular system, and from the cerebral cortex. Thus the cerebellum continuously monitors both sensory and motor information, allowing constant updating of movement patterns and carrying out movements in a smoothly coordinated fashion. The cerebellum, particularly the vermis, also regulates posture as well as patterns of movements such as those involved in walking.

> The cerebellum compares an intended movement or movements with the specific neuromuscular commands issued by the motor cortex and corrects any errors that are detected.

The cerebellum is richly interconnected with the cortex and spinal cord. Current thinking is that the lateral cerebellum, which receives input from the premotor and association cortical areas, acts to preprogram a movement, whereas the vermis acts to update an evolving movement via its input from the sensorimotor cortical and spinal inputs (Kent, 1997a; Nolte, 2002).

Spinal Cord

The spinal cord is the downward continuation of the brainstem and contains the cell bodies for the thirty-one pairs of spinal nerves that run to all the muscles of our body, aside from those of the head and neck. See Figures 12.18 and 12.19.

The spinal cord, like the brain, is enveloped by the meninges, which form a complete protective sheath around the entire CNS. Recall that the dura mater is the outermost layer of the meninges. In the spinal column this layer is separated from the vertebrae by the epidural space. The innermost layer, the pia mater, closely follows the spinal cord itself. As with the brain, the subarachnoid space contains cerebrospinal fluid. The spinal cord is also protected by the vertebral column within which it is situated, as can be seen in Figure 12.20. The spinal cord is one continuous structure, but is divided into several sections: cervical (neck), thoracic (chest), lumbar (lower back), sacral (pelvis), and coccygeal (tail bone).

> The spinal cord is divided into cervical, thoracic, lumbar, sacral, and coccygeal portions and contains the cell bodies for the 31 pairs of spinal nerves.

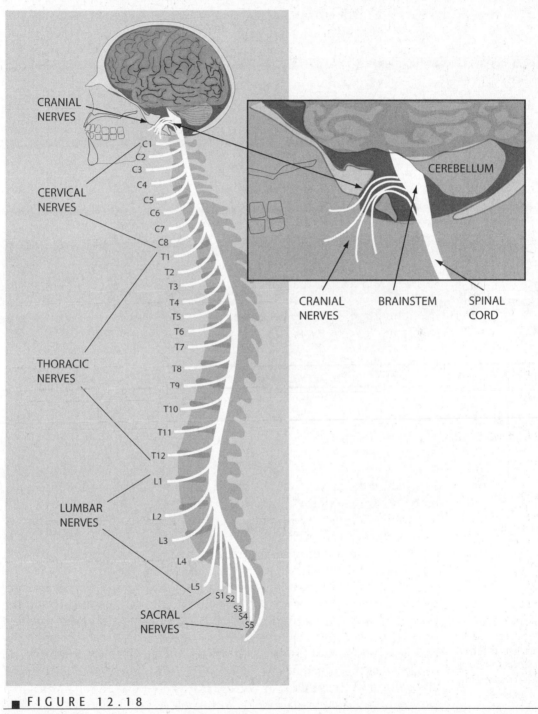

CRANIAL
NERVES

CERVICAL
NERVES

THORACIC
NERVES

LUMBAR
NERVES

SACRAL
NERVES

C1
C2
C3
C4
C5
C6
C7
C8
T1
T2
T3
T4
T5
T6
T7
T8
T9
T10
T11
T12
L1
L2
L3
L4
L5
S1 S2
S3
S4
S5

CEREBELLUM

CRANIAL
NERVES

BRAINSTEM

SPINAL
CORD

■ FIGURE 12.18

Spinal cord.

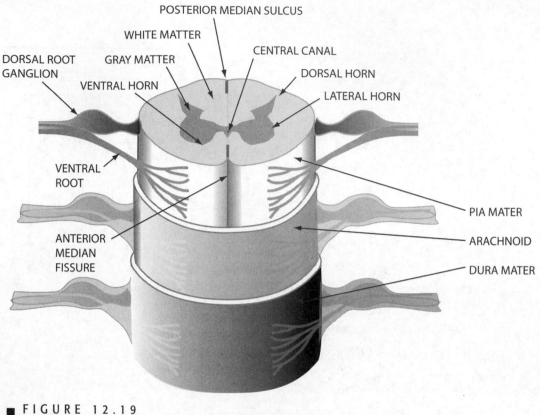

POSTERIOR MEDIAN SULCUS
WHITE MATTER
CENTRAL CANAL
DORSAL ROOT GANGLION
GRAY MATTER
DORSAL HORN
VENTRAL HORN
LATERAL HORN
VENTRAL ROOT
ANTERIOR MEDIAN FISSURE
PIA MATER
ARACHNOID
DURA MATER

■ FIGURE 12.19

Spinal cord detail.

Unlike in the brain, the white matter in the spinal cord forms the outer layer, and the grey matter forms the inner core.

The dorsal (posterior) horns receive sensory information, while the ventral (anterior) horns contain cell bodies for motor nerves.

In an adult the cord is about 42 to 45 cm long and about 1 cm in diameter at its widest point (Nolte, 2002).

Table 12.5 displays the regions of the spinal cord and the areas of the body served by each.

Like the brain, the spinal cord is also made up of areas of grey and white matter. In the brain, as we have seen, the grey matter forms the outer covering and the white matter is located within. This pattern is reversed in the spinal cord, with the white matter on the outside and the grey matter contained within. The shape of the grey matter is often likened to a butterfly with its wings spread. These "wings" actually comprise two sets of horns: the **dorsal or posterior horns** are made up of nerve cell bodies that receive sensory information from all areas of the body, and the **ventral** or *anterior* **horns** contain the cell bodies that project fibers to skeletal muscles. At some levels of the spinal cord there

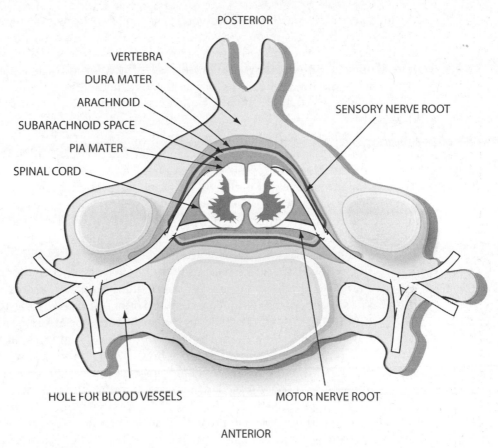

POSTERIOR

VERTEBRA

DURA MATER

ARACHNOID

SUBARACHNOID SPACE

PIA MATER

SPINAL CORD

SENSORY NERVE ROOT

HOLE FOR BLOOD VESSELS

MOTOR NERVE ROOT

ANTERIOR

■ FIGURE 12.20

Spinal cord shown within vertebra.

■ TABLE 12.5

Regions of the Spinal Cord and Areas Served by Each Region

REGION	AREAS SERVED
Cervical (C1-C8)	Back of head, neck, shoulders, diaphragm, arms, hands
Thoracic (T1-T12)	Ribs, back, abdomen
Lumbar (L1-L5)	Lower back, thighs, legs
Sacral (S1-S5)	Thighs, buttocks, legs, feet
Coccygeal (Co1)	Thighs, buttocks, legs, feet

are also lateral horns that are involved in visceral functions. The regions where the anterior and posterior horns meet is called the **intermediate zone**. The white matter surrounding the inner core of grey matter is made up of myelinated sensory and motor pathways bundled into large tracts called funiculi (singular: funiculus). There are four of these funiculi: one dorsal, one ventral, and two lateral. All the pathways, both sensory and motor, are situated within these funiculi.

Sensory pathways within the spinal cord include the spinothalamic tract and the spinocerebellar tract; motor pathways include lateral and anterior corticospinal tracts, the rubrospinal tract, and the lateral vestibulospinal tract.

Major sensory pathways in the spinal cord include the **spinothalamic tract** and the **spinocerebellar tract**. These pathways transmit information about pain, temperature, touch, and proprioception to the thalamus, cerebral cortex, and cerebellum. The major motor tracts include the **lateral corticospinal tract** (also known as the pyramidal tract), the **anterior corticospinal tract**, the **rubrospinal tract**, and the **lateral vestibulospinal tract**. The lateral corticospinal tract originates primarily in the sensorimotor areas of the cerebral cortex. Most of the descending fibers decussate at the pyramids of the medulla (hence the name pyramidal tract) and synapse with the neurons in the anterior horns of the spinal cord. The anterior corticospinal tract is formed by the 10 to 15 percent of descending fibers from the cortical motor areas that do not decussate, but that continue downward on the ipsilateral side to synapse with spinal motor neurons in the anterior horn. The rubrospinal tract originates in the midbrain from a nucleus of cell bodies called the red nucleus, and fibers from each side cross over to synapse contralaterally with anterior horn motor neurons. The cell bodies that give rise to the lateral vestibulospinal tract are located in the vestibular nuclei in the medulla. As with the other motor pathways, fibers synapse with anterior horn motor neurons. Table 12.6 summarizes the sensory and motor pathways of the spinal cord.

■ TABLE 12.6

Selected Funiculi And Pathways of the Spinal Cord

Funiculi	One dorsal
	One ventral
	Two lateral
Sensory pathways	Spinothalamic
	Spinocerebellar
Motor pathways	Lateral corticospinal
	Anterior corticospinal
	Rubrospinal
	Lateral vestibulospinal

Thirty-one pairs of spinal nerves enter and exit the spinal cord by way of spaces between successive vertebrae called intervertebral foramina. All spinal nerves are mixed, that is, they contain both sensory and motor fibers. They are classified on the basis of their origin (for sensory fibers) or target (for motor fibers). Thus, there are four types of spinal nerves: general somatic afferents (GSA) from skin surfaces and proprioceptors; general visceral afferents (GVA) from viscera including digestive tract, respiratory system, etc.; general somatic efferents (GSE) to skeletal muscles; and general visceral efferents (GVE) to viscera including glands, smooth muscles, heart, and so on. Refer to Table 12.7.

Each spinal nerve has both a sensory and a motor branch. The sensory branch exits the spinal cord via the posterior horn, and the motor branch enters the cord via the anterior horn. The two branches converge outside the spinal cord to form the spinal nerve (see Figures 12.19 and 12.20).

The spinal cord functions to institute reflexes. A reflex is an involuntary, stereotyped motor response to a sensory input. Reflexes may be relatively simple and confined to a single cord level (intrasegmental), or complex, involving multiple cord segments (intersegmental) (Haines, Mihailoff, & Yezierski, 2002). A common example of a simple reflex is the knee jerk, or patellar reflex. When the knee tendon is tapped, the front thigh muscle is slightly lengthened. This sensory information travels to the spinal cord via the posterior horn and stimulates the motor portion of the nerve, which in turn causes the involuntary kicking response. Another example is when one puts one's hand too close to a heat source and reflexively pulls it away very rapidly. In this case, the sensory input is the heat. Again, the sensory information travels to the spinal cord and stimulates the motor portion of the nerve to contract the relevant muscles. This process is shown in Figure 12.21. Information is also carried to the thalamus and on to the cerebral cortex, so that the individual becomes aware of his or her motor response a split second after it has occurred.

> All spinal nerves contain both sensory and motor fibers and enter and exit the spinal cord through the intervertebral foramina.

> A reflex is an involuntary, stereotyped motor response to a sensory input.

■ TABLE 12.7

Types of Spinal Nerves, Origins and Destinations

TYPE	MOTOR/SENSORY	ORIGIN/DESTINATION
GSA	Sensory	Skin, proprioceptors
GVA	Sensory	Digestive tract, respiratory system
GSE	Motor	Skeletal muscles
GVE	Motor	Glands, smooth muscles, heart

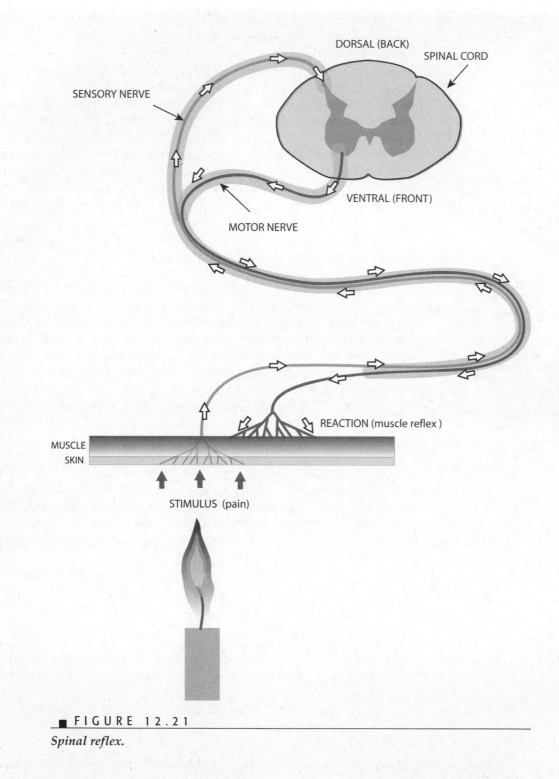

DORSAL (BACK)

SPINAL CORD

SENSORY NERVE

VENTRAL (FRONT)

MOTOR NERVE

REACTION (muscle reflex)

MUSCLE

SKIN

STIMULUS (pain)

■ F I G U R E   1 2 . 2 1

Spinal reflex.

Cranial Nerves

As we have seen, the thirty-one pairs of spinal nerves carry sensory information from the muscles and other sensory receptors of the torso and limbs to the brain and motor commands arising in the central nervous system to the muscles of the torso and limbs. The twelve pairs of cranial nerves transmit information to and from the face and neck regions. The cranial nerves are numbered with roman numerals from I to XII. These nerves are crucial for speech and hearing. Most of the cell bodies of these nerves (III to XII) arise from various levels of the brainstem, as shown in Figure 12.22, and the axons project to muscles in the face, head, ears, and chest. The nerves are numbered according to their order of emergence from the brainstem. Thus CN III emerges at the most superior point in the brainstem, and CN XII emerges at the most inferior point.

The twelve pairs of cranial nerves transmit information to and from the face and neck regions.

We saw that spinal nerves are classified as GSA, GVA, GSE, or GVE. This classification applies also to cranial nerves, but there are some additional categories in the case of cranial nerves: Special somatic afferent (SSA) nerves transmit information from the "special" senses including hearing, equilibrium, vision, and taste. Special visceral efferent (SVE) nerves carry motor commands to voluntary muscles, which develop from an embryological structure called the branchial arch, which gives rise, among others, to the facial muscles. For this reason, SVE fibers are sometimes called branchial motor fibers.

Special somatic afferent nerves transmit information from the special senses, including hearing, equilibrium, vision, and taste; special visceral efferent nerves carry motor commands to the voluntary muscles, which develop from the branchial arches.

While spinal nerves are all mixed (sensory and motor), cranial nerves can be more specialized, containing primarily GSE fibers or primarily SSA fibers, or they can carry a more complex combination of fibers. We will focus on those cranial nerves that are most important for speech and hearing: CN V (trigeminal), VII (facial), VIII (vestibulocochlear), IX (glossopharyngeal), X (vagus), and XII (hypoglossal).

CN V: Trigeminal.   This nerve is made up of three branches, the ophthalmic, maxillary, and mandibular branches (see Figure 12.23).

Both GSA and SVE fibers are found in the nerve. GSA fibers transmit information about touch, pressure, pain, proprioception, and temperature from various areas of the face—the maxillary branch from the upper lip, teeth, and upper jaw; the mandibular branch from the lower lip and teeth, lower jaw, and oral cavity. The SVE component innervates the muscles of mastication, the tensor veli palatini, the tensor tympani, and some of the extrinsic laryngeal muscles.

CN V, the trigeminal, is made up of three branches: ophthalmic, maxillary, and mandibular.

CN VII: Facial.   This is a complex nerve containing GSA, SVA, GVE, and SVE fibers (see Figure 12.24).

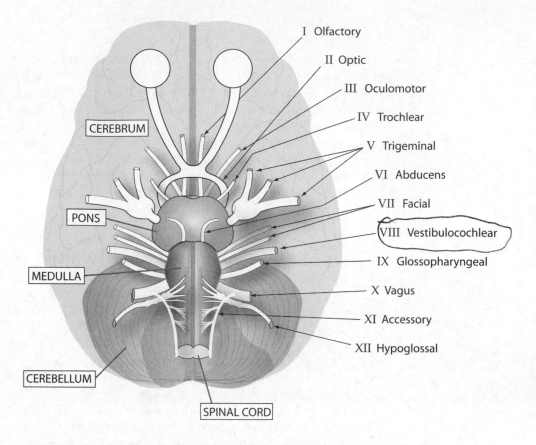

CEREBRUM

PONS

MEDULLA

CEREBELLUM

SPINAL CORD

I   Olfactory

II   Optic

III Oculomotor

IV   Trochlear

V   Trigeminal

VI   Abducens

VII Facial

VIII Vestibulocochlear

IX   Glossopharyngeal

X   Vagus

XI   Accessory

XII Hypoglossal

This schematic view is from the underside (inferior) of the brain looking upward.
The front of the brain (anterior) is at the top of the illustration; the back (posterior)
is at the bottom.

■ F I G U R E 1 2 . 2 2

Brainstem origins of the cranial nerves.

The facial nerve, CN VII,
projects fibers to the
upper face ipsilaterally
and fibers to the lower
face contralaterally.

The largest component consists of the SVE fibers that supply nerve impulses to the muscles of facial expression, the stapedius muscle in the middle ear, and various of the extrinsic laryngeal muscles. Interestingly, innervation patterns to the upper and lower portions of the face differ. Innervation to facial muscles above the eyes is ipsilateral, with axons in the originating motor nuclei in the brainstem projecting to the muscles on the same side. However, projections from the motor neurons to the facial muscles below the eyes are contralateral. This difference in nerve supply may be related to the more linked left and right movements of the forehead and eyes, compared to the relative inde-

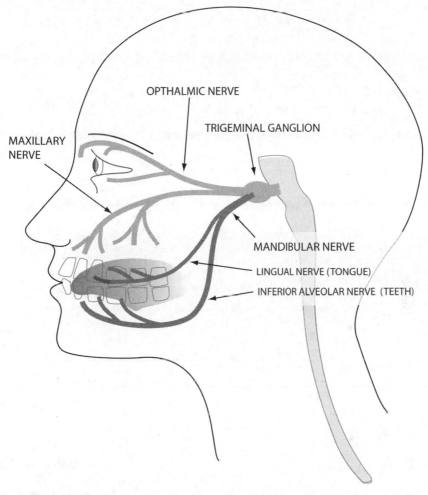

OPTHALMIC NERVE

TRIGEMINAL GANGLION

MAXILLARY
NERVE

MANDIBULAR NERVE

LINGUAL NERVE (TONGUE)

INFERIOR ALVEOLAR NERVE (TEETH)

■ F I G U R E   1 2 . 2 3

Trigeminal nerve.

CN VIII, the vestibulo-
cochlear, has two
branches: vestibular
fibers from the semi-
circular canals and
other structures in the
inner ear and cochlear
fibers from the inner
hair cells in the cochlea.

pendence of right and left side movements of our mouths and lips
(Nolte, 2002). The GSA component of CN VII transmits sensory information from the external ear. Taste information from the anterior two-
thirds of the tongue is carried by SVA fibers. GVE fibers transmit motor
information to the lacrimal (tear) glands and salivary glands.

CN VIII: Vestibulocochlear.   This nerve has two SSA branches, the
vestibular branch and the cochlear branch. The vestibular fibers arise
from the semicircular canals, utricle, and saccule in the inner ear and
relay information to the CNS about balance and head position. The

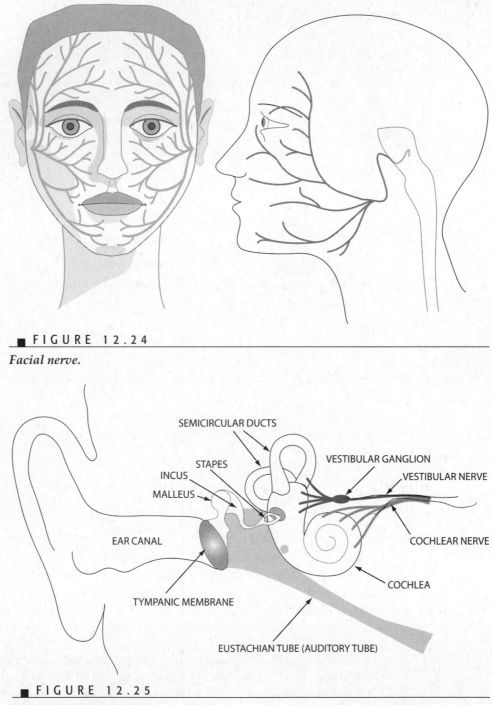

■ FIGURE 12.24

Facial nerve.

SEMICIRCULAR DUCTS

STAPES

VESTIBULAR GANGLION

INCUS

VESTIBULAR NERVE

MALLEUS

EAR CANAL

COCHLEAR NERVE

COCHLEA

TYMPANIC MEMBRANE

EUSTACHIAN TUBE (AUDITORY TUBE)

■ FIGURE 12.25

Vestibulocochlear nerve.

cochlear portion arises from the inner hair cells in the cochlea and transmits auditory information.

The nerve also has a small SVE component with motor information from the brainstem to the inner ear (Webster, 1999).

The glossopharyngeal nerve, CN IX, is involved in taste and swallowing.

CN IX: Glossopharyngeal.

This is another complex nerve with GSA, SVA, GVE, SVE, and GVA fibers (Figure 12.26).

The GSA fibers are associated with sensation from the external ear. The SVA portion is involved with taste from the posterior one-third of the tongue. The GVE fibers transmit motor information to one of the salivary glands in the oral cavity. The SVE fibers carry neural impulses to some of the pharyngeal muscles. The GVA portion transmits sensory information from the Eustachian tube, posterior one-third of the tongue, and pharynx. In general, the motor fibers are involved in swallowing, and the sensory fibers transmit information about taste, as well as pain, touch, and temperature.

CN X, the vagus nerve, has numerous branches involved in visceral function, as well as three branches essential for voice and speech production: the pharyngeal nerve, the superior laryngeal nerve, and the recurrent laryngeal nerve.

CN X: Vagus.

This nerve is not only crucial for phonation, but also plays a vital role in heart rate, endocrine function, and digestion, as seen in Figure 12.27.

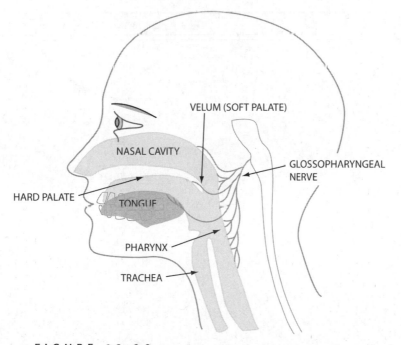

VELUM (SOFT PALATE)

NASAL CAVITY

GLOSSOPHARYNGEAL NERVE

HARD PALATE

TONGUE

PHARYNX

TRACHEA

■ FIGURE 12.26

Glossopharyngeal nerve.

The nerve has many branches, three of which are integral to speech production: the pharyngeal, superior laryngeal, and recurrent laryngeal nerves (Figure 12.28).

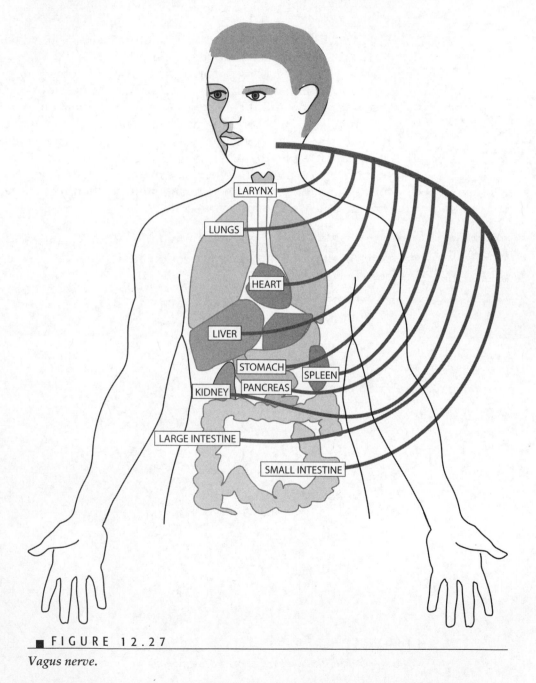

■ F I G U R E 1 2 . 2 7

Vagus nerve.

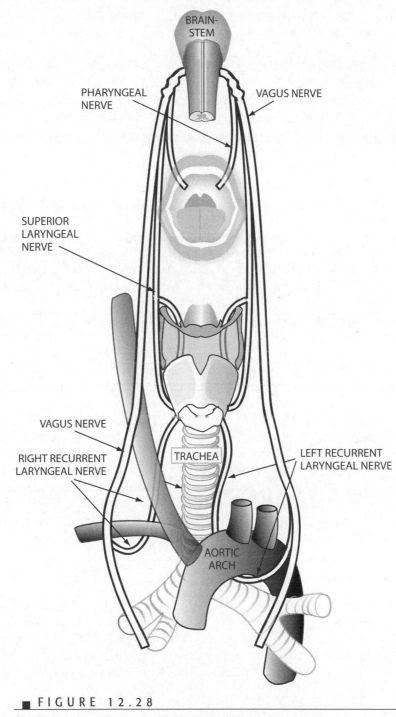

■ FIGURE 12.28

Pharyngeal and laryngeal branches of the vagus nerve.

These three branches are composed of SVE fibers. The pharyngeal nerve innervates the muscles of the soft palate (aside from the tensor veli palatini) and the pharynx. The superior laryngeal and recurrent laryngeal nerves carry neural impulses to the laryngeal muscles. Specifically, the recurrent laryngeal nerve innervates all the intrinsic muscles of the larynx except for the cricothyroid, which is innervated by the superior laryngeal branch. The anatomy of the recurrent laryngeal nerve, unlike other cranial nerves, is not symmetrical on the right and left sides of the body. Before actually entering the larynx, the recurrent laryngeal nerve descends into the chest and then ascends to enter the larynx. Figure 12.28 shows that on the right side the nerve loops under the subclavian artery of the heart before ascending; on the left side, the nerve descends to a lower point in the chest, loops under the aorta of the heart, and then travels upward again to enter the larynx. This difference in the length of the nerve on the right and left sides helps to explain why the left recurrent laryngeal nerve is more prone to injury than the right. This anatomical configuration also accounts for the fact that certain cardiac problems such as congestive heart failure can affect the recurrent laryngeal nerve, resulting in dysphonia.

The vagus also carries GSA fibers from the external ear; SVA fibers from a few taste buds around the epiglottis; and GVE fibers transmitting neural impulses to the heart, smooth muscles in the thorax and abdomen, and various glands. Finally, GVA fibers transmit sensory information from the thoracic and abdominal viscera as well as from the larynx, pharynx, trachea, and esophagus.

CN XII: Hypoglossal. This nerve is composed primarily of GSE fibers innervating intrinsic and extrinsic muscles of the tongue, as well as some of the extrinsic laryngeal muscles (Figure 12.29).

> The hypoglossal nerve, CN XII, primarily innervates muscles of the tongue.

Figure 12.30 illustrates the contributions of the cranial nerves that supply the tongue and larynx, including the trigeminal, facial, glossopharyngeal, and vagus.

Table 12.8 lists the cranial nerves important for speech and hearing, the types of fibers, and their origins and/or destinations.

Blood Supply to the Brain

The brain is crucially dependent on a continuous supply of blood for oxygen and glucose to support the metabolic needs of the nervous tissue. Because the brain does not store these energy-producing elements, the blood supply to the brain cannot be interrupted for more than a few minutes. Longer interruptions can cause permanent brain damage and death as the oxygen supply is cut off and nerve cells start to die.

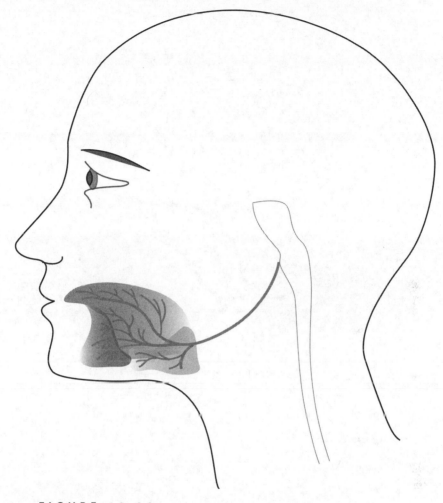

■ FIGURE 12.29

Hypoglossal nerve.

The circle of Willis, located at the base of the brain, is formed by several arteries and their branches, including the internal carotid and the vertebral.

The arteries that supply the brain are patterned in a roughly circular fashion, called the **circle of Willis**. As you can see in Figure 12.31, the arteries that form this circle are the internal carotid and the vertebral, as well as various branches off these major vessels, such as the anterior and posterior communicating arteries. Once it enters the skull, the internal carotid branches into the anterior and middle

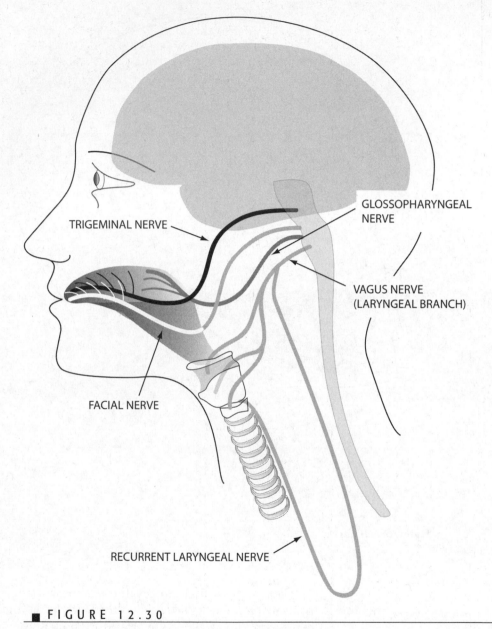

GLOSSOPHARYNGEAL
NERVE

TRIGEMINAL NERVE

VAGUS NERVE
(LARYNGEAL BRANCH)

FACIAL NERVE

RECURRENT LARYNGEAL NERVE

■ F I G U R E 1 2 . 3 0

Nerves that innervate the tongue and larynx.

■ T A B L E   1 2 . 8

Selected Cranial Nerves with Types of Fibers and Innervation

CN NUMBER	NAME	FIBERS	SENSORY/ MOTOR	INNERVATION
V	Trigeminal	GSA	Sensory	Touch, pressure, pain, proprioception, temperature from facial areas
		SVE	Motor	Muscles of mastication, tensor veli palatini, tensor tympani, extrinsic laryngeal muscles
VII	Facial	SVE	Motor	Muscles of facial expression, stapedius, extrinsic laryngeal muscles
		GSA	Sensory	External ear
		SVA	Sensory	Taste from anterior two-thirds of tongue
		GVE	Motor	Lacrimal and salivary glands
VIII	Vestibulocochlear	SSA	Sensory	Balance, head position, sound
		SVE	Motor	Inner ear
IX	Glossopharyngeal	GSA	Sensory	External ear
		SVA	Sensory	Taste from posterior one-third of tongue
		GVE	Motor	Salivary gland
		SVE	Motor	Pharyngeal muscles
		GVA	Sensory	Eustachian tube, posterior one-third of tongue, pharynx
X	Vagus	SVE	Motor	Soft palate, pharynx, larynx
		GSA	Sensory	External ear
		SVA	Sensory	Taste buds around the epiglottis
		GVE	Motor	Heart, thoracic and abdominal smooth muscles, glands
		GVA	Sensory	Thoracic and abdominal viscera, larynx, pharynx, trachea, esophagus
XII	Hypoglossal	GSE	Motor	Intrinsic and extrinsic muscles of tongue, extrinsic laryngeal muscles

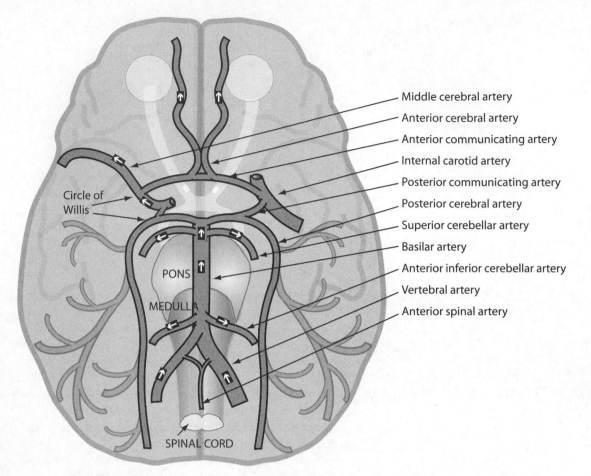

Middle cerebral artery

Anterior cerebral artery

Anterior communicating artery

Internal carotid artery

Posterior communicating artery

Posterior cerebral artery

Superior cerebellar artery

Basilar artery

Anterior inferior cerebellar artery

Vertebral artery

Anterior spinal artery

Circle of Willis

PONS

MEDULLA

SPINAL CORD

■ FIGURE 12.31

Blood supply to the brain.

Within the brain, the anterior, middle, and posterior cerebral arteries (ACA, MCA, PCA), as well as the cerebellar arteries, supply different regions.

cerebral arteries (ACA and MCA) on either side of the brain. The ACA supplies portions of the frontal and parietal lobes, the corpus callosum, the basal nuclei, and part of the internal capsule (Seikel et al., 2004). The MCA provides blood to the temporal lobe, motor strip, and Wernicke's area, among others (Seikel et al., 2004).

The two vertebral arteries, one from each side, join to form the basilar artery, which supplies blood to the brainstem. The basilar artery then branches into the posterior cerebral artery (PCA) and the cerebellar arteries. The PCA provides blood to portions of the temporal and occipital lobes, as well as to the upper midbrain, and the cerebellum. The cerebellar arteries supply the cerebellum.

Motor Control Systems Involved in Speech Production

Speech production, although seemingly effortless for the most part, requires a huge amount of neural processing to occur. The simplest utterance requires neuromuscular signals from numerous areas of the CNS and PNS to numerous muscles involved in respiration, phonation, and articulation. In addition, background postural muscle tone is an important component of the process. Sensory information from muscles, joints, skin, and tendons plays a crucial part in regulating the motor commands that actually cause our structures to in the appropriate sequence, and at the rapid rates involved in speech production.

> Numerous muscles are activated in the production of any phoneme, including respiratory, laryngeal, and articulatory, as well as those involved in the maintenance of appropriate posture and balance.

Think about the simple word *tan.* Just to produce this word, information must be transmitted from the various motor areas of the cerebral cortex along nerve pathways involving the basal nuclei, cerebellum, thalamus, corticospinal and corticonuclear tracts, to the correct spinal and cranial nerves, to the appropriate musculature for each phoneme in the word. Further, the phonemes must be correctly sequenced, so that the utterance emerges as planned, and not as *nat* or *ant.* This involves coarticulating the sounds, moving different articulators almost simultaneously while maintaining the separate identity of each phoneme. For the /t/ sound, the tongue tip must be raised, so neural impulses must arrive via CN XII to the superior longitudinal muscles of the tongue. The velum is raised to direct airflow out the oral cavity, so the levator veli palatini is activated via the pharyngeal branch of CN X. /t/ is voiceless, so the posterior cricoarytenoid muscles of the larynx, innervated by the recurrent laryngeal branch of CN X, are contracted to open the vocal folds, while the lateral cricoarytenoid muscles are relaxed. For the vowel, the vocal folds must close, regulated by the nerve impulses arriving via the recurrent laryngeal nerve at the lateral cricoarytenoids and interarytenoids; the tongue body lowers for the vowel, mediated by neuromuscular commands traveling along CN XII to the vertical muscles. The nasal /n/ requires a lowered velum, so the levator veli palatini relaxes, allowing the velum to drop. Once again the tongue tip is raised, and the vocal folds remain closed and vibrating. Consider that all these neuromuscular commands occur within the space of less than a second, and one begins to see the stunning complexity of the system. Consider also that the appropriate muscles of respiration are activated via the appropriate spinal nerves, changing from the postures for life breathing to those for speech breathing. Simultaneously, the person uttering the word is either sitting or standing or walking, so the appropriate trunk and limb muscles are being regulated as well. In addition, sensory systems of proprioception from joints and muscles, sound from our auditory systems, visual stimuli, and so on, are processed alongside the motor information. Now, take one phoneme and multiply all these neuromuscular events for that phoneme by around 20 or so (we speak at approximately 20 phonemes per second in normal conversational speech), and the importance of the sensorimotor neural control system becomes apparent. Table 12.9 summarizes selected neuromuscular events involved in the production of the word *tan*.

We will look in detail at some of the motor control systems that we use for speech production, including the motor cortex, upper and lower motor neurons, and mechanisms of sensory feedback and feedforward.

Motor Cortex

We have seen that the motor cortex includes primary, premotor, and supplementary motor areas and that each of these areas is equipped with a map, in more or less detail, representing various bodily structures. Far from duplicating each other's functions, however, each motor area regulates movement in different yet complementary ways. The primary motor cortex in area 4 (see Figure 12.10) controls single muscles or small groups of muscles that work synergistically to perform a complex coordinated movement. This area receives extensive sensory input from the thalamus, from the somatosensory cortex, and from the premotor cortex and is thus continuously updated about ongoing and anticipated movement. Research has shown that neurons in M1 regulate the

Primary motor cortex in area 4 controls single muscles or small groups of muscles involved in preparing and carrying out complex coordinated movement.

■ TABLE 12.9

Selected Neuromuscular Events for the Word **tan**

PHONEME	PRIMARY STRUCTURES INVOLVED	PRIMARY NERVE PATHWAYS INVOLVED
/t/	Tongue tip raised by superior longitudinal muscle	CN XII
	Velum raised by levator veli palatini	Pharyngeal branch of CN X
	Vocal folds opened by posterior cricoarytenoids	Recurrent laryngeal branch of CN X
/æ/	Vocal folds closed by lateral cricoarytenoids and interarytenoids	Recurrent laryngeal branch of CN X
	Tongue body lowered by vertical tongue muscles	CN XII
/n/	Velum lowered by relaxation of levator veli palatini	
	Tongue tip raised by superior longitudinal muscle	CN XII
	Vocal folds remain closed by lateral cricoarytenoids and interarytenoids	Recurrent laryngeal branch of CN X

amount of force and the direction needed for the desired movement and that these neurons fire in preparation for (that is, slightly in advance of) an upcoming movement (Mihailoff & Haines, 2002). However, the activity of these neurons can also be modified during a movement, showing that other sensory and motor information coming from many different nervous system locations is processed while a movement is in progress. It is important to note that the primary motor cortex does not initiate movement, but rather collects and channels information about aspects of movement and then transmits this information to the brainstem and spinal cord to be passed along to the appropriate spinal and cranial nerves for execution.

The premotor cortex deals with larger groups of muscles in more widely separated parts of the body and organizes information about upcoming movements based on sensory information.

The premotor and supplementary motor cortices are both located in area 6, anterior to area 4 (see Figure 12.10). The premotor area prepares, plans, and organizes information about upcoming movements based partially on sensory information. The sensory input involves balance and visual information that is needed to enable an individual to assess his or her position in space or the position of relevant structures in space, to judge the direction and force of the movement necessary to reach its target, and to make any adjustments to posture that are necessary to keep one's balance while carrying out the movement. This data is transmitted to M1, as well as to the spinal cord and brainstem. Thus, unlike M1, which regulates relatively small groups of muscles, the premotor cortex deals with larger groups of muscles in more widely separated parts of the body.

The supplementary motor area is involved in the planning of complex movements generated internally, such as those necessary for speech.

The supplementary motor area functions similarly to the premotor cortex. However, while premotor cortex is more involved with movements in response to external environmental stimuli, the supplementary motor cortex plays more of a role in planning complex, internally generated movements (Nolte, 2002). Thus, the supplementary motor area has been implicated in such disorders as stuttering, in which there is a breakdown of the complex, coordinated movements necessary for fluent speech.

Upper and Lower Motor Neurons

The upper motor neuron refers to nerve cells and their axons from various cortical areas that project to the brainstem and spinal cord; the lower motor neuron is the name for nerve cell bodies and axons of the cranial and spinal nerves.

Two components of the motor control system are the **upper** and **lower motor neurons** (UMN and LMN). The UMN comprises the nerve cells and their axons arising from various cortical areas and projecting to the brainstem and spinal cord. The LMN includes nerve cell bodies and axons of cranial and spinal nerves that connect with voluntary muscles. Once motor information from cortical areas has been acted upon by the basal nuclei and cerebellum, the final neuromuscular commands are transmitted by the UMN to the LMN and from there to the target structures for movement execution. Spinal and cranial nerves that make up the LMN are often called, therefore, the final common pathway, since all cortical and subcortical motor information converges onto these nerves.

The two major pathways of the UMN are the corticospinal and corticonuclear (corticobulbar) tracts. The corticospinal tract is a large one, with around 1 million fibers (Nolte, 2002). About a third of the fibers arise in M1, another third in premotor and supplementary motor areas, and the remaining third in the somatosensory cortex in the parietal lobe (see Figure 12.32).

The large corticospinal tract arises from motor and sensory areas in the cortex and its fibers synapse directly onto motor nerve cells in the spinal cord.

Fibers in this tract synapse directly onto motor nerve cells in the anterior horn of the spinal cord, although along the way branches of these fibers project to other locations including the basal nuclei, thalamus, reticular formation, and sensory nuclei (Nolte, 2002). Most fibers in this tract (around 80 to 90%) decussate in the medullary pyramids and continue contralaterally to their spinal targets, while a small percentage of fibers continues ipsilaterally. The crossed fibers on either side form the lateral corticospinal pathways. The anterior corticospinal pathways are made up of the uncrossed fibers.

The corticonuclear tract is still mostly called the corticobulbar tract. The term *bulb* refers to the medulla, although this name is now obsolete. The term *corticobulbar* is not anatomically accurate, but is still used widely to refer to all cortical projections that synapse on motor neurons of cranial nerves in the brainstem. The new term *corticonuclear* was adopted in 1998 by the International Federation of Associations of Anatomists (Mihailoff & Haines, 2002). This term refers specifically to nerve cells and their axons arising from cortical areas and synapsing with motor nuclei of CN V, VII, and XII, as well as the nucleus ambiguus that gives rise to CN X, among other pathways. Only striated muscles that are involved in voluntary movement are supplied by the corticonuclear tract. Whereas fibers in the corticospinal tract arise from several cortical locations, the origin of corticonuclear fibers is more localized to the face and neck portions of the primary motor cortex, as shown in Figure 12.33. The corticonuclear tract innervates the left and right motor nuclei in the brainstem bilaterally, with information from left and right motor cortices traveling ipsilaterally. However, as we have seen, some selected fibers, such as those innervating the lower areas of the face, are contralateral.

The corticonuclear tract arises from fibers in the face and neck portions of the motor cortex and synapse with motor nuclei of CN V, VII, X, and XII.

Direct and Indirect Systems   The corticospinal and corticonuclear tracts together are sometimes referred to as the **pyramidal** or **direct system**. This system is involved in controlling fine, skilled voluntary movements, and damage can result in muscles that are weak or spastic. The **indirect** or **extrapyramidal system** refers to nerve pathways from the cortex to the brainstem or spinal cord that do not synapse directly with the motor neurons, but that travel more circuitously via the basal nuclei and cerebellum before synapsing with spinal

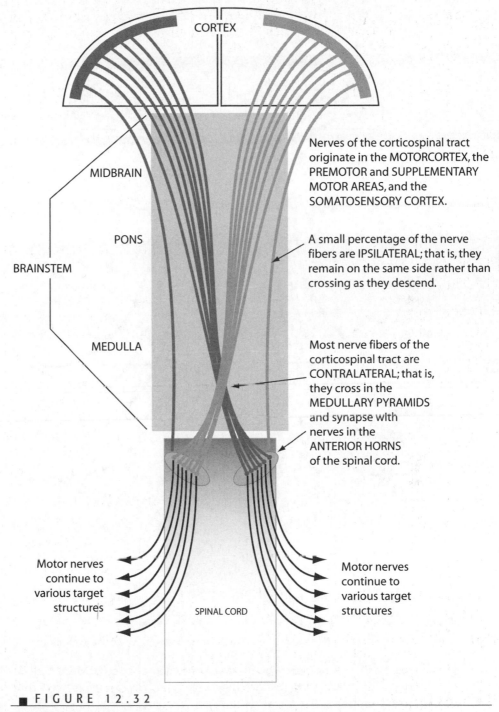

CORTEX

MIDBRAIN

PONS

BRAINSTEM

MEDULLA

Nerves of the corticospinal tract originate in the MOTORCORTEX, the PREMOTOR and SUPPLEMENTARY MOTOR AREAS, and the SOMATOSENSORY CORTEX.

A small percentage of the nerve fibers are IPSILATERAL; that is, they remain on the same side rather than crossing as they descend.

Most nerve fibers of the corticospinal tract are CONTRALATERAL; that is, they cross in the MEDULLARY PYRAMIDS and synapse wIth nerves in the ANTERIOR HORNS of the spinal cord.

Motor nerves continue to various target structures

Motor nerves continue to various target structures

SPINAL CORD

■ FIGURE 12.32

Corticospinal pathway.

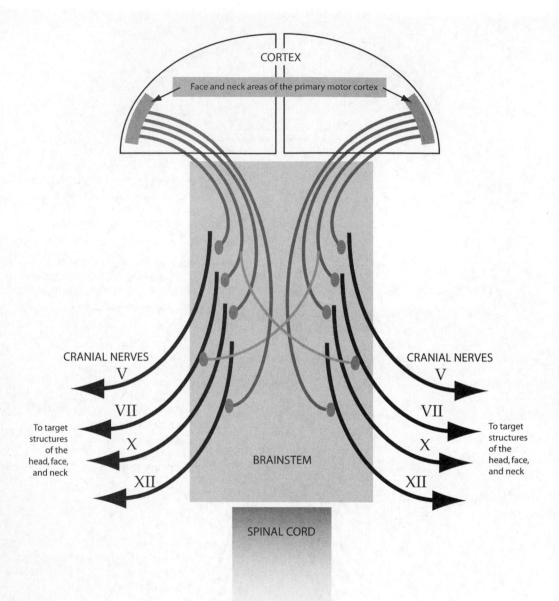

Nerves in the corticonuclear pathway originate in the face and neck areas of the motor cortex. They synapse in the brainstem with CRANIAL NERVES V, VII, X, and XII.

They synapse with the nerves on the SAME SIDE as the hemisphere in which they originate (IPSILATERAL).

An exception occurs in that CN VII fibers also cross over to the opposite side (CONTRALATERAL).

■ F I G U R E 1 2 . 3 3

Corticonuclear pathway.

and brainstem motor nuclei. Damage to the indirect system can result in abnormal involuntary movements such as tics and tremors that interfere with normal voluntary control, as well as postural deficits.

Motor Units   LMN fibers projecting from cranial and spinal motor neurons to voluntary muscles have axonic endings that synapse with muscle fibers. The synapse between an axon and the muscle fiber it innervates is called the neuromuscular junction, myoneural junction, or motor end plate (Figure 12.34).

The neuromuscular junction, or myoneural junction, refers to the synapse between an axon and a muscle fiber.

This junction functions similarly to a nerve-to-nerve synapse. The vesicles of the presynaptic neuron contain the neurotransmitter acetylcholine (ACh), which acts in an excitatory fashion. When the vesicles are stimulated by an action potential, the acetylcholine is released into the synapse, and it generates an EPSP, which causes the muscle fiber to contract. After a very short interval, the acetylcholine is inactivated. Inactivation occurs through several mechanisms. One mechanism is by degrading the chemical into its component parts via an enzyme called **acetylcholinesterase**. Once the ACh is broken down, it can no longer be recognized by the receptor sites, thus stopping its excitatory action. Another mechanism is called reuptake, in which the intact neurotransmitter is recycled back into the vesicles of the presynaptic neuron.

An end-plate potential (EPP) is a small depolarization of a muscle fiber. If the EPP reaches a critical threshold, an action potential is generated, causing the fiber to contract.

The way that muscles contract is essentially the same process as that by which nerves fire. Similar to neurons, which have a resting potential of around −70 mV, the inside of a muscle fiber at rest has negative charge of roughly −95 mV. When the ACh is released into the neuromuscular junction, sodium channels in the membrane surrounding the fiber are opened, allowing sodium ions to diffuse into the fiber. This has the effect of reducing the negative charge within the fiber and creates a small depolarization called an **end-plate potential** (EPP). If the EPP reaches a critical threshold, an all-or-none action potential results, causing the muscle fiber to contract. Once the fiber has contracted, it is followed by a brief refractory period during which it is repolarized and returns to its original resting potential.

The innervation ratio is the ratio of a motor neuron to the number of fibers it innervates.

One motor neuron can innervate varying numbers of muscle fibers. A motor neuron with its associated muscle fibers is called a **motor unit**. The ratio of a motor neuron to the number of fibers it innervates is called the **innervation ratio**. Different structures have motor unit sizes that depend on the function and level of motor control of that structure. For example, large leg muscles that do not require very fine neuromuscular control, but generate a lot of muscular force, have motor units with large innervation ratios. That is, one axon innervates many muscle fibers, around 600 to 1000 fibers per axon (Mihailoff & Haines, 2002). By contrast, smaller structures that do not generate much force

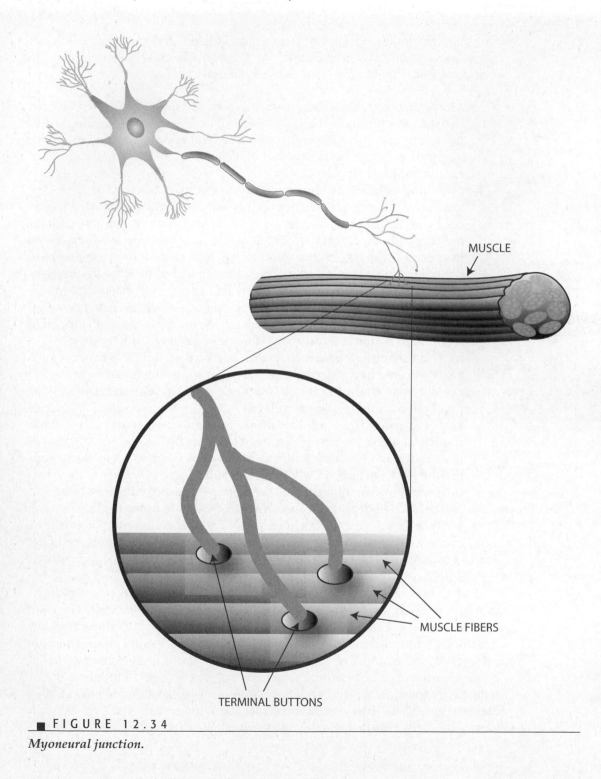

MUSCLE

MUSCLE FIBERS

TERMINAL BUTTONS

■ FIGURE 12.34

Myoneural junction.

Laryngeal muscles have very small innervation ratios, indicating the fine degree of muscular control required for phonation.

and require fine levels of control, such as the laryngeal muscles, have much smaller motor units of 10 to 100 fibers per axon. It is important to note that how strongly a muscle contracts depends on the number of motor units that are activated.

There are three types of motor units, each associated with a different type of muscle fiber. Type S units (slow) are associated with dark red muscle fibers. These fibers do not generate much force, but also do not fatigue easily. They are activated by small diameter motor neurons that, as you recall, have slower conduction rates. These fibers are found in large numbers in muscles that are associated with maintaining posture. These muscles are called slow twitch muscles and can continue to contract for long periods of time. Type FF units (fast fatigable) are associated with light-colored larger fibers that generate large amounts of force for brief amounts of time. They are activated by large diameter, fast conducting nerves and dominate in muscles associated with rapid movements. Muscles innervated by FF units are referred to as fast twitch. Type FR units (fatigue resistant) share characteristics of the other two types. These muscles generate nearly but not quite as much force as fast twitch muscles, but are more fatigue resistant and can therefore sustain contraction for longer periods than can fast twitch muscles.

Slow twitch muscles can contract for long periods of time without fatiguing; fast twitch muscles can generate large amounts of force very rapidly but fatigue quickly.

Motor units differ in size, with S (slow) units being the smallest and FF (fast fatigable) being the largest.

The motor units also differ in terms of size: S units are the smallest in terms of their cell bodies, FF units are the largest, and FR units fall in between. The size difference plays an important role in how we regulate the muscle force needed for smooth movement. As previously discussed, motor neurons fire and trigger an action potential when a critical voltage threshold is reached. Smaller neurons have a lower threshold than larger ones. Thus, the small S units are the first to fire when stimulated. As stimulation becomes more intense, they fire with increasing rapidity. This in turn causes the FR units to fire. Should stimulation continue to increase and FR units fire more rapidly, then FF units are recruited as well and add their force to the movement. This is called the size principle.

Principles of Motor Control

Becoming familiar with neural pathways and brain structures forms the basis for understanding some principles involved in motor control systems. These systems include feedback and feedforward control, efference copy, and motor equivalence.

Feedback and Feedforward   Feedback is an engineering term that refers to the process whereby the output of a particular system is returned to the input in order to influence the ensuing output. Systems can be thought of as being either closed loop or open loop. Closed loop systems return the output back to

Feedback is the process whereby the output of a system is returned to the input in order to influence the ensuing output; in a feedforward system, output from one system becomes the input to a different system.

the original input for purposes of comparison and correction. Open loop systems do not use feedback to modify the output of the system. Speech production relies on both types of systems. In terms of speech production, feedback refers to any type of sensory information available to the speaker, such as auditory information, proprioceptive information, and tactile information. Feedback operates as a control system that allows an individual to detect and correct any errors in his or her speech production. Feedback channels, however, do not operate instantaneously, so that sometimes a speaker has already made an error before he or she becomes aware of it and is able to correct it. In speech production, auditory feedback is probably the most crucial type of information when a child is learning to speak his or her native language. This is clearly evident in the case of prelingually deaf children, who typically have great difficulty in acquiring the appropriate vocal tract positions to generate the phonemes of the language. Auditory feedback becomes less vital once the language has been learned, although there is some evidence that speakers who are deafened later in life may lose some degree of intelligibility due to the hearing loss and lack of auditory feedback. However, most normal speakers do not need a lot of auditory feedback in order to produce intelligible speech, probably because speech is a highly practiced motor skill.

During speech, sensory information from different types of receptors is fed forward to various articulators, allowing rapid "online" adjustments to be made.

Speech production also uses feedforward information. Feedforward refers to the process whereby output from one system becomes the input to another system. In terms of speech production, this may mean that sensory information from the jaw during a particular phoneme may be input to other articulators, such as the lips and tongue, and modifies the activity of these articulators. In this case, the original information from the jaw is not returned to the original source, but acts to influence other articulators. Feedforward mechanisms act much more rapidly than feedback systems. Thus articulatory movements can be modified "online," allowing for a great deal of precision during speech production. Feedforward mechanisms have been demonstrated in experiments in which a subject's articulators are perturbed unpredictably in some way as a subject is producing an utterance. It has been shown that, typically, the acoustic output is not affected, and the subject makes extremely rapid adjustments of the perturbed and unperturbed articulators (tens of milliseconds) in order to maintain the acoustic integrity of the utterance.

Sensory information is crucial for the motor activities of speech production. Barlow (1999) noted that sensory information obtained from proprioceptors, joint receptors, mechanoreceptors, and baroreceptors, as well as auditory, kinesthetic, and cutaneous information, provides important information about muscle systems during speech production. Abbs (1996), as well, noted that sensory projections from the jaw, lips, and tongue are continuously monitored by the nervous system. They are used to regulate and adjust motor output and

Motor equivalence is the ability of the motor system to achieve a particular movement with a great deal of variability in the individual components of the movement.

to coordinate muscular adjustments between articulators. Abbs further noted that while particular motor goals are planned (i.e., specific phonemes or articulator movements), the specific patterns of muscle contractions and joint movements are programmed flexibly based on current sensory and motor information from articulatory, respiratory, and phonatory structures. This is in accordance with the concept of motor equivalence, first described in the early twentieth century. Motor equivalence refers to the ability of the motor system to achieve a particular movement goal or output with a great degree of variability in the individual components of the movement. Speech is a goal-oriented process of moving the articulators into the appropriate position for specific sounds. As long as the correct sound is achieved—that is, the acoustic output is maintained—the precise positioning of the articulators is not important. Experiments using a bite block to fix the mandible in position have shown that even with the jaw fixed, speakers are able to produce an acceptable vowel by slightly adjusting other articulators to compensate for the disruption in normal production. It is likely that feedforward and efference copy mechanisms are involved in making these extremely rapid compensations.

Efference Copy   Efference copy refers to the notion that when a neural motor command signal is sent to a muscle or structure, a second simultaneous "copy" of the signal is transmitted to various sensory systems as well, in order to get the sensory system ready for the anticipated consequences of the motor act (Barlow, 1999). We know that there are many sensory and motor pathways between the sensorimotor areas of the cortex, subcortical structures, and cerebellum. Nerve pathways from the cortex to the cerebellum provide the cerebellum with efference copy signals from the primary motor cortex as well as sensory feedback from the primary sensory cortex (Barlow, 1999). The cerebellum is then in a position to evaluate the ongoing movement and to correct any errors, and projects the new information back to the motor cortex (feedback) as well as to peripheral structures via various nerve pathways (feedforward).

Efference copy refers to the idea that when a neuromuscular command is sent to a muscle, a "copy" of the signal is simultaneously transmitted to various sensory systems.

s u m m a r y

- The nervous system is divided into the central nervous system, which includes the brain and spinal cord, and the peripheral nervous system, which includes the cranial and spinal nerves.
- Neurons are the basic building blocks of the nervous system and consist of cell body, dendrites, and an axon; glial cells perform many metabolic functions.
- Neurons work through a complex electrochemical process by which an action potential is generated and transmitted to other neurons at the synapse.

- The brain is contained within the meninges and is given buoyancy by the cerebrospinal fluid, which is manufactured in the ventricles and circulates around the brain and spinal cord.
- The brain is divided into two hemispheres, connected by the corpus callosum.
- The cortex of the brain is highly convoluted and is divided into frontal, parietal, temporal, occipital, and limbic lobes.
- Within the white matter of the cerebrum are several subcortical structures, including the basal nuclei, thalamus, and hypothalamus.

- The brainstem includes the midbrain, pons, and medulla, which connects to the spinal cord; cranial nerves have their points of origin in various regions of the brainstem.
- The cerebellum is an important structure for coordinating different aspects of movement, such as direction, force, and speed.
- Motor control systems involved in speech production include the motor cortical areas, as well as the upper and lower motor neurons; feedback and feedforward are important components of motor control.

review exercises

1. Identify three types of glial cells and explain the difference between them and neurons in terms of structure and function.
2. Describe the process whereby neurons in a resting state are depolarized and repolarized when stimulated.
3. Identify and describe the areas of the cortex important in the understanding and comprehension of speech.
4. Explain how the subcortical areas and the cerebellum are involved in speech production.

5. Compare and contrast the cranial nerves important for speech and hearing in terms of their origins and effects.
6. Describe the differences and similarities between the corticospinal and corticonuclear nerve pathways.
7. Explain the concepts of feedback, feedforward, efference copy, and motor equivalence with regard to speech production.

chapter 13

Clinical Application
Brain Function Measures

chapter objectives	*After reading this chapter, you will*

After reading this chapter, you will

1. Be familiar with techniques used to image brain structure.
2. Understand methods of imaging brain function.
3. Appreciate how brain-imaging techniques are used to expand knowledge about stuttering.
4. Be familiar with ways in which brain imaging techniques have been used for diagnosis of neurological diseases such as Parkinson's disease and Alzheimer's disease.
5. Appreciate the value of brain-imaging techniques in assessing treatment efficacy in certain neurological diseases.

The way in which the brain functions and the ways in which the brain can malfunction have long fascinated scientists and researchers as well as professionals who work with individuals with brain damage. Methods have been devised over past decades to try to access brain structure and function in order to understand and compare normal and abnormal neural working and to create treatment strategies to restore brain function or to compensate for the damage.

With the advent over the past few decades of sophisticated computerized technology, this objective has become much more attainable. Current brain-imaging techniques allow fine details of brain structures to be visualized, manipulated, and quantified, providing the opportunity for unparalleled understanding of normal and abnormal brain function. These new techniques have also been applied to the study of normal and disordered human communication, allowing for confirmation or rejection of theories, expansion of models, and insight into the efficacy of various surgical, pharmacological, and behavioral treatment techniques.

Much of the information we have about brain function and its relationship to human behavior, including communicative behavior, has come from individuals with various types of neurological disorders or injuries. For example, a lot of what we know about the function of cortical and subcortical areas such as Broca's area and the basal nuclei has been derived by examining the deficits in function of people who have suffered a stroke or other brain injury that affects that region. With current brain-imaging techniques it has now become possible to evaluate normal function from brain-behavior data obtained from neurologically normal individuals. This is preferable, because information derived from individuals with brain damage is often complicated by factors such as age and time post-injury (Plante, 2001), as well as premorbid factors such as education level and socioeconomic status. In addition, relying on correlations between damaged areas and resulting behaviors does not take into account factors such as undamaged brain areas that may, at least partially, compensate for the lost function.

Current brain-imaging techniques can be categorized on the basis of whether they depict brain structure (anatomy) or reflect brain function (physiology). They can also be classified in terms of the type of technology used.

Brain structure is accessed by specialized x-rays and imaging techniques. Brain function is typically indicated indirectly by measuring electrical, biochemical, or physiologic characteristics of the nervous system (Watson & Freeman, 1997). In this chapter we will focus on the primary methods of imaging brain structure, including computerized tomography and magnetic resonance imaging, as well as the main techniques for evaluating function, including functional magnetic resonance imaging, positron emission tomography, single photon emission computerized tomography, and quantitative electroencephalography. We will then explore how the use of these techniques has enhanced our understanding of communication disorders resulting from various neurological causes.

> Current brain-imaging techniques depict either brain structure or brain function.

■ *Techniques for Imaging Brain Structure*

Computerized Tomography

Computerized tomography (CT) is an x-ray technique. Like conventional (planar) x-rays, CT is sensitive to the density of tissues. The denser the tissue, the more radiation energy it absorbs, resulting in a lighter x-ray image. Bone, for example, is extremely dense and shows up as white on x-rays. The difference between planar x-rays and CT is that a CT image is constructed from numerous scans of the brain structure as the x-ray and the x-ray detector rotate around the individual's head (Watson & Freeman, 1997). This results in many different angles at which the structure is scanned, and the resulting scans are combined by a computer into a detailed three-dimensional image of cross sections of selected thicknesses of cortical and subcortical regions of the brain. Current CT scanners are able to image a slices of the target structure very quickly (Haines, Raila, & Terrell, 2002).

Computerized tomography uses x-ray images to create a three dimensional representation of brain structures.

Advantages of CT include the short (1 second per slice) imaging times and widespread availability of the technology. Because of its excellent differentiation between tissues of varying densities the technique allows detection of calcification and hemorrhage (Laughlin & Montanera, 1998). CT is typically used to diagnose tumors, cerebrovascular disease, head trauma, and cerebral atrophy (Watson & Freeman, 1997). The disadvantage, as with any x-ray, is the radiation and resulting potential health risks to the patient.

Magnetic Resonance Imaging

Magnetic resonance imaging (MRI) is a technique that takes advantage of the cellular basis of human tissue. One of the major components of tissue is water, and hydrogen atoms constitute one element of water molecules (H_2O). Over 70 percent of brain tissue is composed of water (Parry & Matthews, 2002). Hydrogen atoms behave like miniature magnets spinning around an axis at a certain frequency. They are normally aligned randomly rather than in specific patterns. During an MRI the patient is exposed to a super-powerful magnet, which causes the hydrogen atoms to line up in parallel with the external magnetic field. A brief radiofrequency wave or pulse (RF) is then directed into the patient. When the frequencies of the RF pulse and the spinning hydrogen protons are close to each other, constructive interference (resonance) occurs, and the proton gains energy. When the radiofrequency wave is turned off, the hydrogen atoms gradually return to their original random alignments, a process called relaxation. As these molecules relax, they release energy in the form of radio waves, which is detected and amplified by a specialized receiver. Different tissues within the brain contain slightly different amounts of water. For example, neurons have higher concentration of water than myelin (Parry & Matthews, 2002). These differences in water and hydrogen content produce the contrasts between different tissues, based on the distribution of hydrogen atoms (Lauter, 1997). This result in radio signals with different amplitudes and different relaxation times. A computer transforms this information into images of the target structure.

Magnetic resonance imaging uses the magnetic properties of hydrogen atoms within human tissue to construct finely detailed images of brain structures.

A major advantage of MRI is that it does not use radiation, and therefore poses no health risks. Because of this, MRI has been used extensively to study the brain not only in people with various disorders and diseases, but also in healthy individuals, resulting in a large body of knowledge of brain structures from infants to geriatrics. Another advantage of MRI is that it can distinguish fine differences between soft tissues such as grey and white matter, cerebrospinal fluid, and vascular structures. With this technique it is also possible to detect differences between normal and abnormal tissue, such as the plaques that occur in multiple sclerosis. Because of the very high degree of spatial resolution that can be obtained with MRI (1 mm), it is even possible to identify individual cranial nerves and subcortical structures (Lauter, 1997). Thus, MRI is a valuable tool for diagnosis of various brain diseases and disorders. There are some disadvantages, however. Imaging times are longer for MRI than for CT, and the cost is higher. Some individuals are not able to undergo MRI because of the presence of metal devices in the body, such as aneurysm clips, pacemakers, or cochlear implants.

> Individuals with metal devices in their bodies such as aneurysm clips, pacemakers, or cochlear implants, are not able to undergo magnetic resonance imaging.

▪ Techniques for Imaging Brain Function

Techniques for imaging brain function are based on blood flow within the brain, brain metabolism of oxygen and glucose, electrical properties of brain physiology, or some combination of these. Whatever technique is used, functional neuroimaging is based on the rationale that the performance of any task places specific information processing demands on the brain, and these demands are met through local changes in neural activity (Fiez, 2001). This results in changes to blood flow within the activated brain area, as well as to metabolism within that region. These changes can then be either directly or indirectly measured in various ways.

> Brain function is imaged by measuring blood flow within the brain, brain metabolism of oxygen and glucose, or electrical brain activity.

Functional Magnetic Resonance Imaging

Functional magnetic resonance imaging (fMRI), like regular MRI, is based on the magnetic properties of hydrogen, as well as on the characteristics of blood flow within the brain. That is, fMRI is an index of changes in the oxygen content of the blood in a particular brain area or region of interest (ROI). It can be used as such because of the way nerves function. After a neuron has fired, we know that neurotransmitter is released into the synapse. Shortly thereafter, the neurotransmitter is either degraded or taken back into the pre-synaptic neuron, a process that needs energy to be completed. The increased energy is provided by increased oxygen, with a corresponding increase in the local

Functional magnetic resonance imaging (fMRI) is based on measurement of increased blood flow, called the hemody-namic response, to specific regions of the brain during the per-formance of some kind of task.

blood flow within the region. This increase in blood flow to a specific area is known as the **hemodynamic response**, and it is this response that is measured in fMRI. The response is correlated with different types of tasks and different brain regions that are activated during these tasks. Thus, fMRI is an indirect measure of brain function, since it is the hemodynamic response that is measured, rather than the actual neuronal function.

A major advantage of fMRI is that it is a safe and noninvasive means of assessing how an individual's brain function changes over time or in different situations. This is valuable when evaluating effects of brain damage on various types of tasks including communicative activities. It is also an excellent diagnostic tool for neurological conditions and can also be useful in assessing recovery patterns with and without treatment interventions. Another advantage is that both fMRI and conventional MRI scans can be obtained together in a single session. This allows both structural and functional components of neurological images to be compared, yielding a rich source of correlated information. In addition, fMRI instrumentation is widely available for medical use.

A disadvantage of fMRI is that, because it is based on the hemodynamic response that occurs around 450 msec after the nerve has fired (Lauter, 1997), the scanning process is relatively slow. Also, the scanner is noisy, which can interfere with auditorily presented stimuli during speech and language tasks.

Positron Emission Tomography

Positron emission tomography (PET) is based on identifying the distribution of an injected or inhaled radioactive substance called a **tracer**, combined with a chemical such as glucose, in a patient's brain. The tracer is eliminated from the individual's body within a relatively short period of approximately 6 to 24 hours. Commonly used tracers include oxygen, nitrogen, carbon, and fluorine. The amount of accumulation of the tracer in a particular brain area depends on the degree of blood flow, which, as discussed above, is related to the amount of neural activity in that region (Borden, Harris, & Raphael, 2003). Areas of the brain that are more active absorb more of the tracer; less active areas absorb less. An index of regional cerebral blood flow (rCBF) is produced with this technology.

Positron emission tomography (PET) reflects brain activity by measuring the distribution of a radio-active substance within an individual's brain, and yields an index of regional cerebral blood flow (rCBF).

The radioactive tracer gradually disintegrates and emits positrons, which are positively charged particles. The positrons collide with electrons, producing gamma rays that are detected and measured by computers. Cross-sectional areas of the brain are scanned from many directions, producing a three-dimensional representation of the scanned area. The PET scanner rotates around the patient, providing sequences of colored three-dimensional

PET scans produce a three-dimensional representation that indicates levels of brain activity in terms of color.

images. The image is interpreted in terms of degree of activity of the various brain regions, represented by different colors. Areas that are red indicate high levels of activity; areas that appear purple or black reflect little or no activity. Activity levels in between are represented by colors in between red and purple.

PET scans are useful for detecting tissue abnormalities such as tumors and for assessing whether tumors are benign or malignant. This technology is helpful in determining whether a brain tumor can be surgically removed.

Current PET technology allows for a much faster scanning time than in previous years, with a time of 40 seconds to scan the entire brain (Lauter, 1997). However, scanning time depends on which type of tracer is used. Radioactive isotopes that have a longer half-life require longer scan times. The shorter the scan time, the more conditions or activities are able to be performed within a single session.

An advantage of the PET technique is the ability to make comparisons within and between individuals in terms of cognitive related changes in blood flow. It is also possible to superimpose PET scans on MRI scans, which allows greater anatomical accuracy in correlating brain structure with brain function.

PET scans can be superimposed on MRI scans, allowing greater anatomical accuracy in correlating brain structure and function in an individual.

There are, however, several disadvantages. One is the radiation to which the individual is exposed, which is around three times that of a conventional chest x-ray. Others are its limited availability and the need to manufacture tracer substances (Plante, 2001). Additionally, compared to CT and MRI, PET produces less detailed images of the structure because of its less fine spatial resolution. Compared to MRI resolution, which can be as fine as 1 mm, PET resolution is approximately 5 mm.

Single Photon Emission Computed Tomography

Single photon emission computed tomography (SPECT) is based on similar principles to PET. The major difference is in the type of radioisotope that is used. In SPECT, the radioisotope creates single photons as the isotope decays, rather than gamma rays, as in PET. These photons are then measured.

Single photon emission computed tomography (SPECT) is based on the same principles as PET.

Like PET scans, SPECT images can also be combined with CT or MRI, allowing the correlation of brain structure with brain function.

The disadvantage of SPECT technology compared to PET is the higher radiation because of the isotopes with longer half-lives that must be used (Lauter, 1997). Both techniques, however, have been used in studies to determine differences in cognitive functioning based on differences in rCBF in groups of people with and without communication disorders.

Electroencephalography and Evoked Potentials

Electroencephalography (EEG) is a technique of recording the electrical potentials generated by the brain. Electrodes are positioned in various locations on the surface of the person's scalp, and the potentials are detected and amplified by specialized equipment. Current EEG techniques use computers to obtain and analyze the data and allow for accurate quantification of information. These techniques are known as qEEG (quantitative EEG), and their development and use has allowed a wider collection of information from several different brain regions simultaneously. The information from several different areas can be correlated to show the degree to which different brain regions coordinate their activity during a particular task (Lauter, 1997). Colored images are also obtained from qEEG, with different colors representing different levels of activity (Kent, 1997b). The brain electrical output is analyzed by means of a Fourier analysis, which produces a display of dominant frequencies occurring within the brain during different types of activities. There are four major frequencies of brain electrical activity: For example, when an individual is very relaxed, the dominant frequency is 8 to 13 Hz (alpha), whereas during deep sleep the primary frequency decreases to a delta frequency of less than 4 Hz. Beta frequency is 13 Hz or higher and occurs when an individual is paying close attention to a task; theta (4 to 8 Hz) occurs when a person is feeling drowsy.

> Quantitative electroencephalographic (qEEG) techniques record brain electrical activity on the surface of the scalp.

A particular category of qEEG technology is known as **evoked potentials** (EP), also called *event-related potentials* (ERP). These are brain electrical potentials that occur in response to some kind of stimulus, which may be tactile, visual, or auditory. As with EEG, electrodes on the scalp are used to obtain and analyze the brain electrical activity occurring before, during, or after the person's response. The resulting waveform typically shows several peaks and valleys, which are labeled in terms of their polarity (positive or negative), and the time that elapsed between their occurrence and the initial stimulus.

> Evoked potentials measure brain electrical activity in response to some kind of stimulus or task and are measured in terms of their latency (how soon after the stimulus they occur) and polarity (positive or negative).

Many behavioral studies have been done to show the relationship between the brain electrical activity, the task that the subject is performing, and the presumed cortical or subcortical area(s) involved in the activity. One of the most studied EPs is the P300. This is a positive peak that occurs approximately 300 msec after an auditory or visual. The stimuli are presented in what is called an "odd-ball" paradigm, in which a few rare or unfamiliar stimuli are randomly presented within a series of standard or familiar stimuli. The peak occurs only in response to the unfamiliar stimuli. This potential has been linked to the way in which individuals process, recognize, and identify important or different stimuli. Both the latency of the P300 in terms of the time it takes for the response to occur after the initial stimulus and

Commonly used evoked potentials include the P300 (linked to recognition and identification of unfamiliar stimuli), N400 (linked to semantic judgment), and Readiness Potential (signals an upcoming motor response).

the amplitude of the resulting response can be measured and provide important information. An increased latency suggests that the person takes longer to process the stimulus. The amplitude of the response has been shown to increase when the stimuli are unpredictable or highly significant to the subject. Thus, this potential is considered to be an index of mental alertness and cognitive activity.

Another evoked potential is the N400, this one occurring around 400 msec after the stimulus and with a negative polarity. This potential has been shown to be linked to semantic judgment. That is, it occurs when there is a mismatch between the meaning of a sentence and the use of a particular word that does not fit with the meaning. An example provided by Hagoort and van Turennout (1997) is the sentence "He spread his warm bread with socks." Other brain potentials signal an upcoming motor response. The Readiness Potential (RP), for example, is a negative potential that starts to occur around one second before an actual voluntary movement and continues through the beginning portion of the movement. This potential reaches its maximum amplitude just after the movement has started to occur. This potential is believed to index cortical preparation for movement (Molt).

The advantage of these techniques is that they allow the timing of brain events to be recorded and interpreted in relation to a specific stimulus. The disadvantage is that because the electrical brain signals are averaged, it is difficult to specify precisely which neural structures are participating in the cognitive activity. Table 13.1 lists the advantage and disadvantage of techniques for imaging brain structure.

Use of Brain-Imaging Techniques in Communication Disorders

The various types of brain imaging techniques discussed in the previous section have wide applicability to disorders involving speech, language, and hearing. The diagnostic evaluation of brain function in neurological disorders such as stroke, Parkinson's disease, Alzheimer's disease, multiple sclerosis, and others has been greatly enhanced by the ability to visualize damaged and undamaged neural structures. The efficacy of treatment techniques for a particular individual can be assessed over a period of time with these tools, and comparisons can be made between different types of therapeutic interventions, including surgical, pharmacologic, and behavioral treatments.

Brain-imaging techniques are valuable in diagnostic evaluation of neurological disorders and in assessment of treatment outcomes.

We will begin with a discussion of brain-imaging techniques that have been used to examine neural function in stuttering. Although stuttering is not an overt neurological disease, it has been believed for

■ TABLE 13.1

Types of Brain-Imaging Techniques, Advantages and Disadvantages of Each Technique

	TECHNIQUES THAT IMAGE BRAIN STRUCTURE	
	Advantages	Disadvantages
CT	Provides detailed 3-D image Differentiates between tissues of different densities Short imaging time Widely available	Possible health risks from radiation
MRI	Distinguishes fine differences between soft tissues Can be used to study disordered or normal structures High degree of spatial resolution No risk of radiation	Longer imaging times than CT Cannot be used with metal devices More costly than CT
	TECHNIQUES THAT IMAGE BRAIN FUNCTION	
	Advantages	Disadvantages
fMRI	Can assess how brain function changes over time or in different situations Safe and noninvasive Can be used in conjunction with MRI	Relatively slow scanning time Scanner is noisy
PET	Good for detecting tissue abnormalities Can compare cognitive related changes in blood flow within and between individuals Can superimpose PET scans on MRI scans	Spatial resolution less than MRI and CT Possible health risks from radiation Scanning time depends on tracer
SPECT	Similar to PET	Higher radiation than PET
qEEG	Excellent temporal resolution Used to index different aspects of cognitive function	Averaging of brain electrical signals prevents precise specification of underlying neural structures

many decades that there is a neurological component to the disorder. We will then look at some of the findings that have been reported for overt neurological diseases such as Parkinson's disease, multiple sclerosis, and Alzheimer's disease.

Stuttering

Since the 1920s researchers have suspected that the root cause of stuttering may be some kind of neurological dysfunction. Travis, in 1928, was the first to

Early brain-imaging studies using EEG indicated that people who stutter have different hemispheric control for verbal tasks than normally fluent speakers.

propose that hemispheric dominance for language in people who stutter (PWS) is different than for normally fluent speakers. Normal speech production is primarily under left hemisphere control. Travis and others suggested that PWS lack this lateralized control, and that it is the lack of clear-cut dominance that results in the stuttered output. Early EEG studies in the 1980s investigated alpha brain wave activity in PWS. These studies (e.g., Moore and colleagues, Boberg et al.) did report findings that were in agreement with the idea of nondominant hemisphere lateralization in stutterers for verbal tasks. What was particularly interesting was that there were reports that after intensive stuttering therapy, the alpha activity normalized (Boberg, Yeudall, Schopplocher, & BoLassen, 1983).

More recent studies using PET, SPECT, and qEEG have confirmed differences in brain activation between fluent and stuttering speakers.

More recently, studies over the past fifteen or so years have used PET, SPECT, and qEEG to investigate brain function in PWS. For example, Finitzo, Pool, Devous, and Watson (1991), using qEEG, found a global reduction of EEG amplitude in the beta frequency range over the right posterior temporal and bi-occipital sites. The same group of researchers (Pool et al., 1991) performed a SPECT study of rCBF in people who do and do not stutter. Stutterers showed reductions in blood flow compared to age- and gender-matched controls in various brain regions of interest in each hemisphere. The stuttering subjects underwent MRIs in order to rule out any vascular problems that might reduce the blood flow, and the authors suggested that the reductions may reflect metabolic or functional anomalies that somehow contribute to the stuttering.

More recent studies using PET to assess rCBF have confirmed differences in brain activation between PWS and fluent speakers, as well in differences in PWS under various speaking conditions. Ingham, Fox, and Ingham (1994) assessed brain activation during solo and choral reading. Choral reading is known to be a fluency-enhancing condition for most people who stutter. The authors reported that the normal speakers showed bilateral (left > right) activation of the primary sensorimotor cortex during both conditions. The stutterers showed increased neural activity during the solo reading condition in the supplementary motor area (left > right) and the superior portion of the premotor cortex (right > left). During the choral reading condition, however, the activation of these regions was either reduced or eliminated.

Brain areas implicated in stuttering include primary motor cortex, premotor cortex, supplementary motor area, Wernicke's area, and cerebellum.

Braun et al. (1997) found that during language formulation tasks normal speakers showed markedly asymmetrical cerebral activity, which lateralized to the left hemisphere. This was not the case for stuttering speakers. During periods of disfluency, the stuttering speakers failed to activate Wernicke's area as well as other areas which are believed to be important in the formulation and expression of spoken language. Ingham, Fox, and Ingham (1997) found that for normal speakers, both solo and choral reading activated brain regions including supplementary motor area, superior lateral premotor cortex, primary motor cortex for mouth,

Broca's area, and cerebellum. Activations were either in the left hemisphere, or bilateral. However, when the stutterers were disfluent in the solo reading condition, the supplementary motor area and the superior lateral premotor cortex were considerably more active than the controls. Further, the superior lateral premotor cortex was lateralized to the right in the stutterers. Similarly, the primary motor cortex in the stutterers was most strongly activated in the right hemisphere. Cerebellar activation was markedly more intense in the stutterers than in the normal speakers, for both solo and choral reading. The stutterers also showed activations in brain areas not seen in the nonstutterers, including the insula, lateral thalamus, and globus pallidus. Interestingly, the stutterers activated Broca's area in the same manner as did the nonstutterers. The authors noted that stuttering, in these subjects, was characterized by extensive hyperactivity of the motor system, with right hemisphere lateralization of primary and extraprimary motor cortices. Normal speakers showed activation of primary auditory area during speech, and this was not the case for the nonstutterers. The authors proposed that this may mean that stutterers do not use auditory monitoring to the same degree as nonstutterers. Similar findings have been reported by Kroll, DeNil, Kapur, and Houle (1997) and Wu et al. (1995).

Hyperactivity of the motor system and right hemisphere lateralization of motor areas have been reported in people who stutter.

Taken together, these findings have led to a suggestion that a complex network of neural structures involved in motor control does not function normally in PWS (Buchel & Sommer, 2004). One hypothesis for this motor control deficit is that there is an excessive amount of dopamine within the CNS. An ongoing study sponsored by the National Institute of Deafness and Other Communication Disorders (NIDCD), which is a branch of the National Institutes of Health (NIH) is testing this hypothesis using PET to measure brain blood flow and the distribution of dopamine in the brains of PWS and normally fluent speakers, as well as MRI to help interpret the anatomical basis of the information (http://www.clinicaltrials.gov/ct/gui/show/NCT00024960).

A hypothesis proposed for the motor control deficit in people who stutter is an excessive amount of dopamine within the central nervous system.

There are exciting clinical implications that can be taken from studies like these. If stuttering, at least in some individuals, is found to be due to excessive dopamine activity, then pharmacological treatments may be effective in eliminating or reducing the motor aspects of the disorder.

Parkinson's Disease

Parkinson's disease (PD), as we know, results from a loss of dopamine in the substantia nigra of the basal nuclei. The major characteristics of this disorder include bradykinesia (slowness of movement), rigidity, and tremor. Brain imaging techniques, primarily using PET, have provided a valuable means of diagnosing and treating this disease. Studies have investigated brain

PET and fMRI studies have been used to investigate brain metabolism in patients with Parkinson's disease and have reported increased activation in the striatum and globus pallidus, but reduced activation in the supplementary motor area and motor cortex.

metabolism in patients with PD both while on and off their medications. Researchers have reported increased metabolism for these patients in the striatum and globus pallidus (Grafton, 2004), both of which are part of the basal nuclei. This increased activity is consistent with the loss of neural inhibition normally provided by the dopaminergic neurons within the substantia nigra. An fMRI study by Grafton (2004) focused on patients in early stages of PD. These individuals showed reduced activation in the supplementary motor area (SMA) and the contralateral motor cortex during a simple finger movement task. Grafton (2004) noted that individuals with PD may show compensation for the decreased activity in the SMA by recruiting the lateral premotor cortex to maintain the movement, a finding that was corroborated by an fMRI showing reduced SMA activation but increased activation of the lateral premotor cortex bilaterally. With L-Dopa medication, however, the hypoactivation in the SMA normalized.

Brain imaging has also been used to identify PD before clinical symptoms have appeared. Clinical symptoms typically only emerge after the loss of dopamine cells has reached a certain level. Thus, there is likely to be considerable degeneration of the substantia nigra, although the actual symptoms shown by the patient may be very mild (Heissa & Hilkera, 2004). Brain imaging, therefore, may provide a way of differentiating PD from other neurological disorders at the early stages, as well for measuring the progression and severity of the disease (Heissa & Hilkera, 2004). This is critically important for providing the most appropriate treatment. PET and SPECT are the preferred techniques to detect loss of neurotransmitter function, as well as brain metabolism and blood flow in patients with PD. For example, Heissa and Hilkera (2004) reported on a PET study that showed the progression of PD in individuals by determining the amount of tracer absorbed by various of the basal nuclei structures. As the disease progressed, a decreasing amount of the tracer was absorbed, demonstrating the decreasing amount of activation in specific basal nuclei components. There was an average decrease per year in the amount of tracer of 8 percent in the striatum and the putamen and 4 percent in the caudate region. PET studies have also been used to demonstrate the effectiveness of different drug therapies as well as of human fetal cell transplantation.

The onset and progression of Parkinson's disease can be measured by brain imaging techniques, allowing for the provision of the most appropriate treatment.

Another avenue for examining changes in PD is via the use of EPs to determine cognitive changes that occur. Cognitive decline is a major feature of PD, with some patients experiencing increasing dementia over the progression of the disease. The P300 potential is a noninvasive way of indexing cognitive function. Prabhakar, Syal, and Srivastava (2000) compared individuals with and without early PD using the P300 "odd-ball" paradigm. Patients with PD did not have any overt clinical signs of dementia. These individuals were

The P300 potential has been used to determine cognitive changes in patients with Parkinson's disease.

tested before starting pharmacological treatment, after fifteen days of treatment, and after three and six months of treatment. The authors found that after the six-month interval, the P300 response was significantly increased in latency in the PD patients, showing decrements in cognitive function, even though the motor symptoms had shown improvement with treatment.

Multiple Sclerosis

Multiple sclerosis (MS) is a progressive disease that affects both the upper and lower motor neurons, but that has a very variable progression in terms of its clinical symptoms. In this disease there is a progressive loss of myelin, which hinders the proper conduction of nerve impulses. However, the loss of motor function does not necessarily correspond to the degree of the demyelinization (Miller, Grossman, Reingold, & McFarland, 1998). This means that MRI imaging of brain structures may not provide a totally satisfactory picture of the patient's neural function, although this methodology does provide an objective and direct assessment of the structural changes that continue to occur in the course of the disease. Researchers at the Dartmouth Brain Imaging Laboratory used both MRI and fMRI to examine how the brains in people with MS reorganized in terms of motor ability and memory in response to the lesion load (that is, the total volume of brain tissue affected by the demyelinization). They found that the brain's neural circuitry does adapt to the damage, which may account for the lack of correspondence between degree of damage and clinical symptoms.

Using a series of MRI studies over time can help to predict which individuals with clinically isolated symptoms of multiple sclerosis will actually go on to develop the full-blown disease.

Several investigators have shown that a series of MRIs over a time period can help to predict which individuals with clinically isolated symptoms of MS will actually go on to develop the full-blown disease (e.g., Brex et al., 2001; Miller et al., 1998). This is important information in order to prescribe the most appropriate drug therapy, and researchers are using MRI to determine the effectiveness of certain medications on lesion load in MS.

Alzheimer's Disease

Alzheimer's disease (AD) is a progressive neurological disease with dementia as its major hallmark. Memory and cognitive abilities decline, and in the late stages of the disease, motor dysfunction also appears. Researchers at various brain imaging labs around the United States are working to find patients at high risk for AD even before they develop symptoms (Ullrich, 2004). For example, investigators at the Medical College of Wisconsin have used fMRI to find a risk marker for AD. This marker measures small changes in blood flow

Identifying individuals with Alzheimer's disease before severe clinical symptoms have developed is vitally important because memory-enhancing drugs are most effective early on in the disease.

in brain areas such as the hippocampus, which, as you recall, is a region involved in memory. Researchers at the Dartmouth Brain Imaging Lab used fMRI to measure the effects of medication on memory. These investigators found that treatment that enhances acetylcholine function can improve memory in patients with mild cognitive impairments. Thus, fMRI studies can be an effective tool in diagnosing AD before the onset of severe symptoms. This is vitally important, because these types of memory-enhancing drugs are most effective early on in the disease (Parry & Matthews, 2002).

Brain imaging has also been useful in determining the neural correlates of other symptoms in AD, such as apathy. Apathy is defined as a lack of motivation in behavior, cognition, and affect (Benoit et al., 2004). Benoit et al. (2004) used SPECT to determine the correlation between apathy and neural function in patients with AD and found abnormal blood flow in the frontal cortex and the anterior cingulate area. The authors noted that the anterior cingulate is important in integrating behaviors that contribute to goal-directed behavior, including emotional, sensory, and vegetative aspects of the behavior.

As well as PET, SPECT, and fMRI, event-related potentials have been used extensively over the past two decades to investigate the cognitive deterioration in AD. In particular, there is a very large body of information based on the P300 potential. For example, Szelies, Mielke, Grond, and Heiss (2002) found that P300 latency was correlated with the degree of severity of the disease, with longer latencies associated with more severe cognitive deficits. Olichney and Hillert (2004) reported that late potentials occurring after approximately 200 msec were abnormal in patients with AD, while earlier occurring potentials that are not dependent on cognitive processing were generally intact. They noted that using the P300 paradigm can help to quantify the effects of drugs that improve attention, such as the cholinesterase inhibitors. These drugs have been shown to improve cognitive function in Alzheimer's disease (AD) and other forms of dementia (Werber, Gandelman-Marton, Klein, & Rabey, 2003). However, as noted by Werber et al. (2003), the efficacy of such treatments has primarily been based on subjective assessment methods such as standardized neuropsychological tests. The authors assessed various pharmacological treatments with cholinesterase inhibitors such as tacrine and donepezil (DPZ) before the initiation of treatment and after twenty-six weeks of treatment with standardized assessment tests as well as the P300 potential. The latency of the potential improved considerably in conjunction with improvements on the standardized cognitive test suggesting that P300 is a reliable instrument for assessment of cognitive response to cholinesterase inhibitor treatment in demented patients. In a similar study, Katada et al. (2003) investigated the effects of donepezil taken daily for six months by patients with AD. P300 latency was reduced after the course of treatment, with a parallel improvement on a standardized test for cognitive function in AD. Thomas

The P300 potential has been used extensively as an objective measure of cognitive function in patients with Alzheimer's disease; it can help to quantify the effects of drugs that improve attention and memory, such as cholinesterase inhibitors.

P300 latency provides very useful information on the progression of Alzheimers' disease, especially in the long-term follow up of patients undergoing various drug treatments.

et al. (2001) likewise evaluated cholinesterase inhibitors using the P300 potential. They compared patients treated with two types of cholinesterase inhibitors (donepezil and rivastigmine) versus those treated with doses of Vitamin E. Those patients treated with either of the cholinesterase inhibitors showed increases in cognitive scores accompanied by decreases in P300 latencies, while patients receiving Vitamin E exhibited worsening cognitive deficits and longer P300 latencies. Thus, several reports have concluded that P300 latency gives very useful information on the progression of AD, especially in the longitudinal follow-up of patients undergoing treatment with cholinesterase inhibitors such as tacrine and DPZ.

The P300 potential, however, does not appear to be sensitive to the specific degree of cognitive decline. Pokryszko-Dragan, Slotwinksi, and Podemski (2003) found that while the mean latency of P300 was significantly prolonged in the entire group of patients with mild and moderate AD, the differences did not distinguish between individuals with mild impairment and those with moderate levels of cognitive deficit. Despite this one drawback, overall, many studies have confirmed that prolonged latencies for P300 may be an accurate, noninvasive, and reliable marker for AD. This is invaluable in the diagnosis of AD, because the latency of the potential is altered in cases of early AD, while overt cognitive degeneration is not yet apparent (Fernandez-Lastra, Morales-Rodriguez, & Penzol-Dias, 2001).

Clinical Study

Background

Rose Ginsberg, an 83-year-old woman living in an assisted-care facility, has lately been complaining that she can't find her car keys, despite the fact that she has not been driving for the last four years. In addition, her daughter has noticed that she has a lot of difficulty in finding words and has a hard time getting to the point of a conversation. Her daughter is concerned that her mother may be showing signs of dementia and has requested that her mother be referred for a neurological exam. Fortunately, the facility is affiliated with a nearby hospital known for its team approach to diagnosis and treatment of neurological disorders.

Clinical Observations

The diagnostic protocol at the center includes a neurological exam with brain imaging techniques as appropriate, a neuropsychological exam, and a speech and language evaluation. During the evaluation, Mrs. Ginsberg appeared oriented to time and place. She was somewhat agitated, but cooperated with all requests.

Findings

An MRI failed to show any structural changes to the brain. The neurologist and neuropsychologist decided to perform an evoked potential test using the P300 potential. The test revealed that P300 latency was significantly lengthened, suggesting early stages of cognitive decline.

The speech and language evaluation substantiated her daughter's reports of significant word-finding difficulties, short-term memory loss, difficulty with topic maintenance, and circumlocution.

Clinical Questions

1. Do you think that a pharmacological approach to this patient might be appropriate? Why, or why not?
2. What would be the role of the speech–language pathologist in Mrs. Ginsberg's case?
3. If the patient is ultimately diagnosed with Alzheimer's disease, what other brain imaging techniques (if any) might be useful to document the progression of the disease?

s u m m a r y

- Current imaging techniques that depict brain structure include computerized tomography (CT) and magnetic resonance imaging (MRI).
- Brain function can be imaged with functional MRI (fMRI), positron emission tomography (PET), single photon emission computed tomography (SPECT), and quantitative electroencephalography (qEEG).

- PET and SPECT studies demonstrate differences in neural function between people who stutter and normally fluent speakers.
- PET studies have been used to identify Parkinson's disease before the appearance of clinical symptoms, as well as to show the progression of the disease.
- The P300 potential has been used extensively in Alzheimer's disease as a marker of cognitive function.

r e v i e w   e x e r c i s e s

1. Explain the importance of obtaining brain-behavior information from healthy individuals with normal brain function, as well as from individuals with neurological diseases or disorders.

2. Identify two advantages and two disadvantages for each of the brain-imaging techniques discussed in the chapter.
3. Explain the relevance of the term *resonance* in MRI.

4. Define *hemodynamic response* and discuss the role of the response in fMRI.
5. Discuss the relationship between PET, SPECT, and rCBF.
6. Identify the characteristics of the P300 potential that make it suitable for indexing cognitive function.
7. Discuss how the theory of cerebral lateralization in stuttering has been advanced by means of current brain-imaging techniques.
8. Describe three ways in which diagnosis and treatment of various neurological disorders is enhanced by brain-imaging techniques.

chapter 14

Models and Theories of Speech Production and Perception

chapter objectives   *After reading this chapter, you will*

1. Understand the differences between theories and models.

2. Be able to describe issues in speech production, such as serial order, degrees of freedom, and context sensitivity.

3. Be familiar with some important theories of speech production, such as target models, feedback and feedforward models, dynamic systems models, and connectionist models.

4. Be aware of issues in speech perception, such as linearity, segmentation, speaker normalization, basic unit of perception, and the specialization of speech perception.

5. Appreciate the different categories of speech perception theories, such as active versus passive, bottom-up versus top-down, and autonomous versus interactive.

6. Be acquainted with some important theories of speech perception, such as motor theory, acoustic invariance theory, direct realism, connectionist theories, logogen theory, cohort theory, fuzzy logical model, and native language magnet theory.

Models and theories are tools that help us to understand and predict the behavior or functioning of a system or some part of a system. Once we understand the various parts of a system, how they are related to each other, and how the system works as a whole, we can predict how the system will work under different conditions, and we can apply this knowledge to understanding how the system or any of its parts breaks down under various conditions. This type of understanding, in turn, can lead to the development of procedures to repair the system.

For example, the systems of speech production and perception are very complex and include many separate subsystems that must work together in a coordinated fashion, such as the respiratory system and the phonatory system. Each of these systems, in turn, is composed of many structures that must also cooperate to achieve the goals and targets of the system. Respiration, for instance, is a system comprised of numerous muscles and other structures that work in a coordinated manner to achieve the goal of inhaling and exhaling. The phonatory system consists of the larynx with all its cartilages, muscles, vocal folds, and so on, all acting to achieve the goal of voice production. And all the systems work together to achieve the final goal, the rapid, meaningful production and perception of speech sounds to encode and decode our thoughts, ideas, and feelings in a linguistically appropriate manner.

Theories are a way of integrating current knowledge about a particular phenomenon; a model is a simplification of a system or its parts that can be manipulated in a controlled manner to test theories.

The speech production and perception systems can break down at any point within any of the subsystems. Because these systems and subsystems are so complex, it is necessary to have theories that integrate current knowledge about them and to make models of the systems to test and extend our knowledge about how they work, how they break down, and how breakdowns can best be compensated for or repaired. The terms *theory* and *model* are often used interchangeably, but there are differences between the two. Very often, models are used to test theories.

■ Theories

A theory is a statement about a particular phenomenon, incorporating the underlying principles and assumptions. A theory is a way of interpreting facts about the phenomenon in an integrated manner. Theories help to explain observed data and information and can be used to make predictions about events related to the phenomenon in question. Because theories are based on incoming information and new research, they are always subject to change. Indeed, as Kent (1997a) has remarked,

Progress in science is marked by the development of new theories, by the rejection of theories that are inadequate to account for the data, and by the modification of theories that account for some but not all of the data. Theories should explain data that have been gathered and should help to guide the collection of important new data. (p. 401)

Theories are not just interesting from a research point of view, they also help to institute changes in practice. These changes can have far-reaching effects in the clinical domain. For example, prior to the late 1970s, most clinicians and researchers in speech pathology believed that spasmodic dysphonia (SD) had a psychological origin, based on certain aspects of the disorder, such as its resistance to traditional voice therapy, its often close association with stressful periods in a person's life, and the fact that many people with this disorder had great difficulty in normal conversational speech, but were able to sing, or whisper, or talk at a higher than normal pitch without trouble. Therefore, the treatment for this disorder was often focused on a combination of speech therapy and psychological counseling. However, in the late 1970s and 1980s, data started accumulating suggesting that spasmodic dysphonia is neurogenic. Many different speech laboratories around the United States gathered experimental data about the neurological aspects of this disorder. By about the mid-1980s, the theory of causation changed from psychogenic to neurogenic.

> Theories of the cause of spasmodic dysphonia started changing several decades ago as experimental data was obtained, resulting in radical changes in treatment strategies.

Based on a neurogenic theory, current treatment techniques have a neurological, rather than a psychological, basis. For instance, injections of botulinum-A toxin (Botox), which affect the neurological functioning of the vocal folds, are often prescribed. This kind of treatment has been shown to be extremely effective in alleviating the symptoms of SD in most patients, whereas previous traditional voice and psychological treatments had not, in general, been successful. Thus, research and theory interact with each other to generate new research, new theories, and new practices.

■ *Models*

A model is a simplification of a system or any of its parts. Models are constructed to represent the system in some way that can then be manipulated in a controlled manner. Modeling a system can be done in numerous ways, such as fashioning a physical or mechanical version of the system to be tested, using specimens for physiological modeling, or applying mathematical and computer algorithms to the system.

> Depending on the type of theory to be tested, models may be mechanical, physiological, mathematical, or a combination of the three.

An example of a mechanical model is one developed by Georg von Békésy, who proposed a theory of hearing based on the traveling wave along the basilar membrane in the cochlea. In his model of the cochlea, a sheet of rubber of varying thickness levels simulated the basilar membrane and was placed in a tank of water representing the endolymph within the cochlea. Waves of different frequencies were introduced into the tank. As von Békésy's theory predicted, at high frequencies the thin part of the rubber sheet vibrated with the highest amplitude, and at low frequencies the thicker part of the sheet responded with the greatest amplitude of vibration. Thus, von Békésy's model of the traveling wave provided support for his theory of hearing.

Physiological models often use specimens taken from animal or human cadavers to determine how a particular structure responds under different conditions. For example, a current theory relating to phonation states that the hydration level of the vocal folds affects vocal fold tissue viscosity, which is proportional to phonation pressure threshold (P_{th}), the minimum subglottal pressure required to set the vocal folds into vibration. This theory has been the basis for clinical management of some laryngeal problems in singers, in which lack of hydration of the vocal folds has been the assumed cause of increased effort in initiating vibration. Based on this assumption, patients are encouraged to increase the humidification of their environments and to drink large amounts of water.

Jiang, Ng, and Hanson (1999) used excised canine larynges to test this theory. The larynges were mounted on a special holder and dehydrated with warm dry air. Air was blown through the vocal folds, causing vibration and sound production to occur, and P_{th} was measured. Within about five minutes of dehydration, vibration and sound production stopped. The larynges were then immersed in a saline solution for 30 minutes, and P_{th} was determined again. P_{th} decreased after the rehydration, allowing sound production to occur with increased efficiency. These findings confirmed clinical impressions that hydration is critical in the physiology of normal phonation.

Mathematical models are an effective means of explaining phenomena and testing theories. For instance, neurological, biomechanical, and aerodynamic factors interact to generate jitter in the human voice. Titze (1991b) was interested in teasing out the effects of neurological sources, such as the number of motor units contributing to muscular contraction and the firing rate of the motor units, on jitter. The application of mathematical models to the activity of the thyroarytenoid muscle allowed Titze to hold certain parameters of muscle function constant, vary other parameters in a systematic manner, and thus isolate the effects on the resulting jitter values. In this way, Titze demonstrated that around 0.2 to 1.2 percent of jitter in the human voice seems to result from neurological sources.

Models and theories abound in trying to explain various aspects of speech production and perception. We will focus on only a few models and theories that attempt to account for the overall processes of production and perception. Kent (1997a) noted that the current understanding of speech behavior is represented by a "mosaic of theories,

Models of speech production attempt to determine the sequencing of speech elements, the regulation of neuromuscular commands involved, and the contextual variation of speech sounds.

most of which pertain to only certain levels of observation or conceptualization." He also pointed out that a major divide exists between theories of speech production and speech perception, which have had largely separate theoretical developments.

Speech Production

Numerous different categories of models and theories of speech production exist, such as target models, feedback–feedforward models, dynamic systems theory, and connectionist theories. However they are categorized, most theories of speech production try to address three major issues related to the organization and regulation of speech motor control. These include how speech is ordered serially, the problem of degrees of freedom, and the question of context sensitivity.

The Serial-Order Issue

Although the output of speech is a continually varying waveform, the linguistic elements that make up speech are produced in a serial order. The order is important for meaning: Although the phonemes /k/, /t/, and /æ/ are used in the words *cat, tack,* and *act,* the order in which they are produced determines how the word will be perceived and recognized. Speech is thus a sequence of elements. The question is precisely which elements are serialized. The elements could be specific features of a sound (e.g., voicing or nasality), phonemes, syllables, parts of syllables, or other larger or smaller elements. Research on this issue continues, with evidence so far favoring a phoneme- or syllable-sized unit of speech organization.

Degrees of Freedom

When we speak, we need to control a huge number of muscles, including those of the respiratory, laryngeal, and articulatory systems. In addition, many structures in these systems can move in different ways, at different speeds, and in different combinations. For example, the lower lip and jaw can move in phase with each other (have the same relative timing) and in the same direction; out of phase with each other (different relative timing), but in the same direction; or in phase with each other, but in opposite directions (Kent, 1997b). Each different potential muscular contraction of each muscle in each system constitutes what is known as a degree of freedom, so the total number of possible number of contractions, or degrees of freedom, is enormous. The speech motor system must somehow regulate all the muscular contractions of all the speech subsystems to ensure that the appropriate structures are moving rapidly and in the correct sequences to generate the target sounds and words.

Many theories have been put forward to explain how the speech motor system achieves this level of control. Some theories propose that the speech motor system "programs" separate neuromuscular signals for each required muscle contraction. Another class of theories organizes muscular control in a hierarchy, with upper levels of the system controlling lower levels. Still other theories suggest that the speech motor system uses various strategies to reduce the total number of degrees of freedom to a smaller number, for instance, by combining muscles into functional groupings that work in a coordinated fashion to achieve a desired goal. In this way, muscles are controlled in groups, rather than individually.

Context-Sensitivity Problem

Theories of speech production need to take into account the fact that sounds vary with the context in which they are produced and are influenced by speaking rate, stress, clarity of articulation, and other factors. Coarticulation is an integral aspect of speech production that results in enormous variability in the production of a target sound. A given speech sound often can be produced in several different ways, and this variability in production is a central factor in speech motor regulation.

Theories of Speech Production

Target Models

Target models describe speech production as a "process in which a speaker attempts to attain a sequence of targets corresponding to the speech sounds he is attempting to produce" (Borden et al., 1994). Some theorists have suggested that these targets are spatial. Spatial target models posit that there is an internalized map of the vocal tract in the brain that allows the speaker to move his or her articulators to specific regions within the vocal tract. The speaker can achieve the targets no matter from what position the articulator(s) begin(s) the movement. The fact that articulators must reach a particular position from different starting points is important, because it means that the movements of the articulator for a specific sound cannot be invariant, but must change depending on the starting point.

Target models describe speech as a series of either spatial or acoustic–auditory targets that a speaker attempts to achieve.

For example, to achieve the velar target for the /k/ sound, the tongue would have to move in a different trajectory depending on the preceding vowel. The path of the tongue would vary, for instance, depending on whether the preceding vowel were /a/, /u/, or /i/. This model proposes that a series of spatial targets are specified in advance by the speaker's brain, with feedback coming from the articulators back to the brain to regulate the fine movements and correct any errors.

Targets have also been specified in acoustic–auditory terms, rather than spatial terms. The goal to be achieved in these models is the acoustic output, while the articulatory movements used to achieve the acoustic output may vary. Thus, a speaker may use different articulatory movements to achieve a particular speech sound, depending on factors such as the adjacent sounds, the speaker's rate of speech, and different patterns of stress.

Both articulatory and acoustic targets form the basis for a framework presented by Perkell, Matthies, and Svirsky (1995) to explain the segmental aspects of speech production. In their framework, morphemes and words consist of sequences of segments, characterized by combinations of what the authors call contrast-defining features. These features form the input to the speech motor programming system and specify how the articulators are to be moved or positioned and/or what acoustic properties are to be achieved by these movements. The generation of a segment usually requires the coordination of movements of several articulators. In the case of a consonant, the segmental description specifies the major articulator (such as the lips, tongue blade, or tongue body) and its positioning, which forms a constriction in the vocal tract.

> Perkell et al. proposed that contrast-defining features specify how the articulators are to be moved or positioned and what acoustic properties are to be achieved by these movements.

Other features specify the action of secondary articulators (such as the glottis and velum). The movements of the secondary articulators must be coordinated with the timing of the primary articulation. The ultimate goals of the articulatory movements are acoustic patterns that will enable the listener to understand what is said. However, for the speaker's production mechanism, the goals are defined as regions in acoustic and articulatory space.

For example, in the utterance /uku/, the acoustic goal for the /u/ may be a region in formant frequency space, and its articulatory goal may be information related to the configuration of the vocal tract. The /k/ has several acoustic goals, including a silent interval and a burst of aperiodic noise. The articulatory goals may be to have the tongue body produce a complete closure with adequate force in the velopalatal region and to build up enough intraoral air pressure to produce a noise burst at the moment of release.

Perkell et al. (1995) noted that the features may be modified in terms of the sizes and locations of their regions in articulatory and acoustic space, depending on context and suprasegmental aspects. For instance, if the sequence /uku/ were embedded in a word, the target region of formant values for the /u/ might be reduced toward those of a more neutral vowel, and the force of contact for the /k/ might be less.

Control of the relative timing of articulatory movements around the acoustic landmarks is programmed, in the model, by a mechanism that uses an

In the early stages of learning speech, tactile and proprioceptive feedback from the articulators is important in acquiring these articulatory–acoustic relationships.

internal model of relations among commands to the articulators, their movements, and the acoustic consequences of those movements. The internal model is acquired and maintained with the use of auditory and somatosensory **feedback** from the articulators (i.e., tactile and proprioceptive feedback). Once speech has been learned, however, auditory feedback is not used in the online, moment-to-moment control of articulatory movements. Somatosensory feedback probably is used online, moment to moment, but at lower levels in a hierarchically organized system of speech motor control. One important purpose of this hierarchical organization is to reduce the number of degrees of freedom that has to be controlled by higher levels.

Feedback and Feedforward Models

Feedback refers to the transfer of part of the output of a system back to the input to regulate and correct any errors in the output. Refrigerators and heating and cooling systems work on a feedback principle.

In terms of speech production, the output is the articulatory or acoustic signal. As we speak, we hear what we are saying through the auditory system, and we also obtain information about the movements of our articulators through proprioceptive, kinesthetic, and tactile channels. In the case of the tongue, the output signal is a specific movement or position of the tongue. Information about the movement is sent to the brain by the feedback loop, including feedback from sensory receptors for touch, position, and movement. The output sent to the brain is compared with the intended movement. If there is a discrepancy between the actual and intended movements, an error signal is generated and sent back to the periphery (i.e., the appropriate muscles) to correct the problem.

Feedback models, however, do not account for several facts about the speech production system. First, feedback channels tend to be relatively slow, whereas the movements involved in speech production are extremely rapid. By the time a movement or auditory error has been detected, the speaker will have already moved on to a different sound. Second, if speech is under feedback control, disruption of feedback channels should have a serious effect on speech production. Many experiments have used different methods to interfere with normal feedback, such as the application of topical anesthesia to target articulators, nerve blocks, noise masking to prevent auditory feedback, and bite blocks of various sizes to immobilize the jaw in various positions. Most of these studies have shown that speech is minimally affected, if at all, by these disruptions. Normal speakers compensate extremely well for disruptions, and typically the compensation occurs almost instantaneously.

Some theorists have proposed **feedforward** models as being more appropriate for speech production. Whereas feedback models depend on a time delay

Feedback is used to detect and correct errors in speech output; feedforward signals are used to make articulatory adjustments online.

during which the signals from the periphery (i.e., vocal tract) return to a central processor in the brain for comparison of the intended and the actual movements, feedforward signals make adjustments at the periphery so that the system is primed to move in an efficient, coordinated manner. Feedforward is therefore a much faster process, which may help to explain why disruptions such as bite blocks do not have much of an effect on speech production. It is likely that both feedback and feedforward are used in the control and regulation of speech production.

Dynamic Systems Models

In this kind of theory, the degrees of freedom problem is addressed by positing that groups of muscles link up together to perform a particular task. These linkages between muscles are not fixed: A muscle might be grouped with a particular set of muscles in what is called a **synergy** or a **coordinative structure** to achieve one particular goal and with a different set of muscles in a different synergy to achieve a different goal. Instead of individual muscles being controlled, an appropriate coordinative structure is selected, comprising a set of muscles that essentially form an integrated unit focused on achieving a particular motor activity. The different muscular responses in a synergy can be adjusted to meet the requirements of a particular task under different conditions.

Coordinative structures refer to flexible groupings of muscles that may change depending on the particular speech output goal.

For example, the lip and jaw muscles function as a coordinative unit in bilabial closure. Typically, the lip and jaw muscles cooperate to close the lips. However, if the person has a bite block clamped between the teeth to immobilize the lower jaw, the upper and lower lips can compensate by increasing the force or extent of their movement. If the lips cannot move for some reason, the jaw by itself can bring the lips together. This theory thus reduces the degrees of freedom required for control, while allowing a great deal of flexibility in the organizational linkages between muscles and structures.

Connectionist Models

Parallel processing models are based on computer models that simulate the non-hierarchical neural processing of the human brain.

Computer models have been developed that simulate the neural processing of the human brain. These models are also known as **spreading activation models** and **parallel-distributed processing models** (PDP). PDP models are based on a way of processing signals that is nonhierarchical. In other words, rather than finishing one step in the process before moving on to the next step, steps are processed more or less in parallel. This kind of processing is somewhat akin to the way that the brain processes information. Indeed, the performance of steps in parallel, or at least with much temporal overlap, is typical of speech production. Consider the case of coarticulation, in which the articulatory movements for ensuing sounds are begun during or concurrently with a preceding sound. For example, in the syllable /ku/, the lips are rounding for the /u/ sound concurrently with the tongue positioning for the /k/ sound.

These kinds of models have been successful in simulating different types of human behavior, including speech production and perception tasks. Connectionist theories are based on computer modeling in which input and output units are linked together in various ways and in various layers of complexity. The input units are programmed to receive information, and the output units are the product generated by the system. More complex systems have layers of hidden units that connect input and output units and that modify the information. The connections between the units can be weighted by the system through excitatory and inhibitory signals, and these weights can be changed by the system as it learns the task.

Many types of tasks have been applied to these networks, including morphological, phonological, and other linguistic applications. Systems have also been taught to produce speech. Interestingly, these networks have shown coarticulatory effects, even though the appropriate coarticulation rules were not supplied to the system's input units.

Speech Perception

As with speech production, many issues in speech perception give direction to the theories attempting to explain how we analyze and perceive the spoken word. Some of these issues are linearity, segmentation, speaker normalization, and the basic unit of speech perception.

Linearity and Segmentation

The linearity principle asserts that a specific sound in a word corresponds to a specific phoneme. The sounds that make up the word are distinct from each other and occur in a particular sequence. The segmentation principle is based on the notion that the speech signal can be divided into discrete units that correspond to specific phonemes.

Speech perception models must take into account the nonlinear correspondence between acoustic signals and linguistic units.

These two principles suggest that speech perception is based on a linear correspondence between the acoustic speech signal and the linguistic phonemic units. An abundance of research, however, has established that this is not the case. For example, acoustic characteristics of a given phoneme vary depending on context. The /k/ in /ku/, for instance, will have somewhat different acoustic cues than the /k/ in /ki/. The same has been shown to be true for the /d/ in /di/ versus /du/.

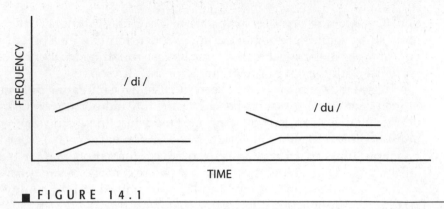

■ FIGURE 14.1

Formant transitions for synthetic /di/ and /du/ for F_1 *and* F_2.

A rising F_2 transition in /di/ and a falling one in /du/ both serve as acoustic cues for /d/. See Figure 14.1.

The frequency of stop bursts also signals different places of articulation depending on context. Research has shown that when a burst is centered at 1440 Hz it is heard as /pi/ before /i/ and /u/, but as /k/ before /a/. Also, because of coarticulation, information is present about the acoustic properties of a specific phoneme, as well as the phonemes that precede and follow it. Consequently, although we perceive speech as a series of separate and distinct phonemes and words, the acoustic boundaries between phonemes are blurred.

Speaker Normalization

As well as the lack of invariance and clear segmentation of phonetic units, theories of speech perception try to take into account other important factors. One of the most puzzling questions in speech perception is that of speaker normalization. That is, how is it that listeners are able to recognize sounds and words despite the large variations in the way that speakers produce them? Speakers vary speech sounds in terms of pitch, loudness, stress, and rate of speech. Speaker age and sex also influence sound production. For example, the same vowel can be produced with very different ranges of formant frequencies from speaker to speaker, and with considerable overlap with other vowels, yet most listeners have no difficulty in vowel recognition. Even infants are able to discriminate speech sounds produced by different talkers with relative ease. Somehow we normalize speech; that is, we seem to be able to ignore irrelevant differences between productions of a given sound, while focusing

> A major issue in speech perception is how listeners are able to recognize sounds and words despite large variations in the way speakers produce them.

on the features that characterize it as a member of that particular phoneme family.

Basic Unit of Perception

Much research effort has also been expended on the question of the basic unit of perception. Do we perceive acoustic–phonetic features, allophones, phonemes, syllables, or larger units of speech? This question remains an issue, although each of these units has some evidence in its support. It may be that individuals rely more on one kind of unit than another depending on the situation and context of the speech to be perceived. For example, in a quiet listening environment with no competing noise, such as background party noise or work-related noise, listeners may pay more attention to smaller units and rely less on the syllabic structure of speech to perceive meaningful information. In a noisy situation, the person may be forced to process at a higher level of linguistic information to supplement and facilitate acoustic–phonetic recognition.

The situation and context in which speech is perceived may influence what kind of units are more salient for a listener.

This issue also has a developmental aspect. There is evidence that infants and young children may process auditory information using larger units such as syllables, whereas older children and adults may rely more on smaller units such as phonemes. Children appear to go through a developmental weighting shift, in which their perceptual strategies change with increasing linguistic experience (Nittrouer, 1996a). Very young children seem to focus more on syllables to process speech information, because with their limited lexicons they do not need to process auditory information at a more detailed level. As the child's lexicon increases, so too does the need for more detailed acoustic–phonetic representation of words to discriminate between the greater number of similar words in the child's memory.

Nittrouer (1996a) suggested that mature language users appear to weight the various components of the signal in ways that they know will lead to correct decisions about phoneme identity, that is, by focusing on the spectral characteristics of the sound wave. Young children focus more on formant transitions between syllables to divide the acoustic signal into syllabic units. As the child matures, he or she begins to weight the more static and more detailed components of the signal more heavily.

Specialization of Speech Perception

Specialization of speech perception is another theoretical question that has been widely studied and that continues to remain an unsolved issue. Speech perception is viewed by some theorists as a specialized process unique to humans. Early findings about categorical perception seemed to corroborate this view. Categorical perception is considered by some scientists to be a mechanism that

Some theorists view speech perception as a specialized human process; others assert that speech signals are perceived in the same way as nonspeech sounds.

humans have developed by which their perceptual system has become specially adapted for the perception of speech. However, experiments with animals such as chinchillas, monkeys, dogs, and birds have shown that these animals are also capable of categorical perception, which therefore cannot be a uniquely human ability. Instead, general auditory perceptual mechanisms common to many mammals may be involved in categorical perception, rather than some specialized speech process.

Nittrouer (1996a) supported the view that speech signals are perceived in the same way as other acoustic events. She noted that "Most sound-producing events result in multicomponent signals. The way in which information from the separate components is combined, and the weight is assigned to each, is determined by what the listener wishes to learn from that signal. Thus, perceptual strategies appear to be specific to the perceptual decisions to be made."

On the other hand, evidence for some specialization of speech perception comes from studies of a phenomenon called the **perceptual magnet effect**. This effect has to do with prototypes of speech stimuli. A prototype is the most representative instance of a category (Hawkins, 1999c). It has been found that certain examples of a sound seem to be better prototypes than others. In other words, individuals are able to identify the best or prototype examples of a vowel compared to poorer or nonprototype examples of that same vowel from a series of acceptable instances of the vowel. The vowels that the person selects as prototypes depend on the person's native language. Infants as young as 6 months old demonstrate this effect, but only for their own language. Research has shown that American and Swedish babies show this perceptual magnet effect for the vowels of their ambient language, but not for the vowels of the non-native language.

The perceptual magnet effect is so called because, figuratively, the prototype "pulls" sounds that are acoustically similar to it toward itself, resulting in poorer discriminability for sounds clustering closely around the prototype. In other words, differences between good representations of a sound are reduced, thus helping individuals to ignore irrelevant differences between members of a category. What makes this effect a possible candidate as evidence of some unique human speech perception abilities is that, unlike categorical perception, this effect is not demonstrated by animals.

Categories of Speech Perception Theories

Numerous theories of speech perception have evolved over the years, and new theories continue to be developed as new information becomes available. The theories have been grouped into three major categories: active versus passive, bottom-up versus top-down, and autonomous versus interactive.

Active versus Passive

Active theories stress the links between speech perception and speech production, which share common properties. In these theories, the individual's knowledge of how sounds are produced is an integral factor in facilitating sound recognition. Passive theories, on the other hand, emphasize the sensory aspects of speech perception. They stress the filtering mechanism of the listener, with knowledge of speech production and vocal tract characteristics playing a minor role and used only in difficult listening situations.

Active theories propose that an individual's knowledge of speech production facilitates sound recognition.

Bottom-Up versus Top-Down

Bottom-up theories are based on the premise that all the information necessary for the recognition of sounds is contained within the acoustic signal. Therefore, the listener does not need to involve linguistic and cognitive processes in decoding sounds. By contrast, top-down theories emphasize higher level linguistic and cognitive operations as playing a crucial role in the identification and analysis of sounds. Most theories are neither completely top-down nor bottom-up, but place more or less weight on acoustic versus linguistic–cognitive contributions to speech perception.

Bottom-up theories focus on the salience of the acoustic signal in speech perception; top-down theories emphasize higher level linguistic and cognitive processes.

Autonomous versus Interactive

Speech perception involves many stages of processing of the acoustic signal. The signal is initially processed at the individual's ear and then goes through many further transformations as it travels to the brain, eventually to be interpreted and understood. Interactive theories posit that information and knowledge from many sources available to the listener are involved at any or all stages of the processing of the signal on its journey through the speech perception system. Autonomous theories propose that the signal is processed in a serial manner, from phonetic to lexical stages, to syntactic stages, to semantic stages, and so on. Other sources of linguistic and cognitive knowledge and contextual information are not brought into play in autonomous theories; rather, the output of one stage of processing provides the input to the next stage.

Interactive theories stress that information and knowledge from many sources are available to a listener at all stages of speech perception.

■ *Theories of Speech Perception*

Motor Theory

An early and still very influential theory of speech perception is the motor theory, developed at the Haskins Laboratory at Yale University. Motor theory is

Motor theory empha-
sizes the link between
speech production and
speech perception in
terms of articulatory
gestures that individu-
als are innately able to
perceive.

an active theory that stresses the link between perception and production of speech. In essence, according to this theory, an individual perceives speech because he or she produces speech. Because listeners
have experience in producing speech sounds themselves, they are
aware, at some level, of the relationship between movements of the articulators, vocal tract configurations, and the acoustic consequences of
these articulator movements and positions. Motor theory assumes that
speech perception is unique, relying on a special processor located
somewhere in the brain to decode speech.

The older version of the theory assumes that there are unchanging, invariant motor commands in the form of neural signals to the articulators to produce the same phoneme in different phonetic contexts. The motor theory has
recently been revised. In the revised theory the acoustic signal is thought to be
perceived in terms of articulatory gestures that individuals are innately able to
perceive, such as tongue backing and lip rounding. The listener does not, however, perceive the actual movements but some kind of abstract articulatory
plan that controls the vocal tract movements that would, ideally, result in a
perfect production of the utterance (Hawkins, 1999b).

In other words, the abstract gestures produce particular constrictions in the
vocal tract, with each constriction being appropriate for a specific phonetic
place and manner of articulation (Hawkins, 1999b). These abstract articulatory
plans are known as **gestures**. A gesture is, according to Hawkins, one of a family of movement patterns that all achieve the same goal, such as a particular
constriction in the vocal tract (e.g., bilabial closure). Gestures for speech can be
thought of as the basic units of speech production, which control and coordinate the cooperative activity of the articulators. The gestures are neuromotor
commands that are specific to speech and therefore to humans. They are phonetic in character, invariant, and accessible only in the specialized phonetic
module in the brain. The theory proposes that listeners somehow retrieve the
intended gesture for the underlying phoneme from the variable acoustic signal
by compensating for the effects of coarticulation.

Research has shown
that prelingual infants
without any productive
experience are able to
discriminate the
phonetic contrasts
between most of the
sounds in most of the
world's languages.

Research, however, does not support many of the assumptions of
motor theory. For instance, Peter Eimas and colleagues (e.g., Eimas,
Miller, & Jusczyk, 1987) carried out research demonstrating that prelingual infants up to about 10 months of age are able to discriminate not
only the phonemes of their ambient language, but, indeed, the phonetic
contrasts between most of the sounds in most of the world's languages.
Clearly, infants do not have experience in producing phonemes and
are not aware of how phonemes are produced by the articulators. The
fact that infants are not able to produce the sounds that they can perceive contradicts the basic tenet of motor theory.

Acoustic Invariance Theory

The acoustic invariance theory assumes that for each distinct phoneme there is a corresponding set of acoustic features. Whenever the phoneme is produced, a core of acoustic properties are always present, regardless of coarticulation and other contextual effects. This core can be thought of in terms of a template against which the listener compares the incoming sound. Stevens and Blumstein (1978) applied this theory to the perception of place of articulation of stops, based on the spectrum of their bursts. The burst for bilabial stops is diffuse and falling. That is, the acoustic energy in the spectrum is mainly concentrated in a few frequency locations across the frequency range, with the amplitude of successive peaks decreasing toward the higher frequencies. Alveolar stops have a diffuse but rising spectrum. Velar stops are characterized by a compact spectrum, with acoustic energy concentrated in one relatively narrow frequency region. See Figure 14.2. Based on a kind of matching process, the listener makes a decision about the similarity in the burst spectrum between the incoming sound and the stored template.

The theory of acoustic invariance assumes a set of core acoustic features for any specific phoneme regardless of coarticulatory or other contextual effects.

Other theorists have suggested that, rather than templates, the basis of acoustic invariance incorporates features such as voicing and nasality. The use of features allows the more than forty phonemes of American English to be broken down into approximately seven essential minimal acoustic contrasts, thus facilitating the process of speech perception (Ryalls, 1996). According to this theory, listeners abstract the essential features of an incoming sound to make a decision about its identity.

Direct Realism

The direct realist theory was developed in the 1980s. This theory is based on the notion that speech perception does not rely on specialized and unique processes, but is similar to other types of perception, such as visual perception. The rationale for this view is that we perceive objects and events directly, rather than reconstructing or interpreting the object or event from the sensory input to the brain. The example often used to illustrate this concept is that of seeing and recognizing a chair. When we perceive a chair, we do so directly, rather than seeing its different angles and lines and patterns of light and shade. This theory is interactive, because it posits that direct knowledge does not stem only from the object or event itself, but also from the experience and activities of the individual doing the perceiving.

The underlying assumption of direct realism theory is that speech perception is similar to other types of perception such as visual perception.

Hawkins (1999c) provides the example of a child looking at a box of cookies. She notes:

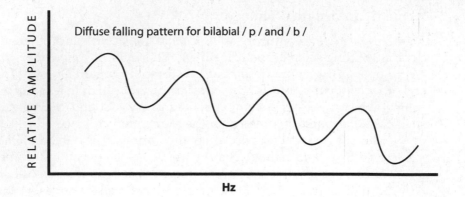

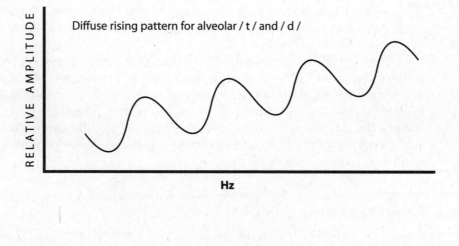

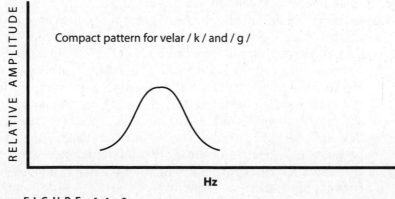

Spectral patterns for stop consonants.

If the child knows what it is, has handled something like it before, it is experienced as a cookie box, as a complete object, knowing its shape even if not all of it can be seen from one position, knowing how much force to use to open it, and so on. If you have never seen a cookie box or its like before, you experience it differently: you may guess but do not know what the shape of the invisible part is, you do not know how heavy it is, and so on. The inexperienced person has a different percept from the experienced person, even though exactly the same set of lines and colors strike both their retinas. (p. 235)

According to direct realism, patterns of light energy or sound energy are only useful in terms of their relationship to the physical environment. In visual terms, we directly perceive an object such as a book or a piano, rather than the different sets of lines, colors, and shadows that make up the stimulus. In terms of speech, we directly perceive the acoustic signal, rather than the gestures of the vocal tract, that is, the place and degree of constriction of the vocal tract by the articulators.

TRACE Model

The TRACE model is a connectionist model that tries to account for the integration and parallel processing of multiple sources of information in speech perception. The basic assumption of connectionist networks is that behavior can be modeled. The network of units that characterizes connectionist models includes phonetic features, phonemes, and words, and there are feedback and feedforward links between the units. The links allow perceptual processing to occur within as well as across the different levels of the system. The connections between upper and lower units allow information to flow in both directions, that is, both top-down and bottom-up. However, the connections within a level are inhibitory, so if a feature or word is present, it will be activated, while competing features or words within that level will be suppressed. The word that is perceived is the one with the greatest amount of activation. The TRACE model is an integrative and interactive system that attempts to explain speech perception and word recognition without relying on specialized mechanisms.

The TRACE model attempts to explain speech perception without relying on specialized mechanisms.

Logogen Theory

Logogen theory is an interactive theory that focuses on word recognition, rather than on acoustic–phonetic aspects of speech perception. A **logogen** is assumed to be some kind of neural processing device associated with each word in a person's vocabulary. All information about the word—its meaning or meanings, its phonetic and orthographic

Logogen theory and cohort theory both focus on larger units of word recognition in speech perception rather than smaller acoustic–phonetic units.

structure, its syntactic functions, and so on—is contained in the logogen. The logogen monitors speech production to detect any information indicating that its particular word is present in the speech signal. If the information is detected and confirmed by appropriate neural activity, the logogen may become activated and result in word recognition.

Cohort Theory

This is another theory focusing on word recognition. Cohort theory differs from logogen theory because it proposes two stages in spoken word recognition: an autonomous stage and an interactive stage. In the autonomous stage, acoustic–phonetic information at the beginning of a word activates all the words in the person's memory having the same word initial information. The words that are activated based on word initial information make up the cohort. For example, a word that begins with *may* would activate all words with that beginning, such as *maybe, mayhem,* and *mayonnaise.* The interactive stage involves eliminating inappropriate words in the cohort, based on the listener's linguistic and cognitive knowledge, as well as the context of the conversation. For instance, if the conversation revolves around lunch, the appropriate word is more likely to be *mayonnaise,* rather than *mayhem.*

Fuzzy Logical Model of Perception

This model assumes that there are three operations in phoneme identification. First, features are evaluated to determine their presence in an interval of sound. However, rather than being rated dichotomously as being present or absent, features are assigned continuous "fuzzy" values ranging from 0 to 1, indicating the degree of certainty that the feature appears in the signal. Zero means that the feature is absent, and 1 means that the feature is definitely present. A value of 0.5 indicates that the signal is completely ambiguous in terms of the feature. The clearest and least ambiguous information has the greatest impact on classification decisions.

The second operation is called prototype matching. At this stage the features that were determined to be present at the first stage are compared with prototypes of phonemes stored in the person's memory. The final operation, pattern classification, determines the best match between candidate phonemes and the input.

The fuzzy logical model is another theory that rejects the notion of specialized processes in speech perception.

This theory rejects the notion of specialized processes in speech perception. The model argues that speech perception is not necessarily categorical, but can be explained by the integration of continuously evaluated features. Thus, continuous information remains available in speech perception, despite the categorical identification and discrimination functions obtained in typical studies.

Native Language Magnet Theory

Native language magnet theory (NLM) has been influential over the past decade in guiding research on speech perception (Frieda, Walley, Flege, & Sloane, 2000). The critical element of this theory is that phonetic categories of a language are organized in terms of prototypes. This organization starts to occur in early infancy. During the first ten months or so of life, infants are able to distinguish between most phonemes of most languages in the world. By age 10 or 11 months, the infant has gone through a reorganization of phonetic categories based on the child's ambient language. By this age the infant can no longer make the distinctions in phonetic contrasts of languages other than its own. NLM theory proposes that these prototypes function as perceptual magnets that assimilate other members of the same phonetic category. Irrelevant perceptual distinctions between members of the same category that are close to the prototype are reduced and can therefore be ignored. Perceptual distinctions between category boundaries, on the other hand, become even more distinct, so the boundaries between phonemes become clearly demarcated. Kuhl and her colleagues, who developed this theory based on their extensive research in infant perception, posited that these perceptual prototypes also serve as speech production targets for infants and young children, thus emphasizing the link between perception and production (Kuhl et al., 1997; Kuhl & Meltzoff, 1996).

In sum, theories of speech perception emphasize different levels of processing of the speech signal. Decoding a spoken message involves the analysis of various-sized components of the signal, including acoustic, phonetic, phonological, lexical, suprasegmental, syntactic, and semantic components. The process of speech perception was nicely summed up by Nygaard and Pisoni (1995), who noted:

> Listeners are able to flexibly alter their processing strategies based on the information available to them in the signal and the information available from their store of linguistic knowledge. On one hand, if the physical signal provides rich, unambiguous information about a phonetic contrast, listeners appear to attend primarily to the physical signal when making their phonetic identifications. On the other hand, if the physical signal is noisy, impoverished, or degraded, as synthetic speech often is, listeners may shift their attention to different levels of processing to assist in phonetic categorization. Thus speech perception appears to be a highly adaptive process in which listeners flexibly adjust to the demands of the task and to the properties of the signal. (p. 82)

Native language magnet theory proposes that phonetic categories of a language are organized in terms of prototypes that function as perceptual magnets and serve as speech production targets for infants and young children.

s u m m a r y

- A theory is a statement about a particular phenomenon, incorporating underlying principles, facts, and assumptions.
- Theories change based on incoming research and effect practice.
- A model is a simplification of a system that can be manipulated in a controlled manner.
- Models can be mechanical, physiological, mathematical, or computer based.
- Speech production theories attempt to account for serial order, degrees of freedom, context sensitivity, and other issues.
- Numerous theories of speech production have been proposed, including target models, feedback and feedforward models, dynamic systems models, and connectionist models.

- Speech perception theories attempt to account for linearity, segmentation, speaker normalization, basic unit of perception, specialization of speech perception, and other issues.
- Theories of speech perception can be categorized as active versus passive, bottom-up versus top-down, and autonomous versus interactive.
- Most theories of perception focus on acoustic–phonetic or phonemic aspects, including motor theory, acoustic invariance theory, direct realism, fuzzy logical models, and connectionist theories; recent theories also attempt to explain word recognition, including logogen theory and cohort theory.

r e v i e w   e x e r c i s e s

1. Differentiate between models and theories and give an example of each to illustrate your points.
2. Explain what is meant by the problem of degrees of freedom and give an example from an area of speech production.
3. List the critical elements in Perkell's articulatory and acoustic target framework of speech production.
4. Describe the reasons why feedback models cannot adequately account for speech production.
5. Compare and contrast dynamic systems models and connectionist models of speech production.

6. Identify and explain the major issues that theories of speech perception try to account for.
7. Give an example of an active theory, a passive theory, an autonomous theory, and an interactive theory of speech perception.
8. Explain the main aspects of motor theory, and compare them with those of acoustic invariance theory.
9. Describe how connectionist models can be applied to both speech production and speech perception.

Appendix

IPA Symbols for Consonants and Vowels

CONSONANTS

/b/	bed, cab	/s/	sun, bus
/d/	dog, red	/t/	toe, pet
/f/	fig, phone, laugh	/v/	valley, leave
/g/	girl, bag	/w/	wave, away
/h/	hat, perhaps	/z/	zoo, buzz
/j/	young, bayou	/ʃ/	ship, bush
/k/	cat, kick	/ʒ/	azure, beige
/l/	love, ball	/θ/	thin, breath
/m/	man, lamb	/ð/	these, breathe
/n/	net, moon	/tʃ/	chime, batch
/p/	pot, top	/dʒ/	jump, judge
/r/	rat, bar	/ŋ/	bang, finger

VOWELS

Front vowels

Back vowels

/i/	she, legal	/u/	shoe, fluke
/I/	hit, inside	/ʊ/	should, book
/e/	cake, ailing	/o/	photo, collate
/ɛˑ/	egg, federal	/ɔ/	awesome, flaw
/æ/	hat, snappy	/a/	hot, hearty

Central vowels

/ə/	about, above
/ɚ/	mother, another
/ɝ/	word, earnest
/ʌ/	up, under

Diphthongs

/ai/	my, admire
/au/	crown, shower
/ɔi/	boy, lawyer
/ei/	say, day
/ou/	show, snow

Glossary

Absolute refractory period   Brief period following an action potential during which the nerve cannot fire, no matter how strong the stimulation.

Absorption   Damping of a wave.

Accelerated speech   Speech that sounds excessively rapid, often occurring in Parkinson's disease.

Accessory muscles of respiration Muscles of the rib cage, back, and neck that may contribute to respiration depending on bodily demands.

Acetylcholinesterase   Enzyme that degrades the neurotransmitter acetylcholine into its component chemicals.

Acoustic reflex   Middle ear reflex that attenuates intense sounds of 80 dB or more; also called the *stapedial reflex.*

Acoustic resonator   Air-filled container in which the air is forced to vibrate in response to another vibration.

Action potential   Wave of depolarization that travels along the length of an axon.

Additive noise   Noise in the vocal signal; also called *spectral noise.*

Adductor spasmodic dysphonia Neurological voice disorder characterized by vocal fold spasms.

Admittance   Measure of how easily energy is transmitted through a system, measured in siemens in the modern metric system (formerly milliohms).

Afferent   Sensory nerve that transmits information from sensory receptors toward the central nervous system.

Alveolar ducts   Openings of the respiratory bronchioles leading into an alveolus.

Alveolar pressure   Pressure of the air within the alveoli of the lungs.

Alveolar ridge   Anterior portion of the hard palate formed by the alveolar processes of the maxilla.

Alveoli   Microscopic thin-walled structures within the lungs filled with air.

Amplitude   Amount of displacement of an object from its rest position.

Amplitude perturbation   Cycle-to-cycle variability in vocal fold amplitude, also called shimmer.

Amygdala   Structure of the limbic system involved in learning and memory.

Amyotrophic lateral sclerosis Progressive neurological disease affecting all voluntary muscles.

Anterior commissure   Location on the thyroid cartilage forming the anterior attachment of the vocal folds.

Anterior corticospinal tract   Motor nerve pathway formed by the fibers of the corticospinal tract that do not decussate at the medulla but that synapse ipsilaterally with neurons in the anterior horns of the spinal cord.

Anticipatory coarticulation A preceding sound modifies the ensuing sound.

Antiformant Same as antiresonance.

Antiresonance Type of acoustic filtering that results in frequencies within a bandwidth being attenuated rather than amplified; on a spectrogram looks like a very weak formant.

Aperiodic Wave in which cycles do not take the same amount of time to occur.

Aphonia Complete absence of voice.

Aponeurosis Broad flat sheet of tendon.

Applied frequency Frequency that acts as an input to a resonator.

Arachnoid mater Middle layer of the meninges.

Articulatory undershoot Articulators fail to achieve the appropriate articulatory target.

Aryepiglottic folds Folds of connective tissue and muscle fibers running from the sides of the epiglottis to the apex of the arytenoid cartilages.

Arytenoid cartilages Paired cartilages of the larynx, forming a joint with the cricoid cartilage.

Aspiration Noise generated by turbulence as air moves through the glottis.

Association nuclei Thalamic nuclei that receive and transmit nerve impulses to and from broad cortical areas.

Astrocytes Most common type of glial cell in the nervous system with projections that connect to blood capillaries and transport nutrients from the blood to the nerve cell.

Attenuation rate Rate in decibels per octave at which a resonator's amplitude of response is attenuated.

Audibility Refers to whether a specific speech cue is presented at a level that a hearing-impaired person can hear.

Axon Projection off the cell body that transmits impulses away from the cell body.

Backward coarticulation An upcoming sound influences the preceding sound.

Band-pass filter Resonator that transmits acoustic energy in a range of frequencies between an upper and a lower cutoff frequency.

Bandwidth Range of frequencies that a resonator will transmit.

Basilar membrane Base of the cochlear duct; basal portion nearest the tympanic membrane is narrow and stiff, with membrane becoming wider and more compliant toward the apical portion farthest from the tympanic membrane.

Bernoulli principle Aerodynamic law stating that air flowing through a constriction increases in velocity and decreases in pressure.

Biphasic closure Type of vocal fold closing pattern commonly seen in pulse register; characterized by partial closure, followed by opening, and then full closure.

Botox injection Procedure in which minute amounts of botulinum toxin are injected into the vocal folds to alleviate spasms.

Boyle's law   Law that states that a volume varies inversely with pressure, given a constant temperature.

Breath group   Utterance produced on one exhalation.

Breathiness   Vocal quality that sounds aspirated due to air loss and turbulence at the glottis.

Broadly tuned   Resonator that transmits a wide range of frequencies.

Bronchi   Structures that branch off the trachea and enter the lungs; part of the lower respiratory system.

Bronchial tree   Part of the respiratory system that includes the trachea, bronchi, and bronchioles.

Bronchioles   Smallest subdivisions of the bronchial system.

Brownian motion   Random high-speed movement of molecules due to their inherent energy.

Cartilaginous glottis   Posterior two-fifths of the glottis; bounded by vocal processes.

Caudate nucleus   Part of the basal nuclei.

Center frequency   Same as natural or resonant frequency.

Central sulcus   Groove on the cortex that divides the brain into anterior and posterior portions.

Cerebellar peduncles   Three nerve pathways (inferior, middle, superior) connecting the cerebellum to the brainstem and thalamus.

Cerebral peduncles   Large bundles of nerve pathways in the midbrain that form a continuation of the internal capsule.

Cerebrospinal fluid   Clear fluid within the subarachnoid space that circulates around the brain and spinal cord.

Cerumen   Waxy substance produced in the external auditory meatus.

cgs system   System of measurement in which c = centimeters, g = grams, and s = seconds.

Chest-wall shape   Positioning of the chest wall for speech production.

Chest-wall system   Part of the respiratory system that includes the rib cage, abdomen, and diaphragm.

Choroid plexus cells   Specialized cells within the ventricles that produce cerebrospinal fluid.

Cilia   Tiny hair-like projections within parts of the respiratory system, such as the trachea and nasal cavities, that help to filter the incoming air.

Circle of Willis   A roughly circular-shaped configuration of arteries that provide blood to the brain; made up of the internal carotid and vertebral arteries as well as branches of these vessels.

Clavicular breathing   Breathing pattern in which the shoulders are raised on inspiration, producing strain in the neck and laryngeal areas.

Closed quotient   EGG measure based on the ratio of the closed phase of the duty cycle to the period of the entire cycle.

Closed-to-open ratio   EGG measure based on the difference in time between the closing and opening phases of the duty cycle, divided by the duration of the closed phase.

Coarticulation   Overlapping of articulatory movements in time so that acoustic characteristics of adjacent sounds influence each other.

Cochlea   Snail-shaped spiral canal housing the nerve receptors for hearing.

Cochlear duct   Structure that divides the cochlea along most of its length; also called the *cochlear partition.*

Cognates   Pairs of sounds with the same manner and place of articulation, but differing in voicing.

Complex sound   Sound with two or more frequencies.

Compliance   The ease with which a body can be displaced or deformed.

Compression   Area of positive pressure.

Conductive hearing loss   Hearing loss caused by problems in the transmission of sound to the inner ear.

Consonant-to-vowel amplitude ratio Relationship of the amplitude of a consonant to the adjacent vowel.

Constructive interference   Waves that combine and increase the amplitude of the resulting wave.

Contact index   EGG measure based on the ratio of the difference in time between closing and opening phases, divided by the duration of the closed phase.

Coordinative structure   Functional linkages between muscles working in synergy to achieve an objective.

Corniculate cartilages   Paired cartilages located at the apex of the arytenoid cartilages.

Corona radiata   Large mass of myelinated nerve fibers from many different brain areas that diverge and flare out in a fan shape as they travel toward the cerebral cortex.

Corpus callosum   Thick band of white matter nerve pathways connecting the right and left hemispheres of the brain.

Cover–body model   Model of the vocal folds that describes their layered structure and different levels of stiffness.

Cricoarytenoid joints   Involved in adduction and abduction of the vocal folds.

Cricoid cartilage   Unpaired ring of cartilage forming the inferior portion of the larynx.

Cricopharyngeus muscle   Muscle located at the inferior border of the pharynx.

Cricothyroid joints   Involved in lengthening and shortening the vocal folds to regulate F_0.

Cricothyroid muscle (CT)   Intrinsic muscle of the larynx composed of oblique and erect parts; elongates and tenses the vocal folds.

Cricotracheal membrane   Sheet of membrane connecting the cricoid cartilage to the trachea.

Crossover   Perceptual boundary between two sounds on an acoustic continuum; related to categorical perception.

Cuneiform cartilages   Small elastic cartilages embedded within the aryepiglottic folds.

Cutoff frequency (F_c)   Frequency at which a resonant system is unresponsive.

Cycles per second   Number of cycles of vibration occurring in one second, equivalent to frequency.

Damping   Decrease in amplitude.

Dead air   Small amount of air not involved in oxygen–carbon dioxide exchange.

Decibel scale   A logarithmic ratio scale that compares the amplitude and/or intensity of a target sound to a standard reference sound.

Dendrites   Projections from the nerve cell body that transmit impulses toward the cell body.

Density   Number of something per unit of space.

Depolarization   Brief reversal of electrical charge within a neuron, going from negative (-70 mV) to positive (30 mV).

Destructive interference   Waves that combine and decrease the amplitude of the resulting wave.

Developmental dyslexia   Disorder in which a person's reading ability is significantly lower than what would be predicted on the basis of age and intellectual ability.

Diaphragm   Muscle that makes up the floor of the thoracic cavity and is instrumental in respiration.

Diplophonia   Perception of two simultaneous pitches in a person's voice.

Direct (pyramidal) system   Motor system comprising the corticospinal and corticonuclear nerve tracts; involved in the control of fine, skilled voluntary movements.

Distocclusion   Condition in which the mandible is retracted due to abnormal occlusion.

Dopamine   Neurotransmittor deficient in Parkinson's disease.

Dorsal horns   Posterior portion of the grey matter of the spinal cord made up of nerve cell bodies that receive sensory information.

Driving pressure   Difference between high- and low-pressure areas that causes air to flow between these areas.

Dura mater   Outermost layer of the meninges; made up of periosteal and meningeal parts.

Duration   Length of time a speech sound lasts.

Duty cycle   Phases of a vocal fold vibratory cycle, including closing, closed, opening, and open.

Dyne   Unit of measure of force and pressure.

Dysphonia   Any kind of vocal dysfunction resulting in a deviant-sounding voice.

Efferent   Motor nerve that transmits information from the nervous system to muscles and glands.

Elasticity   Restoring force that brings an object back to its original size, shape, or position after having been displaced or deformed.

Electroglottography (EGG)   Method of evaluating vocal fold function based on the difference between electrical conductivity of tissue and air; also called *laryngography*.

End-expiratory level   Endpoint of a normal quiet exhalation, equal to resting expiratory level.

End-plate potential (EPP)   Small graded depolarization of a muscle fiber.

Endolymph   Fluid within the membranous canal of the cochlea.

Endotracheal intubation   Process in which a breathing tube is inserted into the trachea through the larynx.

Envelope   Line that connects the frequencies of a complex sound represented on a spectrum.

Epiglottis   Unpaired cartilage of the larynx involved in swallowing.

Epithelium   Type of tissue that lines the inner surfaces of the respiratory system.

erg   Measure of energy in the cgs system.

Esophageal speech   Speech produced by vibrating the superior portion of the esophagus.

Evoked potentials   Also called event-related potentials; brain electrical activity that occurs in response to a controlled stimulus.

Excitatory post-synaptic potential
Occurs when the threshold of the post-synaptic neuron is lowered, making it easier for the neuron to fire.

Expiratory reserve volume   Amount of air that can be exhaled below tidal volume.

External auditory meatus   Channel leading from the pinna to the tympanic membrane; also known as the *ear canal*.

Extrapyramidal system   Collective term for a multisynaptic series of nerve pathways in the central nervous system running from the cerebral cortex and making synaptic connection in the basal nuclei and cerebellum before synapsing with spinal and brainstem motor nuclei.

Extrinsic muscles   Muscles that have one attachment within a given structure (e.g., tongue, larynx) and one outside the structure.

$F_0F_1F_2$ **strategy**   Type of signal-processing strategy used in a cochlear implant, based on estimates of F_1 and F_2 frequencies, at a rate based on the F_0 of the signal or on a random rate around the F_0.

F_0**SPL profile**   Graph that plots phonational frequency range against dynamic range; also called voice range profile or phonetogram.

F_1 **cutback**   Delay of F_1 relative to the beginning of the F_2 transition.

False vocal folds   Also called *ventricular vocal folds*; they lie parallel and superior to true vocal folds.

Falsetto register   A range of very high F_0 with a thin, breathy quality; also called *loft*.

Fasciculi   Nerve pathways formed by long association fibers linking different cortical regions.

Feedback   Transfer of part of the output of a system back to the input to correct any errors in the output.

Feedforward   Signals that make adjustments at the periphery of a system to prime the system.

Fetal cell transplantation   Surgical treatment for Parkinson's disease, designed to replenish missing dopamine.

Final common pathway   Term for the cranial and spinal nerves that supply motor innervation to all the muscles in the body.

Final consonant deletion   Phonological process in which the final consonant of a word is omitted.

Fixed channel strategy   Type of signal processing strategy used in a cochlear implant, in which the acoustic signal is divided into four to twelve frequency bands, and energy in all the bands is transmitted at each cycle.

Flocculonodular lobe   Lobe of the cerebellum.

Flow   Movement of a particular volume of air during an interval of time.

Formant trajectory   Frequency path that a formant follows across an entire segment, such as a vowel.

Formant transition   Shift in formant frequency.

Formants   Resonances of the vocal tract; frequency areas of acoustic energy in vowels and other resonant sounds.

Fourier analysis   Mathematical procedure to identify the individual sinusoids in a complex sound.

Frequency   Rate of vibration of an object.

Frequency perturbation   Cycle-to-cycle variability in vocal frequency, also called jitter.

Frication   Characteristic noise present in fricative sounds.

Fronting   Phonological process in which a sound with a more anterior place of articulation is substituted for one with a more posterior place of articulation.

Functional residual capacity   Amount of air in the lungs and airways at the end of a normal quiet exhalation.

Fundamental frequency (F_0)   Lowest frequency of a complex periodic sound.

Genioglossus muscle   Extrinsic tongue muscle; retracts tongue or draws tongue forward.

Gestures   A family of movement patterns that achieve the same articulatory/acoustic goal.

Glial cells   Term for different types of connective tissues in the nervous system.

Globus pallidus   Part of the basal nuclei.

Glossometry   Technique used to visualize tongue position within the oral cavity using light-emitting diode photosensors mounted on a pseudopalate.

Glottal spectrum   Spectrum of the laryngeal tone before it is modified in the vocal tract.

Glottis   Space between the true vocal folds.

Golgi apparatus   Microscopic organelle within cell cytoplasm that secretes proteins and sugars.

Gyri   Raised surfaces on the cortex of the brain.

Half-power points   Also called 3 dB down points, corresponding to the upper and lower cutoff frequencies of a resonator.

Harmonic frequencies   Frequencies above F_0 in a complex periodic sound.

Harmonic spacing   Distance between harmonic frequencies in a complex sound.

Harmonics-to-noise ratio   Measure, in dB, of the ratio of harmonic energy to noise energy in the voice.

Helicotrema   Point of communication between the scala vestibuli and scala tympani at the end of the cochlear duct.

Hemodynamic response   Increase in local brain blood flow in response to a particular cognitive task.

Hertz (Hz)   Unit of measurement of frequency.

Heteronym   Noun–verb pairs that are contrasted by stress, with a noun receiving stress on the first syllable and a verb receiving stress on the second syllable.

High-pass filter   Resonator that transmits acoustic energy above a specific lower cutoff frequency.

Hippocampus   Structure of the limbic system; involved in learning and memory.

Hoarseness   Vocal quality combining breathy plus rough characteristics.

Homunculus   Caricature representing the differing amounts of neural tissue devoted to motor and sensory representations of different body structures.

Hyoglossus muscle   Extrinsic tongue muscle; pulls the sides of the tongue downward.

Hyoid bone   Bone from which the larynx is suspended; also forms the attachment for the tongue.

Hyothyroid membrane   Sheet of membrane connecting the thyroid cartilage to the hyoid bone.

Hyperadducted   Vocal folds adducted with excessive medial compression.

Hypernasality   Distortion of an oral sound due to excessive nasal resonance.

Hypoadducted   Vocal folds adducted with insufficient medial compression.

Hyponasality   Distortion of a nasal sound due to insufficient nasal resonance.

Identification tasks   Procedure in which listeners transcribe what a speaker says.

Immittance   Measure of how easily a system can be set into vibration by a driving force; includes the admittance and impedance of a system.

Immittance audiometry   Method for diagnosing middle ear problems based on immittance.

Impedance   Measure of the opposition of a system to a flow of energy through it, measured in ohms.

Impedance mismatch   Difference in impedance between two mediums.

Incident wave   Sound wave generated by a vibrating object.

Incus   One of the ossicles of the middle ear; also called the *anvil*.

Indirect (extrapyramidal) system   Multisynaptic motor system comprising nerve pathways that synapse with subcortical and cerebellar neurons before synapsing with motor neurons in the brainstem and spinal cord.

Inertia   Tendency of matter to remain at rest or in motion unless acted on by an outside force.

Inferior colliculi   Two masses of grey matter in the midbrain that project to the medial geniculate nucleus of the thalamus and are involved in auditory processing.

Inferior labial frenulum   Small flap of tissue connecting the inner surface of the lower lip to the midline of the mandible.

Inferior longitudinal muscle   Intrinsic tongue muscle; pulls tip downward, retracts tongue.

Infrahyoid muscles   Extrinsic muscles of larynx; depress the larynx.

Inhibitory post-synaptic potential Occurs when the threshold of the postsynaptic neuron is raised, making it more difficult for the neuron to fire.

Innervation ratio   Ratio of a motor neuron to the number of muscle fibers it innervates.

Inspiratory reserve volume   Amount of air that can be inhaled above tidal volume.

Interarytenoid muscle (IA)   Intrinsic muscle of larynx composed of transverse and oblique fibers; adducts the vocal folds.

Intercostal muscles   Made up of internal and external sets of muscles running between the ribs on both sides.

Interference   Combining of waves in terms of areas of high and low pressure.

Intermaxillary suture   Immovable joint between the palatine processes of the maxilla.

Intermediate zone   Region in the spinal cord where the ventral and dorsal horns join.

Internal capsule   Large mass of myelinated nerve fibers including corticothalamic, thalamocortical, corticonuclear, and corticospinal fibers.

Interneurons   Neurons that connect to each other over short or long distances; most numerous type of neurons in the human nervous system.

Intonation   Variation of F_0 over an utterance.

Ion   Atom or group of atoms that carry a positive or negative electrical charge due to gaining or losing an electron.

Jitter   Cycle-to-cycle variability in frequency of vocal fold vibration; also called *frequency perturbation*.

joule (J)   Measure of energy in the MKS system.

Labial valve   Valve of the vocal tract formed by the lips.

Lamina propria   Sheet of mucous membrane surrounding the body of the vocal folds; has superficial, intermediate, and deep layers.

Laminar flow   Flow of air in which molecules move in a parallel manner at the same speed.

Laryngeal valve   Formed by the true vocal folds.

Laryngeal ventricle   Space between the true and false vocal folds.

Laryngectomy   Surgical removal of all or part of the larynx, usually due to cancer.

Laryngography   More commonly called electroglottography; method of evaluating vocal fold function based on electrical conduction.

Laryngopharynx   Portion of the pharynx behind the larynx.

Laryngospasms   Involuntary spasms of the vocal folds.

Lateral corticospinal tract   Motor nerve pathway also called pyramidal tract; originates in the sensorimotor cortex; most fibers decussate at the medulla and then synapse with neurons in the anterior horns of the spinal cord.

Lateral cricoarytenoid muscle (LCA)   Intrinsic muscle of the larynx; adducts the vocal folds.

Lateral fissure   Deep groove on the cortical surface of the brain that divides the brain into superior and inferior regions.

Lateral geniculate body   Thalamic nucleus that processes visual information and relays it to the visual cortex.

Lateral vestibulospinal tract   Motor nerve pathway that originates in the vestibular nuclei in the medulla and synapses with anterior horn spinal motor neurons.

Levator veli palatini   Muscle that forms a slinglike arrangement and elevates the velum.

Limbic system   Made up of the limbic lobe, hippocampus, amygdala, mamillary bodies, and some thalamic nuclei; involved in emotional, sexual, and visceral functions.

Line spectrum   Graph in which the frequencies in a complex periodic sound are depicted as vertical lines. The height of the line indicates the amplitude of the component frequency.

Linear scale   Scale in which successive units increase by the same amount.

Linearized magnetometer   Instrument used to measure movements of the chest wall.

Lingual frenulum   Band of connective tissue joining the inferior portion of the tongue to the mandible.

Lingual valve   Valve of the vocal tract formed by the tongue and other structures within the vocal tract.

Logarithmic scale   Scale in which successive units increase by increasing amounts.

Logogen   A neural processing device assumed to be associated with each word in a person's vocabulary.

Longitudinal cerebral fissure   Deep groove on the cortex of the brain that divides the brain into two hemispheres.

Longitudinal phase difference   Timing difference between the anterior and posterior portions of the vocal folds as they open and close during vibration.

Low-pass filter   Resonator that transmits acoustic energy below a specific upper cutoff frequency.

Lower cutoff frequency (F_1)   Frequency below F_c at which there is a 3 dB less amplitude of response than at F_c.

Lower motor neuron   Comprised of cranial and spinal nerve cell bodies and their axons that connect with voluntary muscles.

Lower respiratory system   Part of the respiratory system that includes the trachea, bronchial tubes, and lungs.

Lx wave   Waveform generated by electroglottography, with time on the horizontal axis and voltage on the vertical axis.

m-of-n strategy   Type of signal-processing strategy used in a cochlear implant in which n equals the overall number of frequency bands represented in the acoustic signal, and m represents a smaller number of channels with the highest energy peaks in a particular processing cycle.

Mainstem bronchi   Primary bronchi entering the lungs.

Malleus   One of the ossicles of the middle ear; also called the *hammer*.

Malocclusion   Problem in upper and/or lower dental arch relationships.

Manner of articulation   Way in which the articulators relate to each other to regulate the flow of air through the vocal tract.

Manometer   Instrument used to measure static pressures in cm H_2O.

Manubrium   Long section of the malleus, attaching to the tympanic membrane.

Maximum phonational frequency range Complete range of frequencies that an individual can produce.

Mechanical resonator   Resonator that does not contain a body of air.

Medial compression   Force exerted by the LCA and IA muscles to bring the vocal folds to midline.

Medial geniculate body   Thalamic nucleus that processes auditory information and relays it to the auditory cortex.

Median fibrous septum   Divides tongue into right and left sides.

Mel   Unit of pitch on a psychophysical scale.

Membranous glottis   Anterior three-fifths of the glottis; bounded by vocal ligament.

Meninges   Three layers of connective tissues and the spaces between them that form a protective covering for the brain and spinal cord.

Mesiocclusion   Condition in which the mandible protrudes too far forward due to abnormal occlusion.

Microbar   Measurement of dynes per centimeter squared. 1 microbar = 1 $dyne/cm^2$.

Microglia   Type of glial cells in the nervous system that destroy harmful organisms.

Mitochondria   Microscopic organelle within cell cytoplasm involved in cell respiration and energy production.

Mixed hearing loss   Combination of conductive and sensorineural hearing loss.

MKS system   System of measurement in which M = meters, K = kilograms, S = seconds.

Modal register   Most commonly used register for normal conversational speech, encompassing the midrange of F_0.

Motor unit   A motor neuron with the associated muscle fibers that it innervates.

MPEAK strategy   Type of signal-processing strategy used in a cochlear implant, in which electrodes representing F_1 and F_2 are stimulated, as well as two or three other electrodes representing the higher formant regions.

Mucosal wave   Undulating wavelike motion of the vocal folds during vibration, particularly evident in the cover.

Multiphasic closure   Pattern of vocal fold vibration in which there are numerous partial openings and closings prior to complete closure.

Muscular hydrostat   A muscular organ without a cartilaginous or bony skeleton; derives support through selective muscular contraction.

Muscular process   Projection of arytenoid cartilage to which various intrinsic laryngeal muscles attach.

Musculus uvuli   Muscle on the nasal surface of the velum; helps to raise velum.

Myoelastic–aerodynamic theory of phonation   Theory that explains vocal fold vibration in terms of muscular, elastic recoil, and aerodynamic forces.

Narrowly tuned   Refers to a resonator that transmits a narrow range of frequencies.

Nasal formant   High-intensity, low-frequency formant present in nasal sounds.

Nasal murmur   Extra resonances present in nasal sounds due to the coupling of the oral and nasal cavities.

Nasal septum   Cartilaginous and bony plate that separates the nasal cavities.

Nasopharynx   Portion of the pharynx behind the nasal cavities.

Negative pressure   Pressure lower than atmospheric pressure.

Neocortex   Type of cortical tissue that is greatly expanded in humans compared to other primates.

Neuromuscular junction   Synapse between an axon and the muscle fiber it innervates, also known as myoneural junction.

Neutrocclusion   Normal occlusal relationship between upper and lower dental arches.

newton (N)   Unit of measure of force in the modernized metric system.

Nissl bodies   Microscopic organelle within cell cytoplasm that synthesizes proteins.

Nodes of Ranvier   Breaks in the myelin sheath around an axon that serve to increase the nerve's rate of impulse conduction.

Occlusion   Relationship between the upper and lower dental arches and the positioning of individual teeth.

Octave   A doubling or halving of frequency.

Ohm   Unit of electrical resistance.

Oligodendrocytes   Glial cells that form myelin sheaths around nerves in the central nervous system.

Optimum pitch   Range of pitches used by an individual that are produced with minimum vocal effort.

Orbicularis oris   Circular muscle of the lips.

Organ of Corti   Sensory nerve receptor for hearing, consisting of rows of inner and outer hair cells.

Oropharynx   Portion of the pharynx behind the oral cavity.

Oscillation   Back and forth movement of an object.

Ossicles   Series of three small connecting bones in the middle ear.

Otitis media   Middle ear infection.

Otitis media with effusion   Buildup of fluid in the middle ear, caused by infection.

Otoacoustic emissions   Low-intensity sounds originating in the cochlea and transmitted to the external auditory meatus; can be spontaneous or evoked.

Otosclerosis   Formation of spongy bone around the stapes that prevents it from being set into vibration.

Palatal aponeurosis   Broad flat sheet of tendon attaching the velum to the hard palate.

Palatine bones   Bones of the skull that form the posterior one-quarter of the hard palate.

Palatine processes   Projections of the maxilla that form the anterior three-quarters of the hard palate.

Palatoglossus   Muscle that forms anterior faucial pillars; depresses velum or elevates tongue.

Palatometry   Technique for displaying articulatory contacts using electrodes mounted on a pseudopalate.

Palatopharyngeus   Muscles that form the posterior faucial pillars and narrow the pharyngeal cavity.

Parallel distributed processing models   Computer models that simulate the neural processing of the human brain.

Parietal pleura   Membrane lining the inner surface of the thoracic cavity.

pascal (P)   Unit of measure of pressure in the modernized metric system.

Passband   Acoustic resonator that transmits frequencies between the upper and lower cutoff frequencies.

Pattern Playback   Instrument that converts visual patterns into sounds.

Perceptual magnet effect   Notion that individuals are able to identify prototypical examples of a vowel better than nonprototypical examples.

Perilymph   Fluid between the bony canal and the membranous canals of the cochlea.

Period   Amount of time consumed by each cycle in a wave.

Periodic   Wave in which each cycle takes the same amount of time to occur.

Pharyngeal constrictors   Muscles that consist of inferior, middle, and superior fibers; they constrict the pharynx during swallowing.

Phase   Relative timing of compressions and rarefactions of waves.

Phon   Unit of loudness on a psychophysical scale.

Phonation threshold pressure   Minimum amount of P_s needed to set the vocal folds into vibration.

Phonological processes   Strategies used to simplify the motoric complexity of phonetic segments.

Pia mater   Innermost layer of the meninges; closely follows the convolutions of the brain.

Pinna   External portion of the ear, on either side of the head.

Pitch sigma   Frequency variability, in semitones, in a person's voice.

Place of articulation   Location within the vocal tract where articulators contact or approximate each other.

Plethysmograph   Instrument used to measure changes in the cross-sectional areas of the chest wall.

Pleural fluid   Fluid within the pleural space, having a negative pressure.

Pleural linkage   The mechanism by which the lungs and thoracic cavity are linked together to function as a unit.

Pleural space   Small potential space between the parietal and visceral pleurae.

Pneumotachograph   Instrument used to measure airflows.

Pneumothorax   Collapse of a lung due to penetration of the pleural lining.

Positive pressure   Pressure higher than atmospheric pressure.

Postcentral gyrus   Region immediately posterior to the central sulcus containing the primary somatosensory areas.

Posterior cricoarytenoid muscle
Intrinsic muscle of larynx; abducts the vocal folds.

Precentral gyrus   Region immediately anterior to the central sulcus containing the primary motor cortex.

Prephonatory chest wall movements
Positioning of the chest wall that facilitates the generation of pressures for speech production.

Pressure   Force acting perpendicularly on a surface.

Probe tip   Device inserted in the external auditory meatus to measure immittance of the middle ear.

Pseudopalate   Thin acrylic plate custom-designed to cover a person's hard palate and upper teeth.

Pulmonary system   Part of the respiratory system that includes the lungs and airways.

Pulse register   A range of very low F_0 with a creaky quality; also called *glottal fry, vocal fry, creaky voice.*

Pure tone   Sound with only one frequency.

Putamen   Part of the basal nuclei.

Pyramidal system   Collective term for the corticospinal and corticonuclear (corticobulbar) pathways of the central nervous system from the cerebral cortex that synapse directly onto spinal and brainstem motor nuclei.

Quality   Acoustically, the relationship between the harmonic frequencies and their amplitudes in a complex sound; perceptually, the tone or timbre of a sound.

Quarter-wave resonator   Resonator that is open at one end and closed at the other; lowest resonant frequency has a wavelength four times the length of the resonator.

Radiation characteristic   Effect that occurs when the sound traveling through the vocal tract is radiated beyond the mouth into the atmosphere, with the mouth acting like a high-pass filter.

Rarefaction   Area of negative pressure.

Ratio scale   Scale that describes relationships between quantities.

Recoil forces   Forces generated when structures are restored to their original positions after being displaced.

Reflection   Wave that collides with a surface and travels back toward the source.

Register   Perceptually distinct region of vocal quality that can be maintained over a range of F_0.

Rejection rate   Same as attenuation rate.

Relative refractory period   Brief period following the absolute refractory period during which the nerve can only fire with stronger than normal stimulation.

Relaxation pressures   Air pressures generated by the recoil forces of the respiratory system.

Relay nuclei   Thalamic nuclei that receive and transmit nerve impulses to and from specific cortical areas.

Release burst   Burst of aperiodic sound following the silent gap in a stop sound.

Repolarization   Reversal of voltage in a neuron from positive back to negative.

Residual volume   Volume of air remaining in the lungs after a maximum exhalation that cannot be voluntarily expelled.

Resonance curve   Graph displaying the frequency response of a resonant system.

Resonant frequency   Frequency at which an object vibrates depending on its physical characteristics.

Resonator   Object that vibrates in response to another vibration; can be mechanical or acoustic.

Respiratory bronchioles   Subdivisions of the terminal bronchioles.

Respiratory kinematic analysis   Methods of estimating lung volumes from rib cage and abdominal movements.

Resting expiratory level   State of equilibrium in the respiratory system when P_{alv} equals P_{atmos}.

Resting membrane potential   Electrical voltage across the nerve cell membrane at rest with a negative charge of $-70\ mV$ within the cell and a positive electrical charge in the extracellular fluid, resulting in polarization.

Reticular activating system   Part of the reticular formation in the brainstem that controls alertness and consciousness.

Reticular formation   Diffuse network of nuclei that forms the core of the brainstem.

Reverberation   Process generating a sound that lasts slightly longer due to interaction of incident and reflected waves.

Rhotic sounds   Sounds that have /r/ coloring, seen acoustically in a characteristic lowering of F_3.

Rise time   Time it takes for the amplitude envelope or spectrum of a sound to reach its highest value.

Roll-off rate   Same as attenuation rate; also called *slope*.

Roughness   Vocal quality that sounds raspy and low pitched due to aperiodic vocal fold vibration.

Round window   Opening between the scala tympani and the middle ear, covered with membrane.

Rubrospinal tract   Motor nerve pathway that originates in the red nucleus of the midbrain and synapses contralaterally with neurons in the anterior horns of the spinal cord.

Scaling procedures   Procedure in which listeners rate an individual's overall speech intelligibility.

Schwann cells   Glial cells that form myelin sheaths around nerves in the peripheral nervous system.

Secondary bronchus   Subdivision of the mainstem bronchi, supplying the lobes of the lungs.

Sensorineural hearing loss   Hearing loss due to disease or damage to the inner ear or auditory nerve.

Sharply tuned   Resonator that transmits a narrow range of frequencies; also called *narrowly tuned*.

Shimmer   Cycle-to-cycle variability in amplitude of the vocal fold vibration; also called *amplitude perturbation*.

Siemens   Units of electrical conductance, also called millimhos.

Silent gap   Time on a spectrogram of a stop sound during which no sound is seen because pressure is building up.

Simple harmonic motion   A smooth back and forth movement with a characteristic pattern of acceleration through the rest position and deceleration at the endpoints of the movement.

Sinusoid   Pure tone with a sinusoidal shape on a waveform.

Slope   Rate at which a resonator's amplitude of response is attenuated, also known as attenuation rate, roll-off rate, or rejection rate.

Slope index   Measure of a formant transition based on the duration and frequency extent of the transition. Measured in hertz per millisecond (Hz/ms).

Soma   Cell body of a neuron; composed of cytoplasm and nucleus.

Somatotopic organization   Organization of motor control according to body structure.

Sonorants   Class of sounds that are always voiced; airflow is neither completely laminar nor turbulent.

Source-filter theory   Theory describing how the vocal tract filters glottal sound waves to generate different vowels.

Spasmodic dysphonia   Voice disorder characterized by laryngeal spasms.

Spatial summation   Process by which nerve impulses reach the cell body or dendrites at slightly different locations and add together.

Specific language impairment   Disorder in which children show a significant problem with language, in the face of normal hearing, normal nonverbal intelligence, and no known neurological problems.

Spectral noise   Additive noise in the glottal spectrum.

Spectrum   Graph with frequency on the horizontal axis and amplitude on the vertical axis; line spectrum represents periodic sounds, continuous spectrum represents aperiodic sounds.

Spinocerebellar tract   Sensory nerve pathway from the spinal cord to the cerebellum that transmits information about pain, temperature, touch, and proprioception.

Spinothalamic tract   Sensory nerve pathway from the spinal cord to the thalamus that transmits information about pain, temperature, and touch.

Spirometer   Instrument that measures lung volumes; can be wet or dry.

Spreading activation models   Computer models that simulate the neural processing of the human brain. Also called *parallel distributed processing*.

Standard reference sound   Sound with an amplitude of 0.0002 dyne/cm^2 and intensity of 10^{-16} W/cm^2.

Stapedius   Muscle in the middle ear; involved in the acoustic reflex.

Stapes   One of the ossicles of the middle ear; also called the *stirrup*.

Stiffness   Resistance of a structure to being displaced or deformed.

Stress   Emphasis placed on a syllable or word by increasing pitch, intensity, and/or duration.

Striatum   Part of the basal nuclei comprised of the caudate and putamen.

Stridents   Fricatives characterized by intense high-frequency energy.

Styloglossus muscle   Extrinsic tongue muscle; elevates and retracts the tongue.

Subarachnoid space   Space between the arachnoid mater and the pia mater; filled with cerebrospinal fluid.

Subdural space   Space between the dura mater and the arachnoid mater.

Subsonic   Frequencies below the range of human hearing.

Substantia nigra   Part of the basal nuclei, involved in the production of dopamine.

Sulci   Shallow depressions on the cortex of the brain.

Superior colliculi   Two masses of grey matter in the midbrain that project to the lateral geniculate nucleus of the thalamus and are involved in visual processing.

Superior labial frenulum   Small flap of tissue connecting the inner surface of the upper lip to the midline of the alveolar region.

Superior longitudinal muscle   Intrinsic tongue muscle; elevates the tip.

Supersonic   Frequencies above the range of human hearing.

Suprahyoid muscles   Extrinsic muscles of larynx; elevate the larynx.

Suprasegmentals F_0, intensity, and duration changes that occur over a sequence of phonemes, syllables, words, or sentences; they signal linguistic and extralinguistic meanings.

Suprathreshold discriminability   Ability of an individual with hearing loss to recognize a sound when it is presented at an audible level.

Suprathreshold level   Level at which a hearing-impaired person can hear a specific speech signal.

Surfactant   Substance that keeps alveoli inflated by lowering the surface tension of the alveolar walls.

Synapse   Gap between neurons where communication between nerves takes place; may be axo-axonal, axo-somatic, or axo-dendritic.

Synergy   Functional linkages between muscles working to achieve a specific movement goal.

Target undershoot   Failure of articulators to reach the intended vowel target, resulting in a reduction in F_1/F_2 vowel space.

Tectorial membrane   Gel-like membrane forming the roof of the organ of Corti.

Temporal gap   In pulse register, a brief interval during which no acoustic energy is present.

Temporal processing problem   Difficulty in processing the rapid changes in frequency and intensity that are characteristic of speech.

Temporal summation   Process by which nerve impulses reach the cell body within a very short time of each other and add together.

Tensor tympani   Muscle of the middle ear, involved in auditory tube function.

Tensor veli palatini   Muscle of the velum that opens the auditory tube.

Terminal branches   Also known as telodendria; the end point of an axon.

Terminal bronchioles   Subdivisions of the tertiary bronchi.

Terminal buttons   Small sacs on the terminal branches of an axon filled with neurotransmitter molecules.

Tertiary bronchi   Subdivisions of the secondary bronchi, supplying the segments of the lungs.

Thoracic cavity   Chest cavity bounded by the ribs, sternum, vertebral column, and diaphragm, in which the lungs are housed.

Threshold of hearing   Sound that a pair of normal human ears can detect 50 percent of the time under ideal listening conditions.

Threshold of pain   Intensity level of 130 dB, which causes a sensation of pain in the ears.

Thyroarytenoid muscle (TA)   Body of the vocal folds.

Thyroid cartilage   Largest cartilage of the larynx; unpaired.

Tidal volume   Volume of air breathed in and out during a cycle of respiration.

Tonotopic organization   Spatial organization of a structure (e.g., basilar membrane) in terms of frequency distribution.

Torque   A twisting, rotary force.

Torus tubarius   Bulge in the lateral pharyngeal wall caused by the enlargement of cartilage where the auditory tube opens into the pharynx.

Total lung capacity   Total amount of air that the lungs are capable of holding, including residual volume.

Tracer   Radioactive substance used in emission tomography.

Trachea   Membranocartilaginous tube inferior to the larynx; part of the lower respiratory system.

Transducer   Device that converts energy from one form to another.

Transfer function   Same as resonance curve.

Transglottal pressure   Pressure difference across the vocal folds, between tracheal pressure and supraglottal pressure.

Transverse muscle   Intrinsic tongue muscle; pulls edges toward midline.

Transverse palatine suture   Suture between the palatine bones and palatine processes.

True vocal folds   Multilayered structures attached to anterior commissure anteriorly and vocal processes posteriorly; vibrating element of the larynx.

Turbulent flow   Irregular flow with random variations in pressure.

Tympanic membrane   Eardrum.

Tympanogram   Graph of the immittance of the middle ear.

Tympanometer   Instrument that measures and displays the immittance of the middle ear.

Umbo   Tip of the conical surface of the tympanic membrane.

Upper cutoff frequency (F_u)   Frequency above F_c at which there is a 3 dB less amplitude of response than at F_c.

Upper motor neuron   Comprised of nerve cells bodies and their axons arising from various cortical areas and projecting to the brainstem and spinal cord.

Upper respiratory system   Part of the respiratory system that includes the pharynx and the oral and nasal cavities.

Variable resonator   Resonator whose frequency response changes as the resonator changes its shape.

Velopharyngeal passage   Portion of the pharynx between the posterior margins of the oral and nasal cavities.

Velopharyngeal valve   Valve of the vocal tract formed by the velum and posterior portion of the pharynx.

Velum   Soft palate.

Ventral anterior and ventral lateral nuclei   Thalamic nuclei that receive input from the basal nuclei and cerebellum and project to the motor areas of the cerebral cortex.

Ventral horns   Anterior portion of the grey matter of the spinal cord made up of nerve cell bodies that project fibers to skeletal muscles.

Vermis   Midline portion of the cerebellum that connects the two cerebellar hemispheres.

Vertical muscle   Intrinsic tongue muscle; pulls the tongue downward.

Vertical phase difference   Timing difference between the inferior and superior

borders of the vocal folds as they open and close during vibration.

Vestibular membrane   Roof of the cochlear duct.

Visceral pleura   Membrane covering the outer surface of each lung.

Vital capacity   Maximum amount of air that can be exhaled after a maximum inhalation.

Vocal ligament   Portion of the vocal folds consisting of intermediate and deep layers of the lamina propria.

Vocal process   Projection of the arytenoid cartilage to which the vocal folds attach.

Voice bar   Band of low-frequency energy sometimes seen on a spectrogram of a voiced stop or fricative, reflecting vocal fold vibration.

Voice onset time (VOT)   In a stop consonant, time between the release burst to the beginning of vocal fold vibration for the following vowel.

Voicing   Vibration of the vocal folds during phonation.

Volume   Amount of space occupied by something in three dimensions.

Volume velocity   Rate of flow.

Vowel quadrilateral   Diagram representing the tongue positions of height and advancement for vowels.

Vowel reduction   Neutralization of a vowel so its formants look more like a schwa.

Watt (W)   Measure of power.

Wave front   Outermost area of the sound wave propagating spherically through the air.

Waveform   Graph with time on the horizontal axis and amplitude on the vertical axis.

Wavelength   Distance covered by one complete cycle of a wave.

Wet spirometer   Instrument that measures lung volumes and capacities.

White noise   Aperiodic sound that has its energy distributed fairly evenly throughout the spectrum.

References

Abbs, J. H. (1996). Mechanisms of speech motor execution and control. In N. J. Lass (Ed.), *Principles of experimental phonetics* (pp. 93–111). St. Louis: Mosby.

Aerainer, R., & Klingholz, F. (1993). Quantitative evaluation of phonetograms in the case of functional dysphonia. *Journal of Voice, 7*, 136–141.

Ansel, B. M., & Kent, R. D. (1992). Acoustic–phonetic contrasts and intelligibility in the dysarthria associated with mixed cerebral palsy. *Journal of Speech and Hearing Research, 35*, 296–308.

Awan, S. N., & Frenkel, M. L. (1994). Improvements in estimating the harmonics-to-noise ratio of the voice. *Journal of Voice, 8*, 255–262.

Baken, R. J. (1992). Electroglottography. *Journal of Voice, 6*, 98–110.

Baken, R. J. (1996). *Clinical measurement of speech and voice.* San Diego, CA: Singular.

Baken, R. J. (1998). An overview of laryngeal function for voice production. In R. T. Sataloff (Ed.), *Vocal health and pedagogy* (pp. 27–45). San Diego, CA: Singular.

Baken, R., & Cavallo, S. (1981). Prephonatory chest wall posturing. *Folia Phoniatrica et Logopedica, 33*, 193–202.

Baker, K. K., Ramig, L. O., Johnson, A. B., & Freed, C. R. (1997). Preliminary voice and speech analysis following fetal dopamine transplants in 5 individuals with Parkinson disease. *Journal of Speech and Hearing Research, 40*, 615–626.

Barlow, S. M. (1999). *Handbook of clinical speech physiology.* San Diego, CA: Singular.

Behrman, A., & Orlikoff, R. F. (1997). Instrumentation in voice assessment and treatment: What's the use? *American Journal of Speech Language Pathology, 6*, 9–16.

Benjamin, B. (1981). Frequency variability in the aged voice. *Journal of Gerontology, 36*, 722–726.

Bennett, S. (1983). A 3-year longitudinal study of school-aged children's F_0s. *Journal of Speech and Hearing Research, 26*, 137–142.

Benoit, M., Clairet, S., Koulibaly, P. M., Darcourt, J., & Robert, P. H. (2004). Brain perfusion correlates of the Apathy Inventory dimensions of Alzheimer's disease. *International Journal of Geriatric Psychiatry, 19*, 864–869.

Bernstein, L. E., & Stark, R. E. (1985). Speech perception development in language-impaired children: A 4-year follow-up study. *Journal of Speech and Hearing Disorders, 50*, 21–30.

Bertino, G., Bellomo, A., Miana, C., Ferrero, F., & Staffieri, A. (1996). Spectrographic differences between tracheal-esophageal and esophageal voice. *Folia Phoniatrica et Logopedica, 48*, 255–261.

Binder, J. R., Frost, J. A., Hammeke, T. A., Cox, R. W., Rao, S. M., & Prieto, T. (1997). Human brain language areas identified by functional magnetic resonance imaging. *Society for Neuroscience, 17*, 353–362.

Bishop, D. V. M., Bishop, S. J., Bright, P., James, C., Delaney, T., & Tallal, P. (1999). Different origin of auditory and phonological processing problems in children with language impairment: Evidence from a twin study. *Journal of Speech, Language, and Hearing Research, 42,* 155–168.

Blomgren, M., Chen, Y., Ng, M., & Gilbert, H. (1997). *Acoustic, aerodynamic, physiologic, and perceptual properties of modal and vocal fry registers.* Paper presented at the annual convention of the American Speech–Language–Hearing Association, Boston.

Boberg, E., Yeudall, L., Schopplocher, D., & BoLassen, P. (1983). The effects of an intensive behavioral program on the distribution of EEG alpha power in stutterers during the processing of verbal and visuospatial information. *Journal of Fluency Disorders, 8,* 245–263.

Boliek, C. A. (1997). *Respiratory function in voice and speech disorders: Clinical implications.* Paper presented at the annual convention of the American Speech–Language–Hearing Association, Boston.

Boliek, C. A., Hixon, T. J., Watson, P. J., & Morgan, W. J. (1996). Vocalization and breathing during the first year of life. *Journal of Voice, 10,* 1–22.

Boliek, C. A., Hixon, T. J., Watson, P. J., & Morgan, W. J. (1997). Vocalization and breathing during the second and third years of life. *Journal of Voice, 11,* 373–390.

Borden, G. J., Harris, K. S., & Raphael, L. J. (1994). *Speech science primer: Physiology, acoustics, and perception of speech* (3rd ed.). Baltimore: Williams & Wilkins.

Borden, G. J., Harris, K. S., & Raphael, L. J. (2003). *Speech science primer: Physiology, acoustics, and perception of speech* (4th ed.). Philadelphia: Lippincott Williams & Wilkins.

Braun, A. R., Varga, M., Stager, S., Schulz, G., Selbie, S., Maisog, J. M., Carson, R. E., & Ludlow, C. L. (1997). A typical lateralization of hemispheral activity in developmental stuttering: An $H_2^{15}O$ positron emission tomography study. In W. Hulstijn, H. F. M. Peters, & P. H. H. M. Van Lieshout (Eds.), *Speech production: Motor control, brain research and fluency disorders* (pp. 279–292). Amsterdam: Elsevier.

Brex, P. A., Miszkiel, K. A., Riordan, J. I., Plant, G. T., Moseley, I. F., Thompson, A. J., & Miller, D. H. (2001). Assessing the risk of early multiple sclerosis in patients with clinically isolated syndromes: The role of a follow-up MRI. *Journal of Neurology, Neurosurgery and Psychiatry, 70,* 390–393.

Bright, K. E. (1997). Spontaneous otoacoustic emissions. In M. S. Robinette & T. J. Glattke (Eds.), *Otoacoustic emissions: Clinical applications* (pp. 46–62). New York: Thieme.

Broen, P. A., Strange, W., Doyle, S. S., & Heller, J. H. (1983). Perception and production of approximant contrasts by normal and articulation-delayed preschool children. *Journal of Speech and Hearing Research, 26,* 601–608.

Brown, W. S., Jr., Morris, R. J., & Murry, T. (1996). Comfortable effort level revisited. *Journal of Voice, 10,* 299–305.

Buchel, C., & Sommer, M. (2004). What causes stuttering? *PloS Biology, 2,* e46.

Caruso, A. J., & Klasner Burton, E. (1987). Temporal acoustic measures of dysarthria associated with amyotrophic lateral sclerosis. *Journal of Speech and Hearing Research, 30,* 80–87.

Cerny, F. J., Panzarella, K. J., & Stathopoulos, E. (1997). Expiratory muscle conditioning in hypotonic children with low vocal intensity levels. *Journal of Medical Speech–Language Pathology, 5,* 141–152.

Childers, D. G. (1991). Assessment of the acoustics of voice production. In *Proceedings of a conference on assessment of speech and voice production: Research and clinical applications* (pp. 63–83). Bethesda, MD: U. S. Department of Health and Human Services.

Clayman, C. B. (Ed.). (1995). *The human body: An illustrated guide to its structure, function, and disorders.* New York: Dorling Kindersley.

Coleman, R. F., Mabis, J. H., & Hinson, J. K. (1977). Fundamental frequency-sound pressure level profiles of adult male and female voices. *Journal of Speech and Hearing Research, 20,* 197–204.

Colton, R., & Casper, J. K. (1996). *Understanding voice problems: A physiological perspective for diagnosis and treatment* (2nd ed.). Baltimore, MD: Williams & Wilkins.

Cooper, H. (1991). Training and rehabilitation for cochlear implant users. In H. Cooper (Ed.), *Cochlear implants: A practical guide* (pp. 219–239). San Diego, CA: Singular.

Corbett, J. J., Haines, D. E., & Ard, M. D. (2002). The ventricles, choroid plexus, and cerebrospinal fluid. In D. E. Haines (Ed.), *Fundamental neuroscience* (2nd ed.). New York: Churchill Livingstone.

Culpepper, N. B. (1997). Neonatal screening via evoked otoacoustic emissions. In M. S. Robinette & T. J. Glattke (Eds.), *Otoacoustic emissions: Clinical applications* (pp. 233–270). New York: Thieme.

Darley, F. L., Aronson, A. E., & Brown, J. R. (1975). *Motor speech disorders.* Philadelphia: W. B. Saunders Company.

Davis, L. F. (1987). Respiration and phonation in cerebral palsy: A developmental model. *Seminars in Speech and Language, 8,* 101–106.

Davis, P. J., Zhang, S. P., Winkworth, A., & Bandler, R. (1996). Neural control of vocalization: Respiratory and emotional influences. *Journal of Voice, 10,* 23–38.

de Pinto, O., & Hollien, H. (1982). Speaking fundamental frequency characteristics of Australian women: Then and now. *Journal of Phonetics, 10,* 367–375.

Decker, T. N. (1990). *Instrumentation: An introduction for students in the speech and hearing sciences.* New York: Longman.

Denes, P. B., & Pinson, E. N. (1993). *The speech chain: The physics and biology of spoken language* (2nd ed.). New York: W. H. Freeman.

DeVries, S. M., & Newell Decker, T. (1992). Otoacoustic emissions: Overview of measurement methodologies. *Seminars in Hearing, 13,* 15–22.

Dickson, D. R., & Maue-Dickson, W. (1982). *Anatomical and physiological bases of speech.* Austin, TX: Pro-Ed.

Doherty, E. T., & Shipp, T. (1988). Tape recorder effects on jitter and shimmer extraction. *Journal of Speech and Hearing Research, 31,* 485–490.

Dorman, M. F. (2000). Speech perception by adults. In S. B. Waltzman & N. L. Cohen (Eds.), *Cochlear implants* (pp. 317–329). New York: Thieme.

Dromey, C., Ramig, L. O., & Johnson, A. B. (1995). Phonatory and articulatory changes associated with increased vocal intensity in Parkinson's disease: A case study. *Journal of Speech and Hearing Research, 38,* 751–764.

Dubno, J., Dirks, D., & Schaefer, A. (1987). Effects of hearing loss on utilization of short-duration spectral cues in stop consonant recognition. *Journal of the Acoustical Society of America, 81,* 1940–1947.

Dull, C. E., Metcalfe, H. C., & Williams, J. E. (1960). *Modern physics.* New York: Holt, Rinehart and Winston.

Durrant, J. D., & Lovrinic, J. H. (1995). *Bases of hearing science* (3rd ed.). Baltimore, MD: Williams & Wilkins.

Dworkin, J. P. (1991). *Motor speech disorders: A treatment guide.* St. Louis, MO: Mosby Year Book.

Eguchi, S., & Hirsh, L. J. (1969). Development of speech sounds in children. *Acta Otolaryngologica Supplement, 257,* 1–51.

Eimas, P. D., Miller, J. L., & Jusczyk, P. W. (1987). On infant speech perception and the acquisition of language. In S. Harnad (Ed.), *Categorical perception: The groundwork of cognition* (pp. 161–195). Cambridge, UK: Cambridge University Press.

Eisen, A. H., & Ferrand, C. T. (1995). *Disfluencies in college age students with LLD, college age students who stutter, and normally speaking college age students.* Paper presented at the Annual Convention of the American Speech–Language–Hearing Association.

Elliott, L. L., & Hammer, M. A. (1993). Fine-grained auditory discrimination: Factor structures. *Journal of Speech and Hearing Research, 36,* 396–409.

Ertmer, D. J., & Stark, R. E. (1995). Eliciting prespeech vocalizations in a young child with profound hearing loss: Usefulness of real-time spectrographic speech displays. *American Journal of Speech–Language Pathology, 4,* 33–38.

Ertmer, D. J., Stark, R. E., & Karlan, G. R. (1996). Real-time spectrographic displays in vowel production training with children who have profound hearing loss. *American Journal of Speech–Language Pathology, 5,* 4–16.

Eskenazi, L., Childers, D. G., & Hicks, D. M. (1990). Acoustic correlates of vocal quality. *Journal of Speech and Hearing Research, 33,* 298–306.

Fernandez-Lastra, A., Morales-Rodriguez, M., & Penzol-Diaz, J. (2001). Neurophysiological study and use of P300 evoked potentials for investigation in the diagnosis and of follow-up of patients with Alzheimer's disease. *Revistade Neurologia, 6,* 525–528.

Ferrand, C. T. (1995). Effects of practice with and without knowledge of results on jitter and shimmer levels in normally speaking women. *Journal of Voice,* 419–423.

Ferrand, C. T. (1999, November). *Harmonics-to-noise ratios: An index of vocal aging.* Poster presented at the annual convention of the American Speech–Language–Hearing Association, San Francisco.

Ferrand, C. T. (2000). Harmonics-to-noise ratios in prepubescent girls and boys. *Journal of Voice, 14,* 9–14.

Ferrand, C. T., & Bloom, R. L. (1996). Gender differences in children's intonational patterns. *Journal of Voice, 10,* 284–291.

Fiez, J. A. (2001). Neuroimaging studies of speech: An overview of techniques and methodological approaches. *Journal of Communication Disorders, 34,* 445–454.

Finitzo, T., Pool, K. D., Devous, M. D., Sr., & Watson, B. C. (1991). Cortical dysfunction in developmental stutterers. In H. F. M. Peters, W. Hulstijn, & C. W. Starkweather (Eds.), *Speech motor control and stuttering* (pp. 251–262), Amsterdam: Elsevier.

Fisher, K. V., Scherer, R. C., Guo, C. G., & Owen, A. S. (1996). Longitudinal phonatory characteristics after botulinum toxin type A injection. *Journal of Speech and Hearing Research, 39,* 968–980.

Fletcher, S. G., Dagenais, P. A., & Crotz-Crosby, P. (1991a). Teaching consonants to profoundly hearing-impaired speakers using palatometry. *Journal of Speech and Hearing Research, 34,* 929–942.

Fletcher, S. G., Dagenais, P. A., & Crotz-Crosby, P. (1991b). Teaching vowels to profoundly hearing-impaired speakers using glossometry. *Journal of Speech and Hearing Research, 34,* 943–956.

Forrest, K., Weismer, G., Hodge, M., Dinnsen, D. A., & Elbert, M. (1990). Statistical analysis of word-initial /k/ and /t/ produced by normal and phonologically disordered children. *Clinical Linguistics and Phonetics, 4,* 327–340.

Frieda, E. M., Walley, A. C., Flege, J. E., & Sloane, M. E. (2000). Adults' perception and production of the English vowel /i/. *Journal of Speech, Language, and Hearing Research, 43,* 129–143.

Gamboa, J., Jimenez-Jimenez, F. J., Nieto, A., Montojo, J., Orti-Pareja, M., Molina, J. A., Garcia-Albea, E., & Cobeta, I. (1997). Acoustic voice analysis in patients with Parkinson's disease treated with dopaminergic drugs. *Journal of Voice, 11,* 314–320.

Gelfand, S. A. (1997). *Essentials of audiology.* New York: Thieme.

Gill, F. B. (1995). *Ornithology* (2nd ed.). New York: W. H. Freeman.

Glaze, L. E., Bless, D. M., Milenkovic, P., & Susser, R. D. (1988). Acoustic characteristics of children's voice. *Journal of Voice, 2,* 312–319.

Golding-Kushner, K. J. (1997). Cleft lip and palate, craniofacial anomalies, and velopharyngeal insufficiency. In C. T. Ferrand & R. L. Bloom (Eds.), *Introduction to organic and neurogenic disorders of communication: Current scope of practice* (pp. 193–228). Boston: Allyn and Bacon.

Grafton, S. T. (2004). Contributions of functional imaging to understanding parkinsonian symptoms. *Current Opinion in Neurobiology, 14,* 715–719.

Greenberg, S. (1996). Auditory processing of speech. In N. J. Lass (Ed.), *Principles of experimental phonetics.* St. Louis, MO: C. V. Mosby.

Groenen, P., Crul, T., Maassen, B., & van Bon, W. (1996b). Perception of voicing cues by children with early otitis media with and without language impairment. *Journal of Speech and Hearing Research, 39,* 43–54.

Hagoort, P., & van Turennout, M. (1997). The electrophysiology of speaking: Possibilities of event-related potential research on speech production. In W. Hulstijn, H. F. M. Peters, & P. H. H. M. Van Lieshout (Eds.), *Speech production: Motor control, brain research and fluency disorders* (pp. 351–361). Amsterdam: Elsevier.

Haines, D. E., & Mihailoff, G. A. (2002). The medulla oblongata. In D. E. Haines (Ed.), *Fundamental neuroscience* (2nd ed.). New York: Churchill Livingstone.

Haines, D. E., Mihailoff, G. A., & Yezierski, R. P. (2002). The spinal cord. In D. E. Haines (Ed.), *Fundamental neuroscience* (2nd ed.). New York: Churchill Livingstone.

Haines, D. E., Raila, F. A., & Terrell, A. C. (2002). Orientation to structure and imaging of the central nervous system. In D. E. Haines (Ed.), *Fundamental neuroscience* (2nd ed.). New York: Churchill Livingstone.

Hall, K. D., & Yairi, E. (1992). Fundamental frequency, jitter, and shimmer in preschoolers who stutter. *Journal of Speech and Hearing Research, 35,* 1002–1008.

Hardcastle, W. (1976). *Physiology of speech production.* London: Academic Press.

Hardy, S. G. P., Chronister, R. B., & Parent, A. D. (2002). The hypothalamus. In D. E. Haines (Ed.), *Fundamental neuroscience* (2nd ed.). New York: Churchill Livingstone.

Harmes, S., Daniloff, R. G., Hoffman, P. R., Lewis, J., Kramer, M. B., & Absher, R. (1984). Temporal and articulatory control of fricative articulation by speakers with Broca's aphasia. *Journal of Phonetics, 12,* 367–385.

Hartelius, L., Nord, L., & Buder, E. H. (1995). Acoustic analysis of dysarthria associated with multiple sclerosis. *Clinical Linguistics and Phonetics, 9,* 95–120.

Hawkins, S. (1999a). Auditory capacities and phonological development: Animal, baby, and foreign listeners. In J. M. Pickett (Ed.), *The acoustics of speech communication: Fundamentals, speech perception theory, and technology* (pp. 183–197). Boston: Allyn and Bacon.

Hawkins, S. (1999b). Looking for invariant correlates of linguistic units: Two classical theories of speech perception. In J. M. Pickett (Ed.), *The acoustics of speech communication: Fundamentals, speech perception theory, and technology* (pp. 198–231). Boston: Allyn and Bacon.

Hawkins, S. (1999c). Reevaluating assumptions about speech perception: Interactive and integrative theories. In J. M. Pickett (Ed.), *The acoustics of speech communication: Fundamentals, speech perception theory, and technology* (pp. 232–288). Boston: Allyn and Bacon.

Hedrick, M. (1997). Effect of acoustic cues on labeling fricatives and affricates. *Journal of Speech, Language, and Hearing Research, 40,* 925–938.

Hedrick, M. S., & Carney, A. E. (1997). Effect of relative amplitude and formant transitions on perception of place of articulation by adult listeners with cochlear implants. *Journal of Speech, Language, and Hearing Research, 40,* 1445–1457.

Heissa, W. D., & Hilkera, R. (2004). The sensitivity of 18-fluorodopa positron emission tomography and magnetic resonance imaging in Parkinson's disease. *European Journal of Neurology, 11,* 5–12.

Higgins, M. B., & Saxman, J. H. (1991). A comparison of selected phonatory behaviors of healthy aged and young adults. *Journal of Speech and Hearing Research, 34,* 1000–1010.

Hillenbrand, J., & Houde, R. A. (1996). Acoustic correlates of breathy vocal quality: Dysphonic voices and continuous speech. *Journal of Speech and Hearing Research, 39,* 311–321.

Hixon, T. J., Goldman, M., & Mead, J. (1973). Kinematics of the chest wall during speech production: Volume displacements of the ribcage, abdomen, and lung. *Journal of Speech and Hearing Research, 16,* 78–115.

Hoffman, P. R., Daniloff, R. G., Bengoa, D., & Schuckers, G. H. (1985). Misarticulating and normally articulating children's identification and discrimination of synthetic [r] and [w]. *Journal of Speech and Hearing Disorders, 50,* 46–53.

Hoit, J. D. (1995). Influence of body position on breathing and its implications for the evaluation and treatment of speech and voice disorders. *Journal of Voice, 9,* 341–347.

Hoit, J. D., Banzett, R. B., Brown, R., & Loring, S. H. (1990). Speech breathing in individuals with cervical spinal cord injury. *Journal of Speech and Hearing Research, 33,* 798–807.

Hoit, J. D., & Hixon, T. J. (1987). Age and speech breathing. *Journal of Speech and Hearing Research, 30,* 351–366.

Hoit, J. D., Hixon, T. J., Watson, P. J., & Morgan, W. J. (1990). Speech breathing in children and adolescents. *Journal of Speech and Hearing Research, 33,* 51–69.

Hoit, J. D., Shea, S. A., & Banzett, R. B. (1994). Speech production during mechanical ventilation in tracheostomized individuals. *Journal of Speech and Hearing Research, 37,* 53–63.

Hollien, H., & Shipp, T. (1972). Speaking fundamental frequency and chronologic age in males. *Journal of Speech and Hearing Research, 15,* 150–160.

Honjo, I., & Isshiki, N. (1980). Laryngoscopic and voice characteristics of aged persons. *Archives of Otolaryngology, 106,* 149–150.

Horii, Y., & Fuller, B. F. (1990). Selected acoustic characteristics of voices before intubation and after extubation. *Journal of Speech and Hearing Research, 33,* 505–510.

Hutchins, J. B., Naftel, J. P., & Ard, M. D. (2002). The cell biology of neurons and glia. In D. E. Haines (Ed.), *Fundamental neuroscience* (2nd ed.). New York: Churchill Livingstone.

Ingham, R. J., Fox, P. T., & Ingham, J. C. (1994). Brain image investigation of the speech of stutterers and nonstutterers. *ASHA, 36,* 188.

Ingham, R. J., Fox, P. T., & Ingham, J. C. (1997). A H215O positron emission tomography study on adults who stutter: Findings and implications. In W. Hulstijn, H. F. M. Peters, & P. H. H. M. Van Lieshout (Eds.), *Speech production: Motor control, brain research and fluency disorders* (pp. 293–305). Amsterdam: Elsevier.

Jerger, J. F., and Stach, B. (1994). Hearing disorders. In F. D. Minifie (Ed.), *Introduction to communication sciences and disorders* (pp. 603–672). San Diego, CA: Singular.

Jiang, J., Ng, J., & Hanson, D. (1999). The effects of rehydration on phonation in excised canine larynges. *Journal of Voice, 13,* 51–59.

Kamen, R. S., & Watson, B. C. (1991). Effects of long-term tracheostomy on spectral characteristics of vowel production. *Journal of Speech and Hearing Research, 34,* 1057–1065.

Katada, E., Sato, K., Sawaki, A., Dohi, Y., Ueda, R., & Ojika, K. (2003). Long-term effects of donepezil on P300 auditory event-related potentials in patients with Alzheimer's disease. *Journal of Geriatric Psychiatry and Neurology, 16,* 39–43.

Kempster, G. B., Kistler, D. J., & Hillenbrand, J. (1991). Multidimensional scaling analysis of dysphonia in two speaker groups. *Journal of Speech and Hearing Research, 34,* 534–543.

Kent, J. F., Kent, R. D., Rosenbek, J. C., Weismer, G., Martine, R., Sufit, R., & Brooks, B. R. (1992). Quantitative description of the dysarthria in women with amyotrophic lateral sclerosis. *Journal of Speech and Hearing Research, 35,* 723–733.

Kent, R. D. (1994). *Reference manual for communicative sciences and disorders: Speech and language.* Austin, TX: Pro-Ed.

Kent, R. D. (1997a). *The speech sciences.* San Diego, CA: Singular.

Kent, R. D. (1997b). Speech motor models and developments in neurophysiological science: New perspectives. In W. Hulstijn, H. F. M. Peters, & P. H. H. M. van Lieshout (Eds.), *Speech production: Motor control, brain research and fluency disorders* (pp. 13–36). Amsterdam: Elsevier.

Kent, R. D., Dembowski, J., & Lass, N. J. (1996). The acoustic characteristics of American English. In N. J. Lass (Ed.), *Principles of experimental phonetics* (pp. 185–225). St. Louis, MO: C. V. Mosby.

Kent, R. D., Kent, J. F., Weismer, G., Sufit, R. L., Brooks, B. R., & Rosenbek, J. C. (1989). Relationships between speech intelligibility and the slope of second-formant transitions in dysarthric subjects. *Clinical Linguistics and Phonetics, 3,* 347–358.

Kent, R. D., & Read, C. (1992). *The acoustic analysis of speech.* San Diego, CA: Singular.

Kent, R. D., Sufit, R. L., Rosenbek, J. C., Kent, J. F., Weismer, G., Martin, R. E., & Brooks, B. R. (1991). Speech deterioration in amyotrophic lateral sclerosis: A case study. *Journal of Speech and Hearing Research, 34,* 1269–1275.

Klatt, D., & Klatt, L. C. (1990). Analysis, synthesis, and perception of voice quality variations among male and female talkers. *Journal of the Acoustic Society of America, 87,* 820–857.

Kroll, R. M., De Nil, L. F., Kapur, S., & Houle, S. (1997). A positron emission tomography investigation of post-treatment brain activation in stutterers. In W. Hulstijn, H. F. M. Peters, & P. H. H. M. Van Lieshout (Eds.), *Speech production: Motor control, brain research and fluency disorders* (pp. 307–319). Amsterdam: Elsevier.

Kuhl, P. K. (1991). Perception, cognition, and the ontogenetic and phylogenetic emergence of human speech. In S. E. Brauth, W. S. Hall, & R. J. Dooling (Eds.), *Plasticity of development* (pp. 73–106). Cambridge, MA: The MIT Press.

Kuhl, P. K., Andruski, J. E., Chistovich, I. A., Kozhevnikova, E. V., Ryskina, V. L., Stolyarova, E. I., Sunberg, U., & Lacerda, F. (1997). Cross-language analysis of phonetic units in language addressed to infants. *Science, 277,* 684–686.

Kuhl, P. K., & Meltzoff, A. N. (1996). Infant vocalizations in response to speech: Vocal imitation and developmental change. *Journal of the Acoustical Society of America, 100,* 2425–2438.

Lane, H., Perkell, J., Svirsky, M., & Webster, J. (1991). Changes in speech breathing following cochlear implant in postlingually deafened adults. *Journal of Speech and Hearing Research, 34,* 526–533.

Laughlin, S., & Montanera, W. (1998). Central nervous system imaging: When is CT more appropriate than MRI? *Postgraduate Medicine, 104,* 73–90.

Lauter, J. L. (1997). Noninvasive brain imaging in speech motor control and stuttering: Choices and challenges. In W. Hultijn, H. F. M. Peters, & P. H. H. M. Van Lieshout (Eds.), *Speech production: Motor control, brain research and fluency disorders* (pp. 233–257). Amsterdam: Elsevier.

LeDorze, G., Ouellet, L., & Ryalls, J. (1994). Intonation and speech rate in dysarthric speech. *Journal of Communication Disorders, 27,* 1–18.

Leonard, L. B., McGregor, K. K., & Allen, G. D. (1992). Grammatical morphology and speech perception in children with specific language impairment. *Journal of Speech and Hearing Research, 35,* 1076–1085.

Logemann, J. A., Fisher, H. B., Boshes, B., & Blonsky, E. R. (1978). Frequency and cooccurrence of vocal tract dysfunctions in the speech of a large sample of Parkinson patients. *Journal of Speech and Hearing Disorders, 43,* 47–57.

Lynch, J. C. (2002). The cerebral cortex. In D. E. Haines (Ed.), *Fundamental neuroscience* (2nd ed.; pp. 505–520). New York: Churchill Livingstone.

Ma, T. P. (2002). The basal nuclei. In D. E. Haines (Ed.), *Fundamental neuroscience* (2nd ed.). New York: Churchill Livingstone.

Maassen, B., & Povel, D.-J. (1985). The effect of segmental and suprasegmental corrections on the intelligibility of deaf speech. *Journal of the Acoustical Society of America, 78,* 877–886.

Manifold, J. A. Y., & Murdoch, B. E. (1993). Speech breathing in young adults: Effect of body type. *Journal of Speech and Hearing Research, 36,* 657–671.

Martin, D., Fitch, J., & Wolfe, V. (1995). Pathologic voice type and the acoustic predictions of severity. *Journal of Speech and Hearing Research, 38*, 765–771.

Massery, M. (1991). Chest development as a component of normal motor development: Implications for pediatric physical therapists. *Pediatric Physical Therapy, 3*, 3–8.

McAllister, A., Sederholm, E., Sundberg, J., & Gramming, P. (1994). Relations between voice range profiles and physiological and perceptual voice characteristics in ten-year-old children. *Journal of Voice, 8*, 230–239.

McAnally, K. I., Hansen, P. C., Cornelissen, P. L., & Stein, J. F. (1997). Effect of time and frequency manipulation on syllable perception in developmental dyslexics. *Journal of Speech, Language, and Hearing Research, 40*, 912–924.

McFarland, D. H., & Smith, A. (1992). Effects of vocal task and respiratory phase on prephonatory chest-wall movements. *Journal of Speech and Hearing Research, 35*, 971–982.

McGlone R. E., & Shipp, T. (1971). Some physiologic correlates of vocal fry phonation. *Journal of Speech and Hearing Research, 14*, 769–775.

Mendoza, E., Valencia, N., Munoz, J., & Trujillo, H. (1996). Differences in voice quality between men and women: Use of the long-term average spectrum (LTAS). *Journal of Voice, 10*, 59–66.

Metz, D. E., & Schiavetti, N. (1995). Speech breathing processes of deaf and hearing-impaired persons. In F. Bell-Berti & L. J. Raphael (Eds.), *Producing speech: Contemporary issues.* [*For Katherine Safford Harris*] (pp. 187–198). New York: American Institute of Physics.

Metz, D. E., Schiavetti, N., Samar, V. J., & Sitler, R. W. (1990). Acoustic dimensions of hearing-impaired speakers' intelligibility: Segmental and suprasegmental characteristics. *Journal of Speech and Hearing Research, 33*, 476–487.

Meyers, T. A., Swirsky, M. A., Kirk, K. I., & Miyamoto, R. T. (1998). Improvements in speech perception by children with profound prelingual hearing loss: Effects of device, communication mode, and chronological age. *Journal of Speech, Language, and Hearing Research, 41*, 846–858.

Michi, K. -I., Yamashita, Y., Imai, S., Suzuki, N., & Yoshida, H. (1993). Role of visual feedback treatment for defective /s/ sounds in patients with cleft palate. *Journal of Speech and Hearing Research, 36*, 277–285.

Mihailoff, G. A., & Haines, D. E. (2002). Motor system II: Corticofugal systems and the control of movement. In D. E. Haines (Ed.), *Fundamental neuroscience* (2nd ed.). New York: Churchill Livingstone.

Miller, D. H., Grossman, R. I., Reingold, S. C., & McFarland, H. F. (1998). The role of magnetic resonance techniques in understanding and managing multiple sclerosis. *Brain, 121*, 3–24.

Mitchell, H. L., Hoit, J. D., & Watson, P. J. (1996). Cognitive–linguistic demands and speech breathing. *Journal of Speech and Hearing Research, 39*, 93–104.

Molt, L. F. (1997). Event-related cortical potentials preceding phonation in stutterers and normal speakers: A preliminary report. In W. Hultijn, H. F. M. Peters, & P. H. H. M. Van Lieshout (Eds.), *Speech production: Motor control, brain research and fluency disorders* (pp. 363–369). Amsterdam: Elsevier.

Monsen, R. B. (1979). Acoustic qualities of phonation in young hearing-impaired children. *Journal of Speech and Hearing Research, 22*, 270–288.

Morgan, E. E., & Rastatter, M. (1986). Variability of voice fundamental frequency in elderly female speakers. *Perceptual and Motor Skills, 63*, 215–218.

Motta, G., Cesari, U., Iengo, M., & Motta, G. (1990). Clinical application of electroglottography. *Folia Phoniatrica et Logopedica, 42*, 111–117.

Murdoch, B. E., Chenery, H. J., Stokes, P. D., & Hardcastle, W. J. (1991). Respiratory kinematics in speakers with cerebellar disease. *Journal of Speech and Hearing Research, 34*, 768–780.

Nair, G. (1999). *Voice-Tradition and Technology: A state-of-the-art studio.* San Diego, CA: Singular.

Netsell, R., & Hixon, T. J. (1992). Inspiratory checking in therapy for individuals with speech breathing dysfunction (abstract). *ASHA, 34*, 152.

Nittrouer, S. (1996a). Discriminability and perceptual weighting of some acoustic cues to speech perception by 3-year-olds. *Journal of Speech and Hearing Research, 39*, 278–297.

Nittrouer, S. (1996b). The relation between speech perception and phonemic awareness: Evidence from low-SES children and children with chronic OM. *Journal of Speech and Hearing Research, 39*, 1059–1070.

Nittrouer, S. (1999). Do temporal processing deficits cause phonological processing problems? *Journal of Speech, Language, and Hearing Research, 42*, 925–942.

Nolte, J. (2002). *The human brain: An introduction to its functional anatomy.* Philadelphia: Mosby.

Norton, S. J. (1992). Cochlear function and otoacoustic emissions. *Seminars in Hearing, 13*, 1–14.

Nygaard, L. C., & Pisoni, D. B. (1995). Speech perception: New directions in research and theory. In J. L. Miller & P. D.

Eimas (Eds.), *Speech, language, and communication.* New York: Academic Press.

Ochs, M. T., Humes, L. E., Ohde, R. N., & Grantham, D. W. (1989). Frequency discrimination ability and stop-consonant identification in normally hearing and hearing-impaired subjects. *Journal of Speech and Hearing Research, 32*, 133–142.

Olichney, J. M., & Hillert, D. G. (2004). Clinical applications of cognitive event-related potentials in Alzheimer's disease. *Physical and Medical Rehabilitation Clinic of North America, 15*, 205–233.

Orlikoff, R. F. (1990). The relationship of age and cardiovascular health to certain acoustic characteristics of male voices. *Journal of Speech and Hearing Research, 33*, 450–457.

Orlikoff, R. F. (1991). Assessment of the dynamics of vocal fold contact from the electroglottogram: Data from normal male subjects. *Journal of Speech and Hearing Research, 34*, 1066–1072.

Orlikoff, R. F., Kraus, D. H., Harrison, L. B., Ho, M. L., & Gartner, C. J. (1997). Vocal fundamental frequency measures as a reflection of tumor response to chemotherapy in patients with advanced laryngeal cancer. *Journal of Voice, 11*, 33–39.

Pabon, J. P. H., & Plomp, R. (1988). Automatic phonetogram recording supplemented with acoustical voice quality parameters. *Journal of Speech and Hearing Research, 31*, 710–722.

Parry, A., & Matthews, P. M. (2002). *Functional magnetic resonance imaging (fMRI): A "window" into the brain.* Centre for Functional Magnetic Resonance Imaging of the Brain, Department of Clinical Neurology, University of Oxford. Retrieved January 2, 2005, from http://www.fmrib.ox.ac.uk/fmri_intro/fmri_intro.htm

Pederson, M. F., Moller, S., Krabbe, S., Bennett, P., & Svenstrup, B. (1990). Fundamental voice frequency in female puberty measured with electroglottography during continuous speech as a secondary sex characteristic: A comparison between voice, pubertal stages, oestrogens, and androgens. *Journal of Pediatric Otorhinolaryngology, 20,* 16–23.

Pegoraro-Krook, M. I. (1988). Speaking fundamental frequency characteristics of normal Swedish subjects obtained by glottal frequency analysis. *Folia Phoniatrica et Logopedica, 40,* 82–90.

Perkell, J. S., Matthies, M. L., Svirsky, M. A., & Jordan, M. I. (1995). Goal-based speech motor control: A theoretical framework and some preliminary data. *Journal of Phonetics, 23,* 23–35.

Peterson, G., & Barney, H. (1952). Control methods used in a study of the vowels. *Journal of the Acoustical Society of America, 24,* 175–184.

Pickett, J. M. (1999). *The acoustics of speech communication: Fundamentals, speech perception theory, and technology.* Boston: Allyn and Bacon.

Plante, E. (2001). Neuroimaging in communication sciences and disorders. *Journal of Communication Disorders, 34,* 441–443.

Pokryszko-Dragan, A., Slotwinski, K., & Podemski, R. (2003). Modality-specific changes in P300 parameters in patients with dementia of the Alzheimer type. *Medical Science Monitor, 9,* 130–134.

Pool, K. D., Devous, M. D., Sr., Freeman, F. J., Watson, B. C., & Finitzo, T. (1991). Regional cerebral blood flow in developmental stutterers. *Archives of Neurology, 48,* 509–512.

Porter, R. J., Hogue, D. M., & Tobey, E. A. (1995). Dynamic analysis of speech and non-speech respiration. In F. Bell-Berti & L. J.

Raphael (Eds.), *Producing speech: Contemporary issues.* [*For Katherine Safford Harris*] (pp. 169–185). New York: American Institute of Physics.

Prabhakar, S., Syal, P., & Srivastava, T. (2000). P300 in newly diagnosed non-dementing Parkinson's disease: Effect of dopaminergic drugs. *Neurology India, 48,* 239–242.

Prieve, B. A. (1992). Otoacoustic emissions in infants and children: Basic characteristics and clinical application. *Seminars in Hearing, 13,* 37–52.

Raaymakers, E. M. J. A., & Crul, T. A. (1988). Perception and production of the final /s/-ts/ contrast in Dutch by misarticulating children. *Journal of Speech and Hearing Disorders, 53,* 262–270.

Ramig, L. O. (1992). The role of phonation in speech intelligibility: A review and preliminary data from patients with Parkinson's disease. In R. D. Kent (Ed.), *Intelligibility in speech disorders: Theory, measurement and management* (pp. 119–156). Amsterdam: John Benjamin.

Ramig, L. O., Countryman, S., Thompson, L. L., & Horii, Y. (1995). Comparison of two forms of intensive speech treatment for Parkinson's disease. *Journal of Speech and Hearing Research, 38,* 1232–1251.

Ramig, L. O., & Dromey, C. (1996). Aerodynamic mechanisms underlying treatment-related changes in vocal intensity in patients with Parkinson disease. *Journal of Speech and Hearing Research, 39,* 798–807.

Rihkanen, H., Leinonen, L., Hiltunen, T., & Kangas, J. (1994). Spectral pattern recognition of improved voice quality. *Journal of Voice, 8,* 320–326.

Robb, M., & Saxman, J. (1985). Developmental trends in vocal fundamental frequency of young children. *Journal of Speech and Hearing Research, 28,* 420–429.

Robinette, M. S. (1992). Clinical observations with transient evoked otoacoustic emissions with adults. *Seminars in Hearing, 13,* 23–36.

Rosen, S., & Howell, P. (1991). *Signals and systems for speech and hearing.* New York: Academic Press.

Ross, M., Brackett, D., & Maxon, A. B. (1991). *Assessment and management of mainstreamed hearing-impaired children.* Austin, TX: Pro-Ed.

Roy, N., Bless, D. M., Heisey, D., & Ford, C. N. (1997). Manual circumlaryngeal therapy for functional dysphonia: An evaluation of short- and long-term treatment outcomes. *Journal of Voice, 11,* 321–331.

Russell, A., Penny, L., & Pemberton, C. (1995). Speaking fundamental frequency changes over time in women: A longitudinal study. *Journal of Speech and Hearing Research, 38,* 101–109.

Russell, B. A., Cerny, F. J., & Stathopoulos, E. T. (1998). Effects of varied vocal intensity on ventilation and energy expenditure in women and men. *Journal of Speech, Language, and Hearing Research, 41,* 239–248.

Russell, N. K., & Stathopoulos, E. (1988). Lung volume changes in children and adults during speech production. *Journal of Speech and Hearing Research, 31,* 146–155.

Rvachew, S., & Jamieson, D. G. (1989). Perception of voiceless fricatives by children with a functional articulation disorder. *Journal of Speech and Hearing Disorders, 54,* 193–208.

Ryalls, J., Baum, S., & Larouche, A. (1991). Spectral characteristics for place of articulation in the speech of young normal, moderately and profoundly hearing-impaired French Canadians. *Clinical Linguistics and Phonetics, 3,* 165–179.

Sammeth, C. A., Dorman, M. F., & Stearns, C. J. (1999). The role of consonant–vowel amplitude ratio in the recognition of voiceless stop consonants by listeners with hearing impairment. *Journal of Speech, Language, and Hearing Research, 42,* 42–55.

Sapienza, C. M., & Stathopoulos, E. T. (1995). Speech task effects on acoustic and aerodynamic measures of women with vocal nodules. *Journal of Voice, 9,* 413–418.

Sapienza, C. M., Stathopoulos, E. T., & Brown, W. S. (1997). Speech breathing during reading in women with vocal nodules. *Journal of Voice, 11,* 195–201.

Sebel, P., Stoddart, D. M., Waldhorn, R. E., Waldmann, C. S., & Whitfield, P. (1987). *Respiration: The breath of life.* New York: Torstar Books.

Seddoh, S. A. K., Robin, D. A., Sim, H. -S., Hageman, C., Moon, J. B., & Folkins, J. W. (1996). Speech timing in apraxia of speech versus conduction aphasia. *Journal of Speech and Hearing Research, 39,* 590–603.

Seikel, J. A., Drumright, D. G., & Seikel, P. (2004). *Essentials of anatomy and physiology for communication disorders.* Clifton Park, NY: Thomson Delmar Learning.

Seikel, J. A., King, D. W., & Drumright, D. G. (1997). *Anatomy and physiology for speech and language.* San Diego, CA: Singular.

Shanks, J. E., Lilly, D. J., Margolis, R. H., Wiley, T. L., & Wilson, R. H. (1988). Tympanometry. *Journal of Speech and Hearing Disorders, 53,* 354–377.

Shinn, P., & Blumstein, S. E. (1983). Phonetic disintegration in aphasia: Acoustic analysis of spectral characteristics for place of articulation. *Brain and Language, 20,* 90–114.

Silbergleit, A. K., Johnson, A. F., & Jacobson, B. H. (1997). Acoustic analysis of voice in individuals with amyotrophic lateral sclerosis and perceptually normal voice quality. *Journal of Voice, 11,* 222–231.

Silman, S., & Silverstein, C. A. (1991). *Auditory diagnosis: Principles and applications.* San Diego, CA: Academic Press.

Slavin, D. C., & Ferrand, C. T. (1995). Factor analysis of proficient esophageal speech: Toward a multidimensional model. *Journal of Speech and Hearing Research, 38,* 1224–1231.

Smith, A., & Denny, M. (1990). High frequency oscillations as indicators of neural control mechanisms in human respiration, mastication, and speech. *Journal of Neurophysiology, 63,* 745–758.

Smitheran, R., & Hixon, T. J. (1981). A clinical method for estimating laryngeal airway resistance during vowel production. *Journal of Speech and Hearing Disorders, 46,* 138–147.

Sodersten, M., & Lindestad, P. -A. (1990). Glottal closure and perceived breathiness during phonation in normally speaking subjects. *Journal of Speech and Hearing Research, 33,* 601–611.

Solomon, N. P., & Charron, S. (1998). Speech breathing in able-bodied children and children with cerebral palsy: A review of the literature and implications for clinical intervention. *American Journal of Speech Language Pathology, 7,* 61–78.

Solomon, N. P., & Hixon, T. J. (1993). Speech breathing in Parkinson's disease. *Journal of Speech and Hearing Research, 36,* 294–310.

Sorenson, D. N. (1989). A F_0 investigation of children ages 6–10 years old. *Journal of Communication Disorders, 22,* 115–123.

Speaks, C. E. (1992). *Introduction to sound: Acoustics for the hearing and speech sciences.* New York: Chapman and Hall.

Sperry, E. E., & Klich, R. J. (1992). Speech breathing in senescent and younger women during oral reading. *Journal of Speech and Hearing Research, 35,* 1246–1255.

Stark, R. E., & Heinz, J. M. (1996a). Perception of stop consonants in children with expressive and receptive–expressive language impairments. *Journal of Speech and Hearing Research, 39,* 676–686.

Stark, R. E., & Heinz, J. M. (1996b). Vowel perception in children with and without language impairment. *Journal of Speech and Hearing Research, 39,* 860–869.

Stathopoulos, E. T. (1997). *Respiratory function in voice and speech disorders: Clinical implications.* Paper presented at the American Speech–Language–Hearing Association annual convention, Boston.

Stathopoulos, E. T., Hoit, J. D., Hixon, T. J., Watson, P. J., & Solomon, N. P. (1991). Respiratory and laryngeal function during whispering. *Journal of Speech and Hearing Research, 34,* 761–767.

Stathopoulos, E. T., & Sapienza, C. M. (1993). Respiratory and laryngeal function of women and men during vocal intensity variation. *Journal of Speech and Hearing Research, 36,* 64–75.

Stathopoulos, E. T., & Sapienza, C. M. (1997). Developmental changes in laryngeal and respiratory function with variations in sound pressure level. *Journal of Speech, Language, and Hearing Research, 40,* 595–614.

Stathopoulos, E. T., & Weismer, G. (1985). Oral airflow and air pressure during speech production: A comparative study of children, youths, and adults. *Folia Phoniatrica et Logopedica, 37,* 152–159.

Stemple, J. C. (1997). Respiratory function in voice and speech disorders: Clinical implications. Paper presented at the annual convention of the American Speech–Language–Hearing Association, Boston.

Stevens, K. N., & Blumstein, S. E. (1978). Invariant cues for place of articulation in stop consonants. *Journal of the Acoustical Society of America, 64,* 1358–1368.

Strand, E. A., Buder, E. H., Yorkston, K. M., & Olson Ramig, L. (1994). Differential phonatory characteristics of four women with amyotrophic lateral sclerosis. *Journal of Voice, 8,* 327–339.

Strange, W. (1999). Perception of vowels: Dynamic consistency. In J. M. Pickett (Ed.), *The acoustics of speech communication: Fundamentals, speech perception theory, and technology* (pp. 153–165). Boston: Allyn and Bacon.

Subtelny, J. D., Worth, J. H., & Sakuda, M. (1966). Intraoral pressure and rate of flow during speech. *Journal of Speech and Hearing Research, 9,* 498–518.

Sulter, A. M., Schutte, H. K., & Miller, D. G. (1995). Differences in phonetogram features between male and female subjects with and without vocal training. *Journal of Voice, 9,* 363–377.

Summers, W. V., & Leek, M. R. (1992). The role of spectral and temporal cues in vowel identification by listeners with impaired hearing. *Journal of Speech and Hearing Research, 35,* 1189–1199.

Szelies, B., Mielke, R., Grond, M., & Heiss, W. D. (2002). P300 in Alzheimer's disease: Relationship to dementia severity and glucose metabolism. *Neuropsychobiology, 46,* 49–56.

Tallal, P., Miller, S. L., Bedi, G., Byma, G., Wang, X., Nagarajan, S. S., Schreiner, C., Jenkins, W. M., & Merzenich, M. M. (1996). Language comprehension in language-learning impaired children improved with acoustically modified speech. *Science, 271,* 81–84.

Thomas, A., Iacono, D., Bonanni, L., D'Andreamatteo L., & Onofrj, M. (2001). Donepezil, rivastigmine, and vitamin E in Alzheimer disease: A combined P300 event-related potentials/neuropsychologic evaluation over 6 months. *Clinical Neuropharmacology, 24,* 31–42.

Titze, I. R. (1991). A model for neurologic sources of aperiodicity in vocal fold vibration. *Journal of Speech and Hearing Research, 34,* 460–472.

Titze, I. R. (1994). *Principles of voice production.* Englewood Cliffs, NJ: Prentice Hall.

Tjaden, K., & Turner, G. S. (1997). Spectral properties of fricatives in amyotrophic lateral sclerosis. *Journal of Speech and Hearing Research, 40,* 1358–1372.

Trullinger, R. W., & Emanuel, F. W. (1983). Airflow characteristics of stop-plosive consonant productions of normal-speaking children. *Journal of Speech and Hearing Research, 26,* 202–208.

Turner, C. W., Chi, S. L., & Flock, S. (1999). Limiting spectral resolution in speech for listeners with sensorineural hearing loss. *Journal of Speech, Language, and Hearing Research, 42,* 773–784.

Turner, G. S., Tjaden, K., & Weismer, G. (1995). The influence of speaking rate on vowel space and speech intelligibility for individuals with amyotrophic lateral sclerosis. *Journal of Speech and Hearing Research, 38,* 1001–1013.

Tye-Murray, N. (1987). Effects of vowel context on the articulatory closure postures of deaf speakers. *Journal of Speech and Hearing Research, 30,* 99–104.

Tyler, A. A., Figurski, G. R., & Langsdale, T. (1993). Relationships between acoustically determined knowledge of stop place and voicing contrasts and phonological treatment progress. *Journal of Speech and Hearing Research, 36,* 746–759.

Ullrich, D. (2004). Imaging research seeks early detection of Alzheimer's risk. MCW Health News. Retrieved August 5, 2005, from http://healthlink.mcw.edu

Waldstein, R. S., & Baum, S. R. (1991). Anticipatory coarticulation in the speech of profoundly hearing-impaired and normally hearing children. *Journal of Speech and Hearing Research, 34,* 1276–1285.

Watson, B. C., & Freeman, F. J. (1997). Brain imaging contributions. In R. F. Curlee & G. M. Siegel (Eds.), *Nature and treatment of stuttering: New directions* (pp. 143–166). Boston: Allyn and Bacon.

Watson, B. U., & Miller, T. K. (1993). Auditory perception, phonological processing, and reading ability/disability. *Journal of Speech and Hearing Research, 36,* 850–863.

Watson, P. (1997). *Respiratory function in voice and speech disorders: Clinical implications.* Paper presented at the annual convention of the American Speech–Language–Hearing Association, Boston.

Watson, P., & Hixon, T. (1985). Respiratory kinematics in classical (opera) singers. *Journal of Speech and Hearing Research, 28,* 104–122.

Watson, P., Hixon, T., Stathopoulos, E., & Sullivan, D. (1990). Respiratory kinematics in female classical singers. *Journal of Voice, 4,* 120–128.

Webster, D. B. (1999). *Neuroscience of communication* (2nd ed.). San Diego, CA: Singular.

Weismer, G., Martin, R., Kent, R. D., & Kent, J. F. (1992). Formant trajectory characteristics of males with amyotrophic lateral sclerosis. *Journal of the Acoustical Society of America, 91,* 1085–1098.

Werber, E. A., Gandelman-Marton, R., Klein, C., & Rabey, J. M. (2003). The clinical use of P300 event related potentials for the evaluation of cholinesterase inhibitors treatment in demented patients. *Journal of Neural Transmission, 110,* 659–669.

Whitehead, R. L. (1983). Some respiratory and aerodynamic patterns in the speech of the hearing impaired. In I. Hochberg, H. Levitt, & M. J. Osberger (Eds.), *Speech of the hearing impaired* (pp. 97–116). Baltimore: University Park Press.

Winkworth, A. L., Davis, P. J., Adams, R. D., & Ellis, E. (1995). Breathing patterns during spontaneous speech. *Journal of Speech and Hearing Research, 38,* 124–144.

Wolfe, V. I., & Ratusnik, D. L. (1988). Acoustic and perceptual measurements of roughness influencing judgments of pitch. *Journal of Speech and Hearing Disorders, 53,* 15–22.

Workinger, M. S., & Kent, R. D. (1991). Perceptual analysis of the dysarthrias in children with athetoid and spastic cerebral palsy. In C. A. Moore, K. M. Yorkson, & D. R. Beukelman (Eds.), *Dysarthria and apraxia of speech: Perspectives on management* (pp. 109–126). Baltimore, MD: Paul H. Brookes.

Wu, J. C., Maguire, G., Riley, G., Fallon, J., LaCasse, L., Chin, S., Klein, E., Tang, C., Cadwell, S., & Lotenberg, S. (1995). A positron emission tomography [^{18}F]deoxyglucose study of developmental stuttering. *Neurology Report, 6,* 501–505.

Yumoto, E., Gould, W. J., & Baer, T. (1982). Harmonics-to-noise ratio as an index of the degree of hoarseness. *Journal of the Acoustical Society of America, 71,* 1544–1550.

Zemlin, W. R. (1998). *Speech and hearing science: Anatomy and physiology* (4th ed.). Boston: Allyn and Bacon.

Zeng, F. -G., & Turner, C. W. (1990). Recognition of voiceless fricatives by normal and hearing-impaired subjects. *Journal of Speech and Hearing Research, 33,* 440–449.

Ziegler, W., & von Cramon, D. (1983). Vowel distortion in traumatic dysarthria: A formant study. *Phonetica, 40,* 63–78.

Ziegler, W., Hoole, P., Hartmann, E., & von Cramon, D. (1988). Accelerated speech in dysarthria after acquired brain injury: Acoustic correlates. *British Journal of Disorders of Communication, 23,* 215–228.

Index

Feedforward, 363–65
  models, 391–92
Fetal cell transplantation (FCT), 158, 164
$F_0F_1F_2$ strategy, 283
F_1/F_2 plots, 206
  for vowels, 207
F_2/F_1 ratios for vowels, 264
Fibers
  association, 326
  commissural, 325–26
  projection, 326
Filters
  acoustic resonators as, 44–49
  band-pass, 49
  of glottal sound wave, 199–204
  high-pass, 49
  low-pass, 48–49
  parameters of, 48
  types of, 48–49
Final common pathway, 312
Final consonant deletion, 244
Fixed channel strategy, 283
Flocculonodular lobe, 334
Flow, 11, 93
Forced vibration, 42–43
Formant frequencies, 296
  related to oral and pharyngeal volumes,
    201–4
Formants, 197
  steady-state, 208
Formant trajectories, 237, 238
Formant transitions, 208, 216, 265, 269, 287, 289,
    394, 395
Fourcin, Adrian, 149
Fourier, Jean-Baptiste, 26
Fourier analysis, 26, 260, 373
Free vibration, 42–43
Frenulum
  labial, superior and inferior, 169–70
  lingual, 180
Frequency, 33–34
  applied, 43
  average fundamental, 52–54
  center, 48
  cutoff, 46–47
  definition of, 18
  determinants of, 33
  formant, 296

fundamental, 26, 51
  harmonic, 26, 29
  of infants, 55
  lower cutoff, 48
  natural, 48
  resonant, 42, 197, 251
  response, 48
  of sound waves, 17–21
  speaking fundamental, 52
  of speech, 273
  upper cutoff, 48
  variability, 55–56
  variables, 52–57
  vocal, 51–61
  voice fundamental, 132
  vowel formant, 204–6, 263, 265
Frequency perturbation. *See* Jitter
Frication, 220, 224, 239, 287, 288
Fricatives, 27, 98, 106, 182, 190, 194, 220–24, 234,
    238, 243, 247, 268, 270–71, 282, 288, 289
Friction, 22
Frontal lobe, of cortex, 321–22
Front cavity, 214
Fronting, 244
Front vowels, 195–96, 206, 236, 238, 264, 270
F_0SPL profile (voice range profile), 59
Functional articulation disorder, 298
Functional hypokinetic dysphonia, 163
Functional magnetic resonance imaging (fMRI),
    370–71, 379
  advantages of, 371
  disadvantage of, 371
Functional residual capacity (FRC), 86, 106
Functional voice problems
  jitter and shimmer in, 160
Fundamental frequency (F0), 26, 51
  average, 52–54
  speaking, 52–54
Fuzzy logical model of perception, 402–3

G
Gender differences
  in lung volumes, 83
  in rate of breathing, 81
  in registers, 139
  in vocal tract, 196
Genioglossus muscles, 193
Gestures for speech, 398